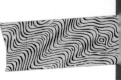

SECOND EDITION

ARRHYTHMIA ESSENTIALS

Brian Olshansky, MD

Professor Emeritus of Medicine
University of Iowa Hospitals
Iowa City, Iowa
Cardiac Electrophysiologist
Mercy Hospital, North Iowa
Mason City, Iowa

Mina K. Chung, MD

Professor of Medicine
Cleveland Clinic Lerner College of Medicine
Case Western Reserve University
Cardiac Electrophysiology and Pacing
Department of Cardiovascular Medicine, Heart and Vascular Institute
Department of Molecular Cardiology, Lerner Research Institute
Cleveland Clinic
Cleveland, Ohio

Steven M. Pogwizd, MD

Featheringill Endowed Professor
in Cardiac Arrhythmia Research
Professor of Medicine, Physiology and Biophysics, and
Biomedical Engineering
Director, Center for Cardiovascular Biology
Associate Director, Cardiac Rhythm Management Laboratory
University of Alabama at Birmingham
Birmingham, Alabama

Nora Goldschlager, MD

Professor of Clinical Medicine
University of California, San Francisco
Chief, Clinical Cardiology
Director, Coronary Care Unit
ECG Laboratory and Pacemaker Clinic
San Francisco General Hospital
San Francisco, California

ELSEVIER

ELSEVIER

1600 John F. Kennedy Blvd.
Ste 1800
Philadelphia, PA 19103-2899

ARRHYTHMIA ESSENTIALS, SECOND EDITION   ISBN: 978-0-323-39968-5

Notices

Knowledge and best practice in this field are constantly changing. As new research and experience broaden our understanding, changes in research methods, professional practices, or medical treatment may become necessary.

Practitioners and researchers must always rely on their own experience and knowledge in evaluating and using any information, methods, compounds, or experiments described herein. In using such information or methods they should be mindful of their own safety and the safety of others, including parties for whom they have a professional responsibility.

With respect to any drug or pharmaceutical products identified, readers are advised to check the most current information provided (i) on procedures featured or (ii) by the manufacturer of each product to be administered, to verify the recommended dose or formula, the method and duration of administration, and contraindications. It is the responsibility of practitioners, relying on their own experience and knowledge of their patients, to make diagnoses, to determine dosages and the best treatment for each individual patient, and to take all appropriate safety precautions.

To the fullest extent of the law, neither the Publisher nor the authors, contributors, or editors, assume any liability for any injury and/or damage to persons or property as a matter of products liability, negligence or otherwise, or from any use or operation of any methods, products, instructions, or ideas contained in the material herein.

Previous edition copyrighted 2012 by Jones & Bartlett Learning, LLC.

Library of Congress Cataloging-in-Publication Data
Names: Olshansky, Brian, author. I Chung, Mina K., author. I Pogwizd, Steven
  M., 1955- author. I Goldschlager, Nora, author.
Title: Arrhythmia essentials / Brian Olshansky, Mina K. Chung, Steven M.
  Pogwizd, Nora Goldschlager.
Description: Second edition. I Philadelphia, PA : Elsevier, [2017] I Preceded
  by: Arrhythmia essentials / Brian Olshansky ... [et al.]. c2012. I
  Includes bibliographical references and index.
Identifiers: LCCN 2016038912 I ISBN 9780323399685 (alk. paper)
Subjects: I MESH: Arrhythmias, Cardiac
Classification: LCC RC685.A65 I NLM WG 330 I DDC 616.1/28–dc23 LC record
available at https://lccn.loc.gov/2016038912

Content Strategist: Maureen Iannuzzi
Content Development Specialist: Stacy Eastman
Publishing Services Manager: Patricia Tannian
Senior Project Manager: Cindy Thoms
Designer: Miles Hitchen

Working together
to grow libraries in
developing countries

www.elsevier.com • www.bookaid.org

Last digit is the print number: 9 8 7 6 5 4 3 2 1

I very much enjoyed reading this text as it represents a tour de force by a group of eminent clinicians and scientists focused on the diagnoses and treatment of cardiac rhythm disorders. The strong points are the beautiful and clear illustrative ECG material together with a methodical and yet practical approach to diagnoses and treatment. The authors are to be applauded for very up-to-date treatment algorithms for a wide variety of arrhythmic disorders, including the genetic arrhythmia syndromes.

This book is easily portable and is of great value for the busy clinician called upon to treat these patients, as well as students and nurses interested in learning more about this rapidly expanding area in medicine. It should also prove of great value to seasoned clinicians eager to gain an authoritative review of the management and treatment of patients with cardiac rhythm disorders.

Melvin Scheinman, MD, FACC
Professor of Medicine
Walter H. Shorenstein Endowed Chair in Cardiology
Chief of Cardiology Genetics Arrhythmia Program
University of California, San Francisco
San Francisco, California

Preface

Arrhythmia Essentials is a comprehensive, yet practical handbook that provides an approach to patients who have cardiac arrhythmias, including those arrhythmias that occur in specific clinical settings. The book is meant to be used to help assess and manage patients with virtually all arrhythmias and related symptoms and includes treatment strategies that may be considered. To this end, we have focused on a step-by-step approach for ease of use. The book is divided into chapters that include sinus node function, bradycardias, tachycardias, heart block, normal and abnormal pacemaker and implantable defibrillator function, and special arrhythmia-related topics such as syncope, palpitations, arrhythmias in the athlete, and other clinical conditions of importance. Also provided is a section that summarizes available drugs useful to treat patients with cardiac arrhythmias. The second edition includes a brand new chapter on managing arrhythmias in pregnancy. Each chapter is accompanied by illustrative electrocardiograms and, where thought to be useful, practical algorithms that help delineate an organized approach to arrhythmia diagnosis and management.

This is the first practical handbook written on this topic that is aimed at practicing clinicians of all specialties, that is based on a contemporary approach, and that focuses on new and advanced therapeutic options and technologies. We believe that the reader will refer to this book often and find it to be compelling, concise, comprehensive, and relevant. It is hoped that this book (in print or on a smartphone or tablet) will find its way to a lab coat pocket, and be available on patient care units rather than sit on the library bookshelf.

Brian Olshansky, MD

Mina K. Chung, MD

Steven M. Pogwizd, MD

Nora Goldschlager, MD

Contents

NORMAL SINUS NODE

Description

Normal sinus rhythm (NSR) is an atrial rhythm caused by electrical activation that originates from the sinus node, a structure located in the area of the junction of the right atrium and superior vena cava. NSR P waves, representing atrial depolarization (but not sinus node activity itself), are upright in leads I and aVL and the inferior leads (II, III, aVF), indicating the high to low atrial activation pattern (Fig. 1.1). The P wave in leads V_1-V_2 may be upright, biphasic, or slightly inverted, whereas the P waves in leads V_3-V_6 tend to be upright, indicating right to left atrial activation. The P-wave morphology may change with alterations in autonomic tone, heart rate, and atrial abnormalities such as hypertrophy. High vagal tone can be associated with a more inferior exit of the impulse from the sinus node, whereas high sympathetic tone can be associated with a more superior exit from the node.

Clinical Symptoms and Presentations

NSR is generally considered to have a rate of 60 to 100 beats per minute (bpm), although 50 bpm is still normal. Rate changes with alterations in autonomic tone; at rest, most individuals have their heart rate regulated by the vagus nerve.

Individuals with high vagal tone (such as those who are in excellent physical condition) may exhibit sinus arrhythmia, a normal rhythm in which the rate varies with respiration (Fig. 1.2). In sinus arrhythmia, inspiration increases the rate and expiration decreases the rate. Sinus arrhythmia is common during sleep and in patients with obstructive sleep apnea, in which the decrease in rate can be substantial.

Various forms of sinus arrhythmia exist, including a non–respiration-dependent form that may indicate sinus node dysfunction (SND).

Ventriculophasic sinus arrhythmia is present when alterations in the sinus rate are due to atrioventricular (AV) block: The P-P intervals enclosing a QRS complex are shorter than P-P intervals not enclosing a QRS complex.

A change in sinus rate can be gradual or abrupt and can occur with change in body position and exercise. Patients who are in good physical condition generally have more gradual acceleration in sinus rate with exercise and a rapid slowing of the sinus rate at the end of exercise,

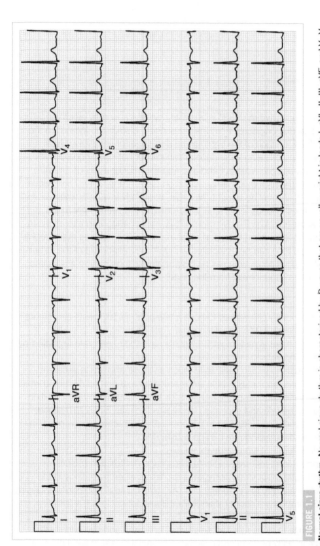

FIGURE 1.1

Normal sinus rhythm. Normal sinus rhythm is characterized by P waves that are usually upright in leads I, aVL, II, III, aVF, and V₃-V₆ at a rate between 60 and 100 bpm.

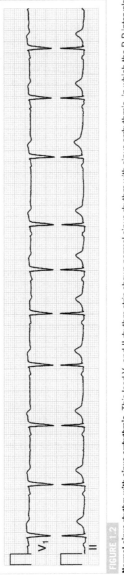

FIGURE 1.2

Normal sinus rhythm with sinus arrhythmia. This lead V_1 and II rhythm strip shows normal sinus rhythm with sinus arrhythmia, in which the P-P intervals vary by greater than 0.16 seconds. Sinus arrhythmia is often related to respiratory cycles.

compared with less physically fit individuals or individuals with heart disease. Higher resting sinus rates have been associated with increased risk for overall mortality.

Wandering atrial pacemaker (WAP) (Fig. 1.3) occurs in association with high vagal tone and is a benign rhythm. In WAP, there are varying exit points of the sinus impulse from the sinus node or impulses that originate from the sinus node and wander from the node to the low atrium and back. WAP is often seen in patients with sinus arrhythmia. WAP should not be confused with "multifocal atrial rhythm" (see Fig. 3.13).

Approach to Management

Although sinus rhythm generally does not require any treatment, an inability to increase the sinus rate appropriately in response to increases in metabolic needs ("chronotropic incompetence") may require permanent rate responsive cardiac pacing when it is documented to cause symptoms. Definitions of chronotropic incompetence are many and varied, and there is no general agreement as to its parameters.

SINUS NODE DYSFUNCTION, INCLUDING SINUS BRADYCARDIA AND TACHYCARDIA-BRADYCARDIA SYNDROME

Description

Sinus bradycardia (SB) (Fig. 1.4) is generally defined as sinus rates of less than 60 bpm, although 50 bpm is likely within the normal range of rate. SB is often a normal finding in young, healthy adults, especially in athletes with high vagal tone. SB frequently occurs at rest and during sleep. In trained athletes or individuals with high vagal tone, sinus rates in the 40s and even at times in the 30s, especially during sleep, are not uncommon. SB may be associated with a narrow QRS complex or, in the presence of bundle branch block (BBB) or intraventricular conduction delay, with a wide QRS complex (Fig. 1.5).

The sinus rate normally slows with age. SND from sinus node degeneration is more frequent in older persons. SND, sometimes termed "sick sinus syndrome," is a very common arrhythmia and includes sinus pauses, sinus arrest, inappropriate SB, chronotropic incompetence, sinoatrial (SA) exit block, combinations of SA and AV conduction abnormalities, and tachycardia-bradycardia (tachy-brady) syndrome (e.g., paroxysmal or persistent atrial tachyarrhythmias with periods of bradycardia or postconversion sinus pauses) (Fig. 1.6).

Associated Conditions

SB is often associated with sinus arrhythmia, escape rhythms (junctional and ventricular), accelerated rhythms (junctional and ventricular), atrial arrhythmias, WAP, or SA or AV Wenckebach-like periods. SB is usually benign but can be associated with certain conditions and diseases, including hypothyroidism, vagal stimulation, carotid sinus hypersensitivity,

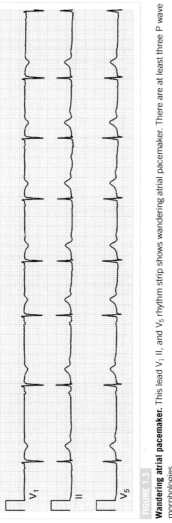

FIGURE 1.3

Wandering atrial pacemaker. This lead V$_1$, II, and V$_5$ rhythm strip shows wandering atrial pacemaker. There are at least three P wave morphologies.

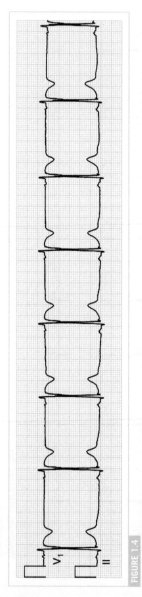

FIGURE 1.4

Sinus bradycardia. This lead II rhythm strip shows SB, which is characterized by sinus P waves (usually upright in leads II, III, aVF) with rate less than 60 bpm.

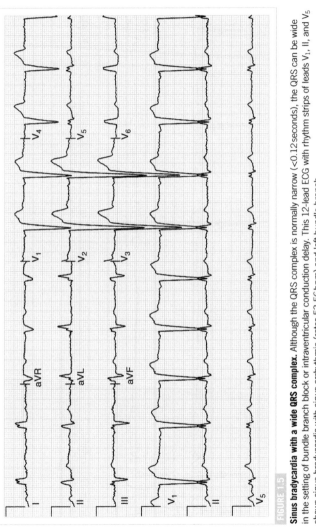

FIGURE 1.5

Sinus bradycardia with a wide QRS complex. Although the QRS complex is normally narrow (<0.12seconds), the QRS can be wide in the setting of bundle branch block or intraventricular conduction delay. This 12-lead ECG with rhythm strips of leads V$_1$, II, and V$_5$ shows sinus bradycardia with sinus arrhythmia (rates 53-56bpm) and left bundle branch.

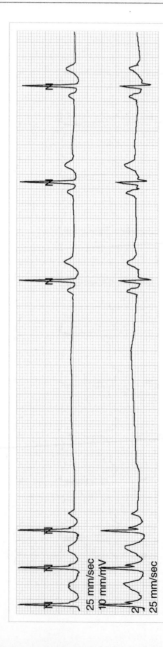

Tachycardia-bradycardia syndrome. This rhythm strip tracing shows an atrial tachyarrhythmia (atrial flutter/tachycardia) that suddenly terminates. The tachycardia is followed by a 3.4-second pause and then sinus bradycardia. The combination of a tachycardia that is suddenly followed by a bradycardia is characteristic of tachy-brady syndrome.

increased intracranial pressure, myocardial infarction (MI), and drugs such as β-adrenergic blockers (including those used for glaucoma), calcium channel blockers, amiodarone, sotalol, clonidine, lithium, and parasympathomimetic drugs. SB occurs in 14% to 36% of MIs and can be associated with AV block. The bradycardia usually resolves without the need for chronic therapy. SB is usually associated with inferior-posterior infarction (caused by increased vagal tone from stimulation of vagal afferents, the Bezold-Jarisch reflex). Clinical syndromes, such as neurocardiogenic syncope and some specific rhythm disorders such as tachy-brady syndrome, can be associated with symptomatic bradycardia as well as symptoms caused by rapid ventricular rates during atrial fibrillation or flutter; severe SB or sinus arrest can occur after spontaneous conversion prior to recovery of the sinus node. SB can be exacerbated by drugs that are used to slow AV node conduction during atrial arrhythmias.

Clinical Symptoms and Presentation

SB is asymptomatic in the vast majority of patients. When present, symptoms may include fatigue, effort intolerance, palpitations, dizziness, lightheadedness, near syncope, syncope, dyspnea, and angina. SND, including chronotropic incompetence, can impair cardiac output or exacerbate heart failure and can be associated with or trigger atrial arrhythmias (e.g., atrial fibrillation) and ventricular arrhythmias (e.g., torsades de pointes). Hemodynamic tolerance of SB is a function of heart rate (a rate of <30 bpm is usually not well tolerated), underlying disease (less tolerated with poor ventricular function), and age (better tolerated in those <50 years old). Tachy-brady syndrome may present with rapid palpitations during atrial arrhythmias and lightheadedness, dizziness, near syncope, and/or syncope during postconversion pauses. SND and/or tachy-brady syndrome can result from cardiac surgery, particularly associated with right atriotomy. SND is relatively common after heart transplantation, as the donor atria can be damaged by ischemia and by atrial anastomoses. The sinus node of the native heart rarely interacts with or affects the transplanted sinus rate. Other causes of SB and/or pauses in heart transplant patients include drugs (rare), trauma, and rejection.

Approach to Management

Evaluation or treatment often is unnecessary if the patient is asymptomatic. Treatment depends on the nature of the rhythm disturbance and is usually directed toward prevention of symptoms. Asystole can be life-threatening, but more often it causes symptoms and is due to vagal surges or SND. Asystolic pauses in a young, otherwise healthy person are generally due to vagal surges related to a neurocardiogenic response. An asystolic response after cardioversion, after a tachycardia, and in a patient who is older or has heart disease is often due to SND. Because SND can be subclinical but exacerbated by medical therapy, rate-slowing drugs should be avoided if possible.

A heart rate less than 30 bpm is an indication to evaluate further for treatment. Symptoms caused by SND can be difficult to assess. Exercise testing (if feasible with a temporary pacemaker if a previous exercise test showed inappropriate heart rate response) can help distinguish the cause of symptoms. If severe SND (i.e., SB associated with sinus exit block, sinus pauses, and sinus arrest) is suspected but cannot be documented by physical examination, telemetry monitor strip, or electrocardiogram (ECG), it can be evaluated further with a Holter monitor (low sensitivity), event monitor, implantable loop recorder, or electrophysiology test (low sensitivity and specificity).

The timing of the pauses or the bradycardia is important. It is not uncommon for a patient to develop SB or asystolic episodes during sleep. Although often caused by enhanced vagal tone, this may in some patients be related to sleep apnea. If pauses are seen during sleep on telemetry or Holter monitoring, sleep apnea should be considered and ruled out.

Short-term monitoring is used for the acute setting in the hospital. Such monitoring is capable of detecting all rhythm disturbances over a period of time. Admitting a patient with symptoms suggestive of bradycardia and then placing the patient on a monitor are usually unproductive steps unless the patient is having frequent and severe episodes. Thus, the first-line approach is long-term monitoring, as long as this approach is considered safe. External event recorders can document episodes of symptomatic SB, but their yield will depend on the frequency of the episodes. In some instances, these events can be difficult to capture because of their episodic nature; in these cases, an implantable loop recorder that continuously records and erases the cardiac rhythm (but has memory) may be optimal. This leadless implant can record and save episodes automatically or can be triggered manually.

The Holter monitor, a continuous 24-hour ambulatory monitor, has the advantage of determining all heart rhythms, symptomatic or asymptomatic, during the recording period and therefore helps determine the presence or absence of SND; however, correlative information relating rhythm and symptoms is often lacking.

Electrophysiology testing can be used to determine SND. The test includes a measurement for SA conduction time and sinus node recovery time. Both of these measurements have a low degree of sensitivity, and the specificity is essentially unknown. Thus, the utility of the electrophysiology test is relatively uncertain, and it is not routinely used to diagnose or exclude the arrhythmia.

Autonomic testing is generally not performed to determine the effect of parasympathetic and sympathetic activation as a cause for changes in heart rate. In patients with syncope in whom a neurocardiogenic reflex is suspected but not diagnosed with certainty, the tilt table test may be helpful in determining its presence. The tilt table test has an unclear specificity and sensitivity, and there is no gold standard to determine the presence or absence of the neurocardiogenic reflex and the relationship of this reflex to SB or asystole. The accuracy with which this test predicts the cause of syncope is dependent on both the protocol and the patient. In a patient with apparent asystolic episodes caused by suspected SND, the tilt table test may be helpful in distinguishing an autonomic reflex from SND.

For the patient with recent syncope or severe symptoms thought to be due to SND, hospital admission is required, especially for those with multiple medical problems, those who have been injured, and those who are older. Acute treatment is needed if there are severe symptoms or serious sequelae of bradycardia (Tables 1.1 and 1.2).

TABLE 1.1

SINUS NODE DYSFUNCTION AND SINUS BRADYCARDIA MANAGEMENT

Setting	Therapy
Asymptomatic	• No therapy required. There is some relationship between the presence of sleep apnea and sinus node dysfunction; some reports have suggested that permanent pacing, even in asymptomatic patients, may benefit sleep apnea.
	• Identify and treat associated medical conditions such as hypothyroidism.
	• Avoid rate-slowing drug if feasible.
Symptomatic—acute	• Treat reversible causes. Consider drugs as the cause (β-adrenergic blockers, calcium channel blockers, and digoxin, antiarrhythmic drugs [sotalol, amiodarone, flecainide, and propafenone]). A drug may be a contributor, but until the problem resolves, treatment will be required.
	• Atropine 0.6-2 mg intravenous every 5 min, up to a total of 2 mg. Low doses and slow infusion may cause paradoxical bradycardia due to increase in sinus rate and degree of AV block. Atropine will not work for heart transplant patients. This is only a short-term solution.
	• Isoproterenol 1-5 mcg/min is effective but can exacerbate myocardial ischemia. Do not give to patients with unstable coronary artery disease. Isoproterenol is rarely indicated and should only be considered in extreme conditions when a temporary pacemaker is not available.
	• Temporary pacemaker (preferably atrial, if AV conduction is intact and the bradycardia is not due to high vagal tone) when unstable and episodes are prolonged, persistent, highly symptomatic, recurrent, or unresponsive to acute medical therapy, such as atropine or isoproterenol, or with bradycardia-associated ventricular arrhythmias (e.g., torsades de pointes). Temporary pacing may be used if permanent pacing is not possible, not indicated, or dangerous (such as the presence of an ongoing infection). Temporary pacing can be accomplished by epicardial wires (after cardiovascular surgery) or by temporary balloon-tipped catheters placed percutaneously with or without fluoroscopy (unreliable) or a temporary bipolar lead (screw in or not) that is more reliable. Placement of a temporary pacemaker can be associated with adverse events. It should be undertaken only if there is a long-term need to pace but there is no immediate permanent pacemaker placement availability (e.g., patients with recurrent syncope who on monitoring have pauses of 5 s or more, symptomatic or not). Temporary pacing is not indicated if there are prolonged pauses caused by neurocardiogenic reasons (e.g., vasovagal syncope, suctioning, endoscopy, vomiting, and cough).

Continued on following page

SINUS NODE DYSFUNCTION AND SINUS BRADYCARDIA MANAGEMENT (Continued)

Setting	Therapy
	• Transcutaneous pacing may be used emergently prior to placement of a temporary pacing lead. It is highly unreliable and painful. It is not very effective over time and is hardly ever indicated. It could be used for a patient who has precipitous hemodynamic collapse due to persistent or recurrent asystole. It has not been shown to reduce the risk of death but occasionally can be used until an adequate temporary pacemaker is placed. Most patients with episodic asystole do not fit into the category of having a life-threatening arrhythmia, but patients with prolonged and recurrent asystole might fit into this category, especially if the patient is older and has underlying heart disease. Transcutaneous pacing is not stable over time because of impedance changes between the large electrodes and myocardium; moreover, adequate sedation is usually necessary to prevent pain.
Symptomatic—chronic	• Permanent pacemaker: ○ Class I (ACC/AHA recommended) indications: Documented symptomatic SB, including frequent pauses that cause symptoms; symptomatic bradycardia occurring as a consequence of essential long-term drug therapy at a dose and type for which there are no acceptable alternatives; symptomatic chronotropic incompetence. ○ Class IIa (ACC/AHA accepted, not mandatory, well substantiated) indications: Sinus node dysfunction from necessary drug therapy with HR <40 bpm when a clear association between presence of bradycardia and significant symptoms has not been documented; syncope of undetermined origin with major abnormalities in sinus node dysfunction found at electrophysiology (EP) study. ○ Class IIb (ACC/AHA accepted, not mandatory, less well substantiated): Minimally symptomatic patients with chronic awake HR <40 bpm. • Temporary transvenous pacemaker, if severe symptoms associated with HR <30 bpm, unresponsive to acute medical therapy (e.g., atropine, isoproterenol) or bradycardia-associated ventricular arrhythmias (e.g., torsades de pointes). Temporary pacing is rarely indicated for chronic symptomatic problems unless there are frequent recurrences of symptomatic pauses or bradycardia.

ACC, American College of Cardiology; *AHA*, American Heart Association; *AV*, atrioventricular; *HR*, heart rate; *SB*, sinus bradycardia.

Permanent cardiac pacing is the treatment of choice for symptomatic SB (including chronotropic incompetence) if there is no transient (such as vasovagal bradycardia) or reversible cause or if the SB occurs as a result of essential drug therapy. Patients with tachy-brady syndrome may require permanent pacing to facilitate drug treatment of their atrial arrhythmias, as drug therapy for rapid atrial arrhythmias may aggravate the bradyarrhythmias.

Pacing may be indicated for specific patients in whom the relationship between the bradycardia and hemodynamic compromise can be demonstrated.

SINUS NODE DYSFUNCTION MANAGEMENT IN SPECIFIC CLINICAL CIRCUMSTANCES

Setting	Therapy
MI	• Common causes for SB in setting of an acute MI: β-adrenergic blockers, calcium channel blockers, amiodarone, morphine, lidocaine, chronic antiarrhythmic drugs, pain, increased vagal tone (especially with inferior MI), atrial ischemia. Usually resolves.
	• In addition to symptomatic SB, additional indications for treatment of SB include recurrent or worsening ischemia (evident by ST segment changes on the ECG), poor cardiac output, hypotension, or bradycardia-related ventricular arrhythmias. These are more common in the first 3-5 days after infarction.
	• Temporary pacing if there is symptomatic SB (despite stopping medications, including β-adrenergic blockers), prolonged pauses (>3 s recurrently or occasional ones >5 s), hypotension, heart failure symptoms. Permanent pacing is rarely needed. In some instances, a wait of 5-7 days may not be long enough to know if there is complete resolution of bradycardia. In that case, a permanent pacemaker is indicated when there are continued pauses or heart rates <40 per minute. Treadmill exercise testing can be used to ascertain chronotropic competence after MI.
Pre-op	• Atropine should be available, especially at induction of anesthesia and during intubation when vagal tone is high.
	• SB is very common intraoperatively due to maneuvers that increase vagal tone such as intubation. If hypothermia is planned, SB can be expected. No treatment is required.
	• Even if asymptomatic, patients who cannot increase cardiac output because of SB may require temporary pacing.
Post-op	• SB is common, often due to pain, opiates, or effect of surgery itself, and is usually not treated.
	• Temporary pacing (preferably atrial but with ventricular backup pacing if there is a vagal component) at 80-100 bpm can be used in cases of hemodynamic decompensation. Permanent pacing should be considered if SB does not resolve after 3-5 post-op days.
Heart transplant	• One to three weeks after transplant, SND, including SB, may resolve and require no chronic therapy.
	• Acutely, isoproterenol is first-line therapy, as opposed to atropine, which will not work in the denervated heart.
	• Theophylline 150-200 mg PO bid may work in the subacute setting. Although effective in the short term, it has not been proven effective over the long term.
	• After 10-20 days, if persistent, symptomatic, and not expected to resolve, SND may require treatment with a permanent pacemaker. An atrial pacing device might be considered to avoid tricuspid valve damage (patient may need repeated biopsies that may dislodge pacing leads), but make sure it is secure in the transplanted donor (not recipient) atrium, such that paced atrial beats will conduct intrinsically to the ventricles.

bid, Twice daily; *ECG,* electrocardiogram; *MI,* myocardial infarction; *PO,* per os; *SB,* sinus bradycardia; *SND,* sinus node dysfunction.

After cardiac surgery, sinus node function that fails to recover may also necessitate a permanent pacemaker. Because it can take 5 to 6 weeks before full return of sinus node function, frequently a decision is made to implant a pacemaker by the fifth to seventh post-op day before hospital discharge. It is best to make that decision while temporary pacing wires are still in place so that temporary pacing can be instituted if it is necessary.

SINOATRIAL EXIT BLOCK

Description

SA exit block results from a block in conduction from the sinus node to the atria. It usually appears on the ECG as the absence of a P wave, with the pause duration being a multiple of the basic P-P interval. In first-degree SA block, conduction of sinus impulses to the atrium is delayed, but a 1:1 response is maintained; because impulse formation in the sinus node is not visible on the ECG, it is impossible to diagnose, as it looks like sinus rhythm. Second-degree SA block takes the form of type I or type II (analogous to AV block); some sinus impulses fail to depolarize the atria (i.e., intermittent absence of a P wave). Type I (Wenckebach pattern) SA block (Fig. 1.7) is characterized by normal P-wave morphology and axis consistent with a sinus node origin and group beating with (1) progressive shortening of the P-P interval leading up to a pause in P-wave rate, (2) constant PR interval, and (3) P-P pauses less than twice the normal P-P interval.

Type II SA block (Fig. 1.8) is characterized by a constant P-P interval followed by a pause that is a multiple (e.g., 2 times, 3 times) of the normal P-P interval. The pause may be slightly less than twice the normal P-P interval but is usually within 0.1 seconds of this interval. Third-degree SA block indicates complete failure of SA conduction but cannot be differentiated from a sinus pause.

Associated Conditions

SA exit block is usually related to drug therapy (digoxin, calcium channel blockers, β-adrenergic blockers), vagal stimulation, SND with degenerative disease of the sinus node and atrium, or hyperkalemia. It is unusual after MI but may be caused by vagal excess (Bezold-Jarisch reflex) from an inferoposterior MI. If unrelated to an acute cause that is reversible or transient, SA exit block may cause progressive bradycardia.

Clinical Symptoms and Presentation

SA exit block may be asymptomatic or associated with mild palpitations because of pauses and the irregularity of heart rate; however, most symptoms are similar to those listed under SB.

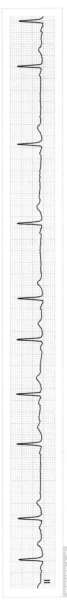

Sinoatrial exit block type I. This is a lead II rhythm strip of sinus rhythm with slight P-P interval shortening followed by a pause that is less than twice the prevailing P-P interval. This represents SA exit block (type I) in a patient who has sinus node dysfunction.

FIGURE 1.7

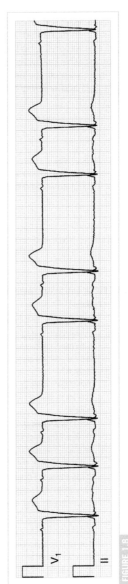

Sinoatrial exit block type II. This is a rhythm strip of leads V_1 and II showing sinus rhythm (rate 67 bpm) with sinus pauses that are twice the prevailing P-P interval. There is also left bundle branch block.

FIGURE 1.8

Approach to Management

Patients should be assessed for potentially reversible causes (e.g., drugs) and then monitored, and any inciting stimulus should be removed. If asymptomatic, no therapy is indicated, although close follow-up for progressive bradycardia should be maintained. Treatment is indicated only if symptomatic and involves the avoidance of precipitating factors and possibly atrial pacing for persistent symptoms (Table 1.3; Algorithm 1.1).

SINUS PAUSE/ARREST

Description

Sinus pause or sinus arrest, caused by transient failure of impulse formation at or exit from the SA node, is manifested on the ECG as absent P waves with or without an escape rhythm (Fig. 1.9).

Associated Conditions

Most commonly associated conditions include paroxysmal elevation in vagal tone, intrinsic SND, and drug therapy. Antiarrhythmic drugs,

---

TABLE 1.3

SINOATRIAL EXIT BLOCK AND SINUS PAUSE MANAGEMENT

Setting	Therapy
Type I or II second-degree block	• If asymptomatic, no therapy is required.
	• If symptomatic bradycardia, for acute cases, use atropine; for chronic cases (rare), use permanent single chamber rate adaptive pacemaker or dual chamber rate adaptive pacemaker cardiac pacing (see sinus bradycardia).
	• Discontinue responsible drugs (e.g., digoxin), if possible. If not possible, and there are episodes of symptomatic bradycardia, a permanent pacemaker is indicated.
	• Exclude hyperkalemia.
Myocardial infarction	• If symptomatic bradycardia, for acute cases, use atropine; note, however, that atropine can occasionally produce increased sinus node firing rate, increased sinoatrial exit block, and paradoxical slowing of atrial and ventricular rate.
	• Usually transient. External pacing if pauses are prolonged and cause hemodynamic embarrassment.
Pre-op	• If asymptomatic, no specific therapy required. External pacer available.
	• If elective surgery and symptomatic with no reversible cause, use atrial or dual chamber (AAI[R] or DDD[R]) pacemaker before surgery.
	• If urgent surgery and symptomatic, use atropine and assure availability of a temporary external or transvenous endocardial pacemaker.
	• Vagal stimulation due to intubation, Foley catheter placement, and so forth may worsen block but may respond well to atropine.
Post-op	• Usually no treatment, but pace temporarily if symptomatic or hypotensive.

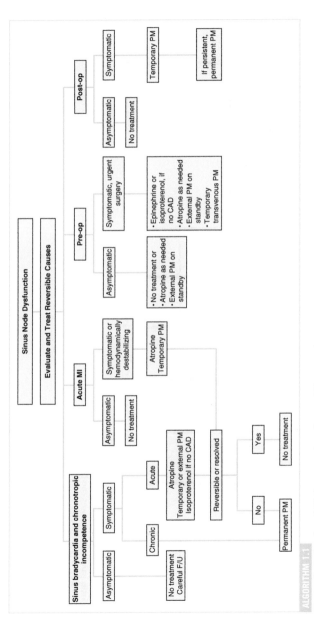

ALGORITHM 1.1

Sinus node dysfunction. *CAD,* Coronary artery disease; *PM,* pacemaker.

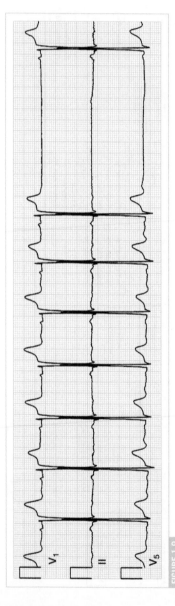

FIGURE 1.9

Sinus pause. Sinus pauses can be prolonged, in which case they can be referred to as sinus arrest. In this lead V₁, II, and V₅ rhythm strip, following 7 beats of sinus rhythm (rate ~68 bpm), there is a 3-second sinus pause, followed by a sinus beat.

including quinidine, procainamide, digoxin, propafenone, flecainide, amiodarone, β-adrenergic, calcium channel blockers, and sotalol, can worsen SND (which may have been occult on the ECG initially). Sinus pauses or arrest may result from degenerative changes of the sinus node, acute MI, excessive vagal tone or stimuli, digitalis toxicity (rare), sleep apnea, stroke, neurocardiogenic syncope, carotid sinus hypersensitivity, or tachy-brady syndrome.

Clinical Symptoms and Presentation

Symptoms may include syncope, heart failure, angina, weakness, fatigue, dizziness, confusion, or shortness of breath. It is crucial to correlate symptoms with the arrhythmia, as symptoms may be due to other causes. Sinus pauses tend to progress if not due to a reversible cause.

Approach to Management

Patients should be evaluated for sleep apnea, carotid hypersensitivity, and vagal excess (consider tilt table test if documentation is lacking). Any identified underlying causes that may be exacerbating sinus pauses should be treated. These include drugs, ischemia, neurocardiogenic causes, and hyperkalemia. A pacemaker is indicated when the patient is highly symptomatic and the underlying cause is not treatable by removing the inciting stimulus or when pauses are long and frequent (Algorithm 1.2).

SINUS TACHYCARDIA

Description

Sinus tachycardia (ST) is characterized by a sinus P wave at a rate of more than 100 per minute, usually followed by a QRS complex that is usually narrow (but may be wide in the presence of an underlying BBB) (Fig. 1.10). ST is common and ubiquitous. It is present during exercise but can occur at rest when associated with any number of conditions. Atrial tachycardia or atrial flutter with 2:1 block may be mistaken for ST but usually does not have distinct upright P waves evident in leads II, III, aVF (Fig. 1.11). ST with first-degree AV block may be difficult to diagnose if the sinus P wave is buried in the T wave (Fig. 1.12). Sinus node reentry tachycardia, generally an uncommon form of supraventricular tachycardia, can mimic ST in P-wave morphology. Consider carotid sinus massage or adenosine to distinguish sinus node reentry tachycardia (which will usually terminate) from ST (which will only slow without terminating).

Associated Conditions

The differential diagnosis for ST is extensive and includes some severe and potentially life-threatening disorders. Potential underlying causes that should be considered include drugs, such as cocaine, amphetamines (and amphetamine-like drugs such as methylphenidate), catecholamines (isoproterenol, epinephrine, dopamine, ephedrine), β-adrenergic

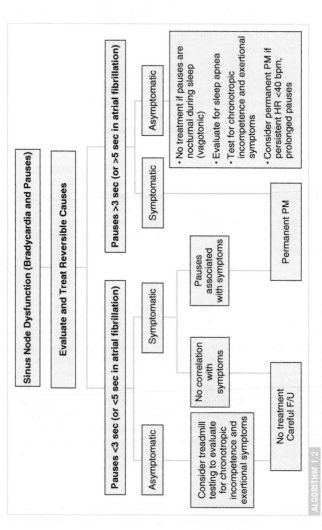

ALGORITHM 1.2
Sinus node dysfunction (bradycardia and pauses). *HR,* Heart rate; *PM,* pacemaker.

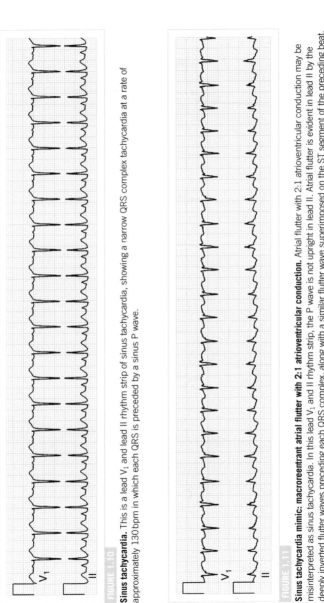

FIGURE 1.10

Sinus tachycardia. This is a lead V₁ and lead II rhythm strip of sinus tachycardia, showing a narrow QRS complex tachycardia at a rate of approximately 130 bpm in which each QRS is preceded by a sinus P wave.

FIGURE 1.11

Sinus tachycardia mimic: macroreentrant atrial flutter with 2:1 atrioventricular conduction. Atrial flutter with 2:1 atrioventricular conduction may be misinterpreted as sinus tachycardia. In this lead V₁ and II rhythm strip, the P wave is not upright in lead II. Atrial flutter is evident in lead II by the deeply inverted flutter waves preceding each QRS complex, along with a similar flutter wave superimposed on the ST segment of the preceding beat.

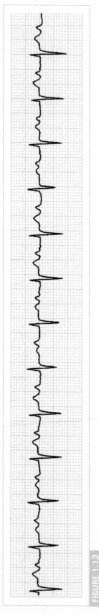

FIGURE 1.12

Sinus tachycardia with first-degree atrioventricular block. In this rhythm strip the P and T waves are close together, but examination of the preceding T waves show the distinct P waves and first-degree AV block.

blocker withdrawal, and anticholinergics (atropine, scopolamine); tobacco; caffeine; alcohol; fever; infection; anemia; hypovolemia; pulmonary embolism; hyperthyroidism; congestive heart failure (CHF); hypoglycemia; pneumothorax; or persistent pain. ST may also be caused by dysautonomias, postural orthostatic tachycardia syndrome (POTS), and anxiety. ST occurs in up to approximately one-third of patients with acute MIs (anterior most common) and may be due to left ventricular (LV) dysfunction, persistent pain, hypoxemia due to pulmonary edema, hypovolemia, atrial infarction, catecholamine infusion, pericarditis, pulmonary embolism, cardiac rupture with tamponade, aortic insufficiency, or mitral regurgitation from papillary muscle dysfunction. ST can occur after ablation of AV node reentrant tachycardia due to vagal denervation and can last for months. Anxiety is a diagnosis of exclusion for ST at rest.

Less than 5% of ST is due to abnormal or inappropriate ST (IST) in which there is no specific or explainable cause. IST is a condition in which the heart rate is faster than expected. Heart rate at rest and even in a supine position may be faster than 100 bpm, and in some individuals, minimal activity causes a rapid and substantial increase in heart rate. Patients can become highly symptomatic and can be restricted from doing any kind of physical activity. The mechanisms responsible for IST are not completely understood. It is important to distinguish IST from appropriate ST and from POTS. It is important to rule out reversible causes of tachycardia. IST may be due to excess sympathetic stimulation of the sinus node or unusual electrophysiologic properties of the sinus node. The genetics and family history of this condition are not well known. Treatment can be as simple as physical training but also may require medication such as β-adrenergic blockers; even in high doses, however, β-adrenergic blockade is often ineffective (the I_f channel blocker [ivabradine] has been shown to be effective). In some instances, sinus node modification may be required, but this has limited efficacy and may cause asystolic episodes and is generally not recommended.

Clinical Symptoms and Presentation

Palpitations are the most common complaint, but dizziness, lightheadedness, and near syncope can occur. Many are asymptomatic. ST is usually self-limited; however, ST may be particularly hazardous in patients with mitral stenosis (decreased diastolic filling may precipitate pulmonary edema), hypertrophic cardiomyopathy (decreased LV filling time with consequent decreased LV volume worsens LV outflow tract obstruction), and myocardial ischemia (decreased diastolic coronary perfusion intensifies ischemia). Patients with IST may have persistent tachycardia for prolonged periods. Impaired LV function could potentially develop from persistent high rates, causing a tachycardia-induced cardiomyopathy, but the incidence of this is rare.

It is important to look hard for an underlying cause, as one nearly always exists, may be severe, and may need to be treated. In cases of suspected IST, evaluation to exclude hyper-β-adrenergic states should be performed, including thyroid function tests; 24-hour urine tests for catecholamines, metanephrine, vanillylmandelic acid (VMA), 5-hydroxyindoleacetic acid (5-HIAA); and possibly drug screening. Herbal supplement use should also be investigated as potential causes of occult stimulant ingestion. Treatment is directed toward the underlying cause. Treatment directed at slowing the sinus rate is reserved for severely symptomatic patients (before treatments for the underlying cause become effective) and for symptomatic patients with IST. In selected patients with highly symptomatic IST refractory to medical therapies, sinus node modification/ablation using catheter ablation techniques may be beneficial (Table 1.4).

TABLE 1.4

SINUS TACHYCARDIA MANAGEMENT

Setting	Therapy
Asymptomatic	• No specific therapy. Therapy is directed at underlying cause.
	• IST, in which no specific cause can be found, and which is asymptomatic and chronic without any measurable effect on cardiac function, usually does not require specific therapy.
Symptomatic	• No specific therapy indicated unless all physiologic causes are excluded.
	• Treatment for IST is indicated if symptoms impair the patient's ability to function normally. Initial therapy: β-adrenergic blockers (preferably cardioselective, β1). Titrate slowly over several days. Doses may need to be high (e.g., atenolol 200 mg/day, metoprolol 200 mg bid, or acebutolol 400-800 mg/day). Calcium channel blockers (e.g., diltiazem, verapamil) can be tried if β-adrenergic blockers are ineffective or not tolerated. The I_f blocker ivabidine 5-7.5 mg bid alone or in combination with a β-adrenergic blocker can be effective. If medical therapy and an exercise program do not help, catheter ablation or modification of part of the sinus node can be considered for severely symptomatic, refractory cases. Rule out POTS prior to considering ablation.
MI	• β-Adrenergic blockers may decrease heart rate in patients with ST during MI. They can also decrease myocardial oxygen demand and improve prognosis; however, β-adrenergic blockers may need to be deferred or avoided when pulmonary edema, severe LV dysfunction, or AV block is present.
	• Correct alterations in fluid status (fluid depletion, fluid overload). Right ventricular infarcts can cause sinus tachycardia by decreasing LV filling and often respond to treatment with intravenous fluid.
	• Inotropes (e.g., milrinone, dopamine) can cause sinus tachycardia and should be suspected if increase in heart rate occurs (whether or not there is improvement in the signs and symptoms of heart failure). In this case, decreasing the dose or stopping the inotropic drug may be beneficial.

TABLE 1.4

SINUS TACHYCARDIA MANAGEMENT (Continued)

Setting	Therapy
	If sinus tachycardia presents after thrombolytic drugs or angioplasty, consider other causes (e.g., LV failure or bleeding). β-Adrenergic blockers may exacerbate heart failure and worsen LV dysfunction, and should be used with caution.
	In the setting of persistent sinus tachycardia associated with severe pulmonary edema, hypotension, or recurrent ischemia, evaluation for possible revascularization or for mechanical complications should be considered.
Pre-op	Sinus tachycardia is common in this setting. It is often due to anxiety, and treatment is not required; however, it is important to consider an organic condition precipitating sinus tachycardia that may interfere with the induction of anesthesia, with the surgical procedure, or with recovery from the surgery. It is also very important that pulmonary edema and acute myocardial ischemia are ruled out.
Post-op	Sinus tachycardia is common after noncardiac as well as cardiac surgery. Approximately 15% of patients will have persistent sinus tachycardia at the time of discharge following CABG.
	Common causes of sinus tachycardia in this setting should be considered and include pain, hypovolemia, anemia, pulmonary edema, myocardial ischemia, pneumothorax, hemothorax, pulmonary embolus, sepsis, and infection.
	If no cause can be found, no treatment is necessary. If it persists by time of hospital discharge and no cause is found, a β-adrenergic blocker for 4-6 weeks can be used.
Pregnancy	Sinus tachycardia is a common physiologic response to pregnancy, with heart rate progressively increasing from first to third trimesters. Thus, sinus tachycardia typically does not warrant specific therapy during pregnancy.
	Pregnant women with sinus tachycardia and findings suggestive of heart failure should be evaluated for potential peripartum cardiomyopathy. Findings suggestive of heart disease include paroxysmal nocturnal dyspnea, jugular venous distension, hepatomegaly, rales, RV heave, and an abnormal cardiac impulse that is displaced and sustained.
	β-Adrenergic blockers could be considered for symptomatic sinus tachycardia, but would be preferable to avoid, particularly nearer to delivery.

AV, Atrioventricular; *bid*, twice daily; *CABG*, coronary artery bypass graft; *IST*, inappropriate sinus tachycardia; *LV*, left ventricular; *MI*, myocardial infarction; *POTS*, postural orthostatic tachycardia syndrome; *RV*, right ventricle; *ST*, sinus tachycardia.

POSTURAL ORTHOSTATIC TACHYCARDIA SYNDROME

Description

POTS is a condition in which there is a rapid and sustained increase in heart rate with minimal change in blood pressure while going from a supine to a sitting or standing position. Various definitions exist, but generally the increase in heart rate is at least 30 bpm (or an increase in sinus rate to more than 120 bpm) with minimal change in blood pressure and occurs after several minutes of standing from a supine position. This is due to an autonomic condition probably related to changes in peripheral or splanchnic vascular tone in which the heart rate increases to prevent a drop in blood pressure; however, the exact mechanisms are not completely understood. This condition may be overdiagnosed in some instances, as there may be a reversible cause for the problem, such as dehydration or bleeding. As such, POTS is a diagnosis of exclusion.

Clinical Symptoms and Presentation

POTS can occur in a variety of different clinical situations. It commonly occurs in young females and is associated with lightheadedness, palpitations, fatigue, confusion, chest pain, and headaches. Only rarely does syncope occur.

POTS is characterized as being primary or secondary. The primary form is a partial dysautonomic form, which may be related to a postviral syndrome or could be merely related to aging. There is also a hyperadrenergic form. Diabetes, a paraneoplastic syndrome, and joint hypermobility syndromes have been described as possible etiologies in secondary forms. There are potential poorly defined psychiatric problems, including anxiety neuroses, that are present in individuals with POTS.

In primary dysautonomic POTS, there is inadequate vascular resistance with orthostatic stress. This is more common in females than males. It tends to occur after viral illnesses, pregnancy, surgery, sepsis, and trauma. It has an acute onset and generally resolves. Hyperadrenergic POTS is due to excess norepinephrine spillover with evidence for inappropriate sympathetic stimuli. Migraine headaches are common. Orthostatic hypertension tends to occur. There is a family history and a gradual onset. Many mechanisms have been postulated as a cause for POTS, including peripheral denervation with supersensitivity, acetylcholine receptor autoantibodies that are due to a postviral illness, central hyperadrenergic state, norepinephrine transporter deficiency, decreased baroreceptor gain, and idiopathic hypovolemia (due to altered aldosterone, renin, and angiotensin II activity). POTS has also been associated with mast cell activation.

Secondary POTS is due to peripheral autonomic denervation and can occur with diabetes, amyloidosis, sarcoidosis, lupus, heavy metals, alcoholism, chemotherapy, and Sjögren's syndrome. It can occur in pure autonomic failure or multiple system atrophy and paraneoplastic syndromes. In the latter, it may be due to autoantibodies to acetylcholine receptors of the ganglia similar to postviral POTS.

The differential diagnoses include dehydration, hyperthyroidism, drugs, supplements such as guarana, caffeine, IST, supraventricular tachycardia, pheochromocytoma, anemia, pulmonary emboli, and panic disorder.

Approach to Management

Management first requires a determination that the syndrome is indeed POTS. Reversible causes must be excluded. The type of POTS (primary or secondary) should be determined. Consider nonpharmacological interventions such as lifestyle changes, with drug therapy as necessary.

No treatments are proven to be effective. Management strategies may include simply avoiding triggers, exercise (particularly supine exercise like rowing), water, salt, thromboembolic deterrent (TED) hose, fludrocortisone, midodrine, and even β-adrenergic blockers. Other drugs that have been tried include serotonin reuptake inhibitors, clonidine, erythropoietin, oral vasopressin, yohimbine, methylphenidate, methyldopa, phenobarbital, octreotide, pyridostigmine, modafinil (for "brain fog"), and ivabradine (not approved for this indication). Droxidopa, indicated for neurogenic orthostatic hypotension and not rigorously tested in POTS, may work for this condition.

Drugs to avoid include vasodilators, diuretics, opiates, nitrates, tricyclic antidepressants, phenothiazines, ethanol, angiotensin-converting enzyme (ACE) inhibitors, β-adrenergic blockers, α-blockers, calcium channel blockers, ganglionic blockers, hydralazine, sildenafil, monoamine oxidase (MAO) inhibitors, and bromocriptine.

Chapter 2

Bradyarrhythmias— Conduction System Abnormalities

Atrioventricular (AV) block occurs when an atrial impulse either is not conducted to the ventricle or is conducted with delay. This assumes that the impulse occurs at a time that conduction would be expected to occur based on normal conduction and refractory period properties. Conduction block assumes that the rate of the atrial rhythm is in the normal physiological range and is regular. For example, a premature atrial impulse that is not conducted ("blocked") is not considered to be AV block (AVB). AVB is classified on the basis of severity into three types. First-degree AVB is characterized by conduction of all sinus impulses but with a prolonged PR interval more than 0.20 seconds. In second-degree AVB, intermittent block of AV conduction occurs, manifesting as some nonconducted or blocked P waves, but with evidence of AV conduction on other beats. Second-degree AVB can be further categorized into Mobitz types I and II, 2:1, or high-degree (advanced) AVB. In third-degree AVB, there is complete absence of AV conduction when it would be expected.

First-Degree Block

Description

First-degree AVB (Fig. 2.1) represents delay in conduction from the atria to the ventricles and manifests as a prolonged PR interval of more than 0.20 seconds, but all impulses are conducted. The PR interval represents the time from the onset of atrial depolarization due to sinus node activation to the onset of ventricular repolarization (i.e., conduction time from the atrium → AV node [AVN] → His bundle → Purkinje system → ventricles). However, it does not reflect conduction from the sinus node to the atrial tissue. The conduction delay may occur in the atria, AVN, His bundle, and His-Purkinje system. If the QRS complex is narrow and normal appearing, the greatest AV delay usually occurs in the AVN. If the QRS is wide, the conduction delay or block is more likely to occur in the His-Purkinje system than it would be if the QRS were narrow. However, block in the AVN can manifest as a prolonged PR and wide QRS if preexisting bundle branch block (BBB) or rate-dependent aberrancy is present. Diagnosis is usually easy, based on the surface electrocardiogram (ECG) showing a prolonged PR interval. On the ECG during first-degree AVB, the P wave may be

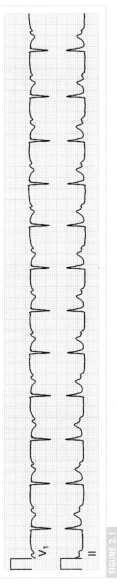

FIGURE 2.1

Sinus rhythm with first-degree atrioventricular block. In this lead V_1 and II rhythm strip, the P and T waves begin to merge, but close examination of the preceding T waves shows the superimposed P waves and first-degree AV block.

buried in the previous QRS complex (especially during sinus rhythm) or the previous T wave and can be difficult to distinguish from a junctional rhythm. If block is in the His-Purkinje system, first-degree AVB is usually associated with BBB.

Associated Conditions

Spontaneous causes of first-degree AVB include intrinsic disease of the AVN and/or His-Purkinje system), high vagal tone, or dual AV nodal pathways (in which two separate populations of PR intervals may be seen). Other causes include drugs that slow AVN conduction, such as calcium channel blockers, β-adrenergic blockers, or digoxin. Isolated first-degree AVB can occur with anterior or inferior myocardial infarctions (MIs). First-degree AVB is generally self-limited and not associated with progression to complete heart block (CHB), but it may be associated with poorer prognosis in those with heart disease. Exceptions include rheumatic fever (for which it is a sign of acute carditis) and endocarditis (for which it may suggest the presence of a valve ring abscess, especially involving the aortic valve), in which first-degree AVB may presage the development of higher levels of block.

Clinical Symptoms and Presentation

First-degree AVB does not usually cause symptoms; however, if the PR interval is markedly prolonged (more than 300 to 600 ms), a loss of optimal AV synchrony may reduce the atrial contribution to ventricular filling, therefore decreasing cardiac output, especially in patients with diastolic dysfunction, and lead to symptoms of heart failure. Rarely the PR interval may be sufficiently long to cause nearly simultaneous contraction of the atria and ventricles, resulting in pacemaker syndrome–like symptoms (fatigue, shortness of breath, near syncope, neck fullness, chest pain).

Approach to Management

There is no specific therapy for first-degree AVB, unless the PR interval is so prolonged as to lead to symptoms. If permanent pacing is considered for symptomatic, very prolonged first-degree AVB, a dual-chamber pacemaker programmed to DDD mode of function but with or without rate response, is the recommended pacing system. His bundle pacing is an option if the level of block is at the AVN. Right ventricular pacing should be minimized because it can cause left ventricular (LV) dyssynchrony; however, His bundle pacing may not be achievable in some patients because it is technically more difficult to achieve than right ventricular apical or outflow tract pacing and is not available in all centers. If the level of block is infra-Hisian, His bundle pacing is not indicated. Another option, not well tested for isolated first-degree AVB, is cardiac resynchronization therapy (CRT) pacing, in which both right and left ventricles are paced. This approach is preferable especially if there is a longstanding need for ventricular pacing for hemodynamic purposes and there is ventricular dysfunction (Table 2.1, Algorithm 2.1).

FIRST-DEGREE ATRIOVENTRICULAR BLOCK MANAGEMENT

Setting	Therapy
Asymptomatic	Usually benign and requires no therapy.
	If due to drugs, no need to discontinue.
Symptomatic, PR very long (300-400 ms)	Because such symptoms as lightheadedness and dizziness are nonspecific and common, especially in older persons, it is essential to exclude other causes before ascribing symptoms to first-degree AVB.
	A rare indication for a DDD pacemaker. Shortening the PR interval to 150-200 ms may improve weakness, fatigue, and shortness of breath by restoring optimal AV synchrony. Consider His bundle pacing if the conduction prolongation is at the level of the AVN.
	If patient is hospitalized and with refractory low cardiac output, consider temporary AV sequential pacing to improve hemodynamics and symptoms and to determine the benefit of permanent pacing.
MI	No therapy usually required (possible exception if the PR is very long).
	May be due to drugs to treat MI (e.g., β-adrenergic blockers, calcium channel blockers, digoxin). If asymptomatic, no medication changes are usually required. If symptomatic or PR very long, consider reducing dosage.
	Consider atrial infarction or elevated atrial pressures as the cause and treat appropriately.
Preoperative	No specific therapy.
	No need for temporary prophylactic pacing as it does not presage higher degrees of AVB.
	If due to a drug, decrease the dose or stop using the drug if it is not essential.
Postoperative	If PR is markedly prolonged (300-400 ms) and hemodynamic compromise is suspected, dual-chamber pacing (at PV or AV interval of 150-200 ms) may improve hemodynamics.
	This may be instituted if temporary pacing wires are present after cardiac surgery.
	If first-degree AVB appears for the first time after aortic valve surgery, it may indicate damage to the His-Purkinje system (usually associated with left bundle branch block in these cases).
	Prolonged PR intervals can cause hemodynamic problems after cardiac surgery since the timing of the "atrial kick" may be more important during this time in which diastolic dysfunction is possible.
Endocarditis	Carefully evaluate for the presence of aortic insufficiency, consider TEE.
	Acute development of first-degree AVB, especially if it occurs with a new bundle branch block (transient or persistent), is highly suspicious for the presence of a valve ring abscess.
	Requires surgical treatment.
	Consider TEE.
	Transfer patient to a unit with cardiac telemetry (if not already there), as progression to higher levels of AVB can occur.

Continued on following page

TABLE 2.1

FIRST-DEGREE ATRIOVENTRICULAR BLOCK MANAGEMENT (Continued)

Setting	Therapy
Rheumatic fever	• First-degree AVB is a sign of rheumatic carditis and may presage the development of higher levels of AVB, including complete heart block.
	• May be an indication for steroids.
Infiltrative and restrictive cardiomyopathies	• If PR is markedly prolonged (>300 ms), dual-chamber pacing (at PV or AV interval of 150-200 ms) may improve hemodynamics and symptoms.
	• Ventricles with severe diastolic dysfunction are especially dependent on atrial kick to maximize cardiac output.
	• If prolongation is at the level of the AV node, consider His bundle pacing.

AV, Atrioventricular; *AVB*, atrioventricular block; *AVN*, atrioventricular node; *MI*, myocardial infarction; *TEE*, transesophageal echocardiography.

Second-Degree Atrioventricular Block—Mobitz Type I

Description

Periodic failure of conduction from the atria to ventricles (with regular atrial activation) characterizes second-degree AVB. In typical Mobitz type I second-degree AVB (Wenckebach AVB), there is progressive lengthening of the PR interval followed by one nonconducted P wave (P wave not followed by a QRS complex). Mobitz type I second-degree AVB often is associated with group beating with a constant P-P interval and changing (usually—and classically—shortening) R-R intervals with the cycle ending with a P wave not followed by a QRS complex. The R-R interval enclosing the nonconducted P wave is classically less than twice the preceding R-R interval. The more classic periodicity of Mobitz type I second-degree AVB is most common with shorter AV conduction ratios (e.g., 4:3 and 3:2) and can be atypical with longer AV conduction ratios (e.g., 9:8 and 10:9). Wenckebach AVB can occur at resting rates or with faster sinus rates. All AVNs demonstrate this normal physiologic behavior at fast enough rates (usually around 180 to 200 bpm). Mobitz type I second-degree AVB almost always occurs in the AVN. Only rarely is this rhythm due to AVB in the His bundle or His-Purkinje system. Infra-Hisian Wenckebach block may be present if AV Wenckebach occurs with a widened QRS complex (over 120 ms) (Fig. 2.2). Infra-Hisian block is associated with a higher risk of progression to CHB, but typical Mobitz type I second-degree AVB with a narrow QRS (Fig. 2.3) rarely progresses to advanced or CHB. Carotid sinus massage can help to distinguish block occurring in the AVN from infra-Hisian block: carotid massage will enhance the Wenckebach conduction in the AVN but have an opposite effect if the block is below the His bundle. In contrast, increasing the sinus rate by increasing sympathetic tone or decreasing vagal tone (e.g., with walking, exercise, or intravenous atropine) is expected to enhance AVN conduction but may worsen infra-Hisian block.

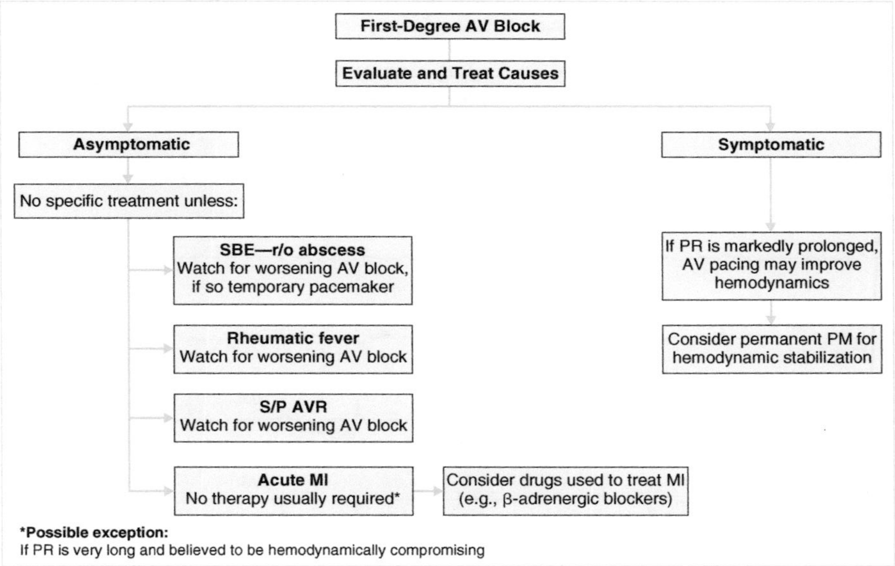
First-Degree AV Block
Evaluate and Treat Causes
Asymptomatic
No specific treatment unless:
SBE—r/o abscess
Watch for worsening AV block, if so temporary pacemaker
Rheumatic fever
Watch for worsening AV block
S/P AVR
Watch for worsening AV block
Acute MI
No therapy usually required*
Consider drugs used to treat MI (e.g., β-adrenergic blockers)
Symptomatic
If PR is markedly prolonged, AV pacing may improve hemodynamics
Consider permanent PM for hemodynamic stabilization
*Possible exception:
If PR is very long and believed to be hemodynamically compromising

ALGORITHM 2.1

First-degree AVB. *AVB,* Atrioventricular block; *AVR,* aortic valve replacement; *MI,* myocardial infarction; *PM,* pacemaker.

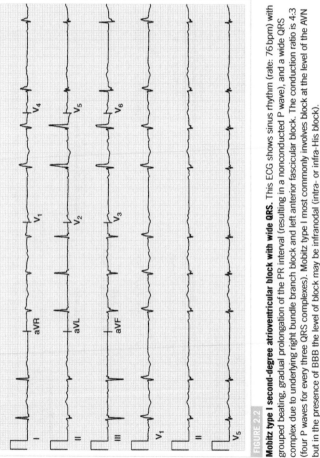

FIGURE 2.2

Mobitz type I second-degree atrioventricular block with wide QRS. This ECG shows sinus rhythm (rate: 76 bpm) with grouped beating, gradual prolongation of the PR interval (resulting in a nonconducted P wave), and a wide QRS complex due to underlying right bundle branch block and left anterior fascicular block. The conduction ratio is 4:3 (four P waves for every three QRS complexes). Mobitz type I most commonly involves block at the level of the AVN but in the presence of BBB the level of block may be infranodal (intra- or infra-His block).

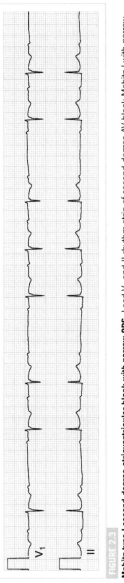

FIGURE 2.3

Mobitz type I second-degree atrioventricular block with narrow QRS. Lead V_1 and II rhythm strip of second-degree AV block Mobitz I with narrow QRS. This is from a patient after cardiac surgery. There is ST elevation in lead II, consistent with pericarditis.

Associated Conditions

Intermittent Mobitz type I second-degree AVB occurs in up to 6% of healthy individuals. Atrial pacing to rates of 180 to 200 bpm will cause AV Wenckebach in 90% of individuals. Mobitz type I second-degree AVB is more common in the older population, in which it may be an isolated finding. "Vagotonic" AVB can mimic Mobitz type I second-degree AVB but is not a true Wenckebach phenomenon because the sinus rate in these cases is not regular and often slows prior to the nonconducted P wave. Vagotonic AVB is common in athletes and during sleep in healthy people. Long episodes with substantial slowing of ventricular rate may occur during sleep; there is no need for therapy. This rhythm is also not uncommon in sleep apnea patients, especially if they are obese. Pathologic causes include intrinsic disease in the AV conducting system (almost always in the AVN), drugs that block conduction or lengthen refractoriness in the AVN (digoxin, not necessarily at toxic levels, β-adrenergic blockers, calcium channel blockers), Lyme disease, the Bezold-Jarisch reflex (caused by inferior MI and the effect of increased vagal tone on the AVN), myocarditis, and rarely after radiofrequency ablation of the AV junction in an attempt to terminate AV nodal reentry.

Clinical Symptoms and Presentation

Symptoms are usually absent during this rhythm; however, especially if the AV conduction ratio is low (e.g., 3:2), it may occasionally cause severe symptoms at rest, including syncope, fatigue, weakness, lightheadedness, or palpitations, symptoms similar to that of pacemaker syndrome.

Approach to Management

Asymptomatic Mobitz type I second-degree AVB due to block in the AVN does not generally require any treatment, and permanent pacemaker implantation is not indicated because progression to advanced or complete AVB or asystole is rare. However, if Mobitz type I second-degree AVB is associated with a wide QRS complex, the level of the block may be in the His-Purkinje system and culminate into CHB. Symptomatic Mobitz type I second-degree AVB may require treatment, which is generally limited to stopping any offending drug or awaiting the effects of ischemia, infarction, or other injury to resolve. Permanent pacing is indicated if symptoms or hemodynamic compromise can be directly attributed to this rhythm (Table 2.2).

Second-Degree Atrioventricular Block—Mobitz Type II

Description

Mobitz type II second-degree AVB is characterized by single nonconducted ("blocked") P waves with constant P-P and PR intervals (no change in the PR > 0.025 seconds) before and after the nonconducted P waves. This is generally due to block below the AV junction infranodal and in the His bundle (intra-His block) or lower in the His-Purkinje system (infra-His block) but not the AVN. Because the block is usually infra-Hisian, Mobitz type II second-degree AVB is associated with a high rate of progression to advanced or CHB. The QRS complex is typically wide (Fig. 2.4) or demonstrates BBB,

TABLE 2.2

MOBITZ TYPE I SECOND-DEGREE ATRIOVENTRICULAR BLOCK MANAGEMENT

Setting	Therapy
Outpatient— Asymptomatic	• Treadmill testing will help assess chronotropic competence (if this rhythm is not related to myocardial ischemia), as well as enhance AVN conduction, thereby reducing the degree of Wenckebach block (e.g., from 5:4 to 8:7 or producing first-degree AVB only).
	• Holter monitoring can assess the degree and level of AVB and the persistence of the problem during activities of daily living and any diurnal variation.
	• If the QRS duration is wide and Holter monitoring or stress testing suggests infranodal block, an electrophysiology study may help to confirm the level of AVB.
	If block is demonstrated to be intra- or infra-Hisian, permanent pacemaker implantation is reasonable, even in an asymptomatic patient.
	On occasion, intra-Hisian block can be demonstrated in a patient with a narrow, normal-appearing QRS complex by the production of higher degrees of AV block during treadmill testing with the increase in sinus rate.
	• No therapy.
	If not due to reversible cause (e.g., drugs or transient damage to the AV node from Lyme disease) and the QRS duration is normal, as more advanced or complete heart block rarely develops.
	There may be increased risk of syncope and symptoms in the future.
Outpatient— Symptomatic	• Some AV nodal blocking drugs (digoxin, β-adrenergic blockers, calcium blockers) may be the cause and should be reduced or stopped if possible, and then only if severe symptomatic bradycardia occurs.
	• If older or at high risk for structural heart disease, consider an echocardiogram to assess LV function (even if no physical findings are present).
	• If due to a correctable cause such as AV nodal blocking drugs, stop the drug if possible.
	• If there is a wide QRS or bundle branch block, it is possible that Wenckebach can be due to block below the AV node (in the His-Purkinje system).
	In this case, permanent pacemaker implantation is indicated.
	• Acutely, intravenous atropine or oral theophylline usually increases conduction through the AV node.
	These may paradoxically decrease ventricular rate and increase the degree of block if the block is below the bundle of His.
	• Permanent pacemaker implantation is indicated if symptomatic second-degree AVB is not otherwise correctable.
MI	• Is often reversed during thrombolysis or angioplasty.
	May also appear for the first time concomitantly with these procedures.
	Transient in nature.
	• Temporary DDD pacing for the following:
	Persistent low heart rate (<40 bpm)
	Low cardiac output
	Ischemia

Continued on following page

TABLE 2.2

**MOBITZ TYPE I SECOND-DEGREE ATRIOVENTRICULAR BLOCK
MANAGEMENT** (Continued)

Setting	Therapy
	◦ Refractory hypotension
	◦ Symptoms of lightheadedness and dizziness
	• Atropine or theophylline may reverse the block but can cause unwanted tachycardia during drug administration.
	◦ These drugs are only rarely indicated except at the time of presentation of the patient.
	• Atypical AV block is more common in inferior-posterior MIs due to the Bezold-Jarisch reflex and the effect of increased vagal tone on the AV node.
	◦ This is usually transient, and unless there is hemodynamic collapse, there is no need for a temporary pacemaker.
	◦ Rarely is there a need for a permanent pacemaker—this is true even if transient third-degree (complete) AV block occurs, as high degrees of block tend to resolve over 5-7 days.
	• If the AV block does not resolve but the ventricular rate is >40 bpm, no therapy is required if patient is asymptomatic.
	• If the block does not resolve after 7 days and/or ventricular rate < 40 or if patient is symptomatic, a permanent pacemaker is indicated.
Preoperative	• Assess drugs given and their need; stop offending drugs that enhance vagal tone, if possible.
	• If no symptoms, no therapy.
	• If symptomatic and no reversible causes, provide temporary pacing before surgery.
	◦ Need for permanent pacing can be accomplished in the postoperative setting.
	• Atropine or isoproterenol may be given to increase AV node conduction if symptomatic or hemodynamically significant.
Postoperative	• Rare after CABG but, if it occurs, consider an offending drug or transient ischemia to the AV node.
	◦ No therapy is generally needed.
	• If associated with wide QRS complex, consider block below the His.
	◦ If it persists, consider an EP study to assess the level of the block.
	• If patient is asymptomatic and block is above His, no need for permanent pacemaker.
	• If patient is symptomatic or block is below the His, permanent pacemaker is indicated.
	• If the block is associated with valve (especially aortic) surgery, consider direct damage to the AV node.
	◦ If persistent, a pacemaker is indicated for symptoms or persistent slow rate (<40 bpm or no increase in rate with exercise).

AV, Atrioventricular; *AVB,* atrioventricular block; *CABG,* coronary artery bypass graft; *EP,* electrophysiology; *LV,* left ventricular; *MI,* myocardial infarction.

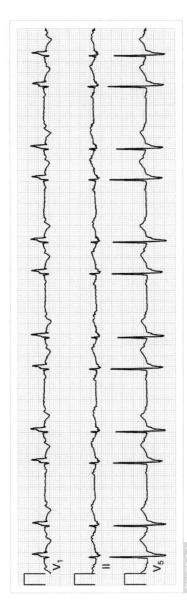

FIGURE 2.4

Mobitz type II second-degree atrioventricular block with a wide QRS. This lead V_1, II, and V_5 rhythm strip shows sinus rhythm with Mobitz type II second-degree AVB with 3:2 conduction (three P waves for every two QRS complexes). There is no progressive PR interval lengthening prior to the nonconducted P wave. Block is likely to be infranodal.

although rarely a narrow QRS complex is observed. In patients with 2:1 AVB, or intermittent "dropped" P waves, when the QRS complex is narrow, a Wenckebach pattern, gradually prolonging the PR interval before the nonconducted P wave (i.e., Mobitz type I second-degree AVB), should be sought in recorded rhythm strips or ECGs because the block may be in the AVN and have a much more benign prognosis. In contrast to Mobitz type I second-degree AVB, in Mobitz type II second-degree AVB, carotid sinus massage may have a paradoxical effect of improving 1:1 AV conduction due to slowing of the sinus rate; however, increasing the sinus rate (e.g., with walking, exercise, or intravenous atropine) may worsen Mobitz type II infra-Hisian block or elicit 2:1 AVB due to the early arrival of atrial impulses at the infranodal conduction system while it is still refractory.

Associated Conditions

Causes include intrinsic degenerative disease in the His-Purkinje system, drugs that slow or block conduction in the His-Purkinje system (e.g., propafenone, flecainide, procainamide, quinidine, disopyramide), coronary artery disease (CAD) including MI, myocarditis, infiltrative disease such as amyloid, sarcoidosis, Lyme disease, neuromuscular diseases, and ablation of the AV junction. It can be exacerbated by exercise and by drugs that increase AV nodal conduction and the sinus rate, such as atropine. When occurring in the setting of acute MI, Mobitz type II second-degree AVB is usually due to anterior MI due in turn to left anterior descending coronary artery obstruction with its distribution involving the septal perforator branch.

Clinical Symptoms and Presentation

Symptoms include lightheadedness, near syncope, and syncope, although many patients are asymptomatic, depending on the AV conduction ratio. Nevertheless, Mobitz type II second-degree AVB is associated with a high rate (>50%) of progression to CHB, which may be sudden and unpredictable in onset.

Approach to Management

It is important to exclude vagotonic block and Mobitz type I second-degree AVB in the AVN. Extensive review of rhythm strips and ECGs is particularly important if the QRS complex is narrow because attribution of the level of block to the AVN in an asymptomatic patient requires no therapy, whereas diagnosis of block in the His-Purkinje system indicates a need for permanent pacemaker implantation. A wide QRS complex or BBB supports the level of block being in the His-Purkinje system. Carotid sinus massage or exercise can help to confirm the diagnosis; an electrophysiology (EP) study can be performed when there remains significant doubt as to the localization of the site of block. Because of the high risk of progression to CHB, Mobitz type II second-degree AVB is an indication for permanent pacemaker implantation (Table 2.3, Algorithm 2.2).

MOBITZ TYPE II SECOND-DEGREE ATRIOVENTRICULAR BLOCK MANAGEMENT

Setting	Therapy
Outpatient— Asymptomatic	• Risk for complete heart block and death is significant (approximately 50%).
	• A dual-chamber permanent pacemaker is recommended as the pacing system of choice.
	• Admit the patient for a permanent pacemaker and place on a cardiac monitor.
	• In the absence of symptoms or progressive (higher-degree AVB), there is no need for a temporary pacemaker before permanent pacemaker implantation.
	• Avoid atropine.
	• Evaluate for the presence of underlying cardiac disease, such as infiltrative processes (e.g., amyloid), or MI.
Outpatient— Symptomatic	• Dual-chamber permanent pacemaker implantation is indicated.
	• Admit the patient and place on a cardiac monitor.
	• If symptomatic or hemodynamically detrimental ventricular bradycardia is present, a temporary pacemaker is indicated if a permanent system cannot be placed expeditiously.
	• Do not give atropine because this may worsen the AVB and produce a slower ventricular rate.
	• Exercise, sinus tachycardia, and catecholamines also can worsen the degree of block by enhancing AV nodal conduction and impinging on the refractory period of the His-Purkinje system.
MI	• Place temporary pacemaker.
	• Mobitz type II second-degree AVB is associated with a high rate of heart failure in this setting.
	• A permanent pacemaker is indicated if the AVB is persistent because the risk of complete heart block is >50%.
	• Long-term prognosis may not be improved.
	• Avoid the use of antiarrhythmic drugs (including lidocaine) in the absence of a pacemaker, unless there is sustained ventricular tachyarrhythmia, as these drugs may worsen the degree of AVB.
	• Do not give atropine.
	• Mobitz type II second-degree AVB has a lower (albeit not known with certainty) incidence in the current early revascularization era but if present or of new onset may improve with time, but this is rare. After being present and persistent, a pacemaker will likely be needed.
Preoperative	• Place permanent pacemaker.
	• If urgent or emergent surgery, place a temporary pacemaker with the plan for a permanent pacemaker after surgery.
	• If CABG, epicardial atrial and ventricular wires can be placed, with temporary pacing as standby, until a permanent transvenous pacemaker can be placed.

Continued on following page

TABLE 2.3

MOBITZ TYPE II SECOND-DEGREE ATRIOVENTRICULAR BLOCK MANAGEMENT (Continued)

Setting	Therapy
	• It is best to place the permanent pacemaker after CABG or other cardiac surgery as leads otherwise tend to dislodge.
	• If endocarditis, temporary pacemaker until infection resolves and after cardiac surgery.
	○ Avoid antiarrhythmic drugs and atropine.
Postoperative	• If bradycardia, temporary pacing (via epicardial wires, if present, after cardiac surgery).
	• Temporary Mobitz type II AV block may resolve after cardiac surgery.
	○ It may be due to trauma near the His-Purkinje system (e.g., with aortic valve surgery, where left bundle branch block is a not infrequent accompaniment).
	• Persistent (e.g., more than 3-5 days) Mobitz type II block will require permanent pacing.
	• No antiarrhythmic drugs should be given unless an adequate backup ventricular pacing is available.
	• Endocarditis with abscess near the septum can destroy the His-Purkinje system.
	○ Despite surgical repair, permanent pacing will likely be required.
	• For patients having tricuspid valve replacement, an endocardial lead can occasionally be placed across a porcine bioprosthesis without producing tricuspid regurgitation but should be avoided if there is a mechanical valve.
	○ Tricuspid valve repair (e.g., annuloplasty) should not pose a problem in positioning a right ventricular lead.

AV, Atrioventricular; *AVB*, atrioventricular block; *CABG*, coronary artery bypass graft; *MI*, myocardial infarction.

Second-Degree Atrioventricular Block—2:1
Atrioventricular Block

Description

2:1 second-degree AVB occurs when every other P wave is conducted to the ventricles but alternate P waves are not. AVB may be occurring at the level of the AVN, within the His bundle, or in the His-Purkinje system. If the QRS is narrow (Fig. 2.5) and normal appearing, the level of the block is most likely in the AVN (which is more benign). If the QRS is wide (Fig. 2.6) because of BBB or other nonspecific, intraventricular (IV) conduction delay, block in the AVN is still often more common, but block in the His-Purkinje system (infra-AV nodal) is more frequent than when the QRS complex is narrow. To help to define the level of the block, observation of a long monitored strip can be helpful because 2:1 AVB frequently does not persist. If and when the AV conduction ratio changes, the other forms of AVB (Mobitz type I or II) should then become apparent. Rhythm monitoring

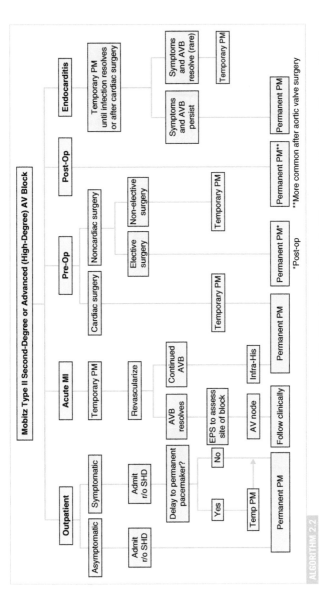

ALGORITHM 2.2

Mobitz type II second-degree or advanced (high-degree) AVB. *AVB*, Atrioventricular block; *EPS*, electrophysiology study; *MI*, myocardial infarction; *PM*, pacemaker; *SHD*, structural heart disease (no overt evidence of myocardial, valvular, congenital or coronary heart disease).

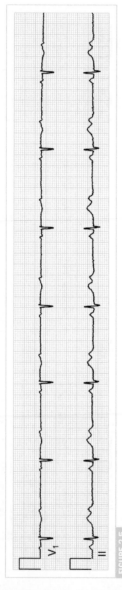

FIGURE 2.5

2:1 Atrioventricular block, narrow QRS. This rhythm strip of leads V_1 and II shows sinus rhythm (rate: 84 bpm) with 2:1 AVB (ventricular rate: 42 bpm) that could represent either Mobitz type I or type II second-degree AVB. The narrow QRS complexes suggest that block is most likely to be in the AVN and that the nature of the 2:1 AVB is most likely to be Mobitz type I second-degree AVB. In general, a narrow QRS and 2:1 AV conduction is likely to be Mobitz type I second-degree AVB, whereas a wide QRS in 2:1 AV conduction is more likely to be infra-AV nodal block (Mobitz type II). Changing the AV conduction ratio (e.g., atropine) will help to define the site of block. Another way to help distinguish the level of the block is to exercise the individual and/or do continuous or long-term monitoring to determine if the 2:1 AV block is associated with other types of AV block (e.g., Mobitz type I or II second-degree AV block).

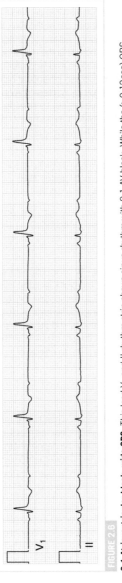

FIGURE 2.6

2:1 Atrioventricular block, wide QRS. This lead V$_1$ and II rhythm strip shows sinus rhythm with 2:1 AV block. While the (>0.12 sec) QRS complexes, consistent with right bundle branch block, suggest that Mobitz type II second-degree AV block is likely, this rhythm is simply called 2:1 AV block.

while the patient does some form of exertion (e.g., arm exercise, standing, and walking) may also help to demonstrate the level of block. Block at the level of the AVN should improve with the decrease in vagal tone and increase in adrenergic tone, but block below the AVN in the His-Purkinje system may worsen, with consequent slowing of ventricular rate, as AV nodal conduction improves and increases the frequency of inputs to the His-Purkinje system. Likewise, atropine and isoproterenol may improve AV conduction through the AVN but worsen infranodal block. Carotid massage may also help to distinguish the two by worsening AV nodal block but improving block in the His-Purkinje system by slowing the sinus and AV nodal inputs to the His-Purkinje system, allowing the His-Purkinje system to recover from its refractory state between inputs.

Associated Conditions

2:1 AVB occurs in the same conditions as those associated with Mobitz type I (Wenckebach) or type II second-degree AVB.

Clinical Symptoms and Presentation

Symptoms include lightheadedness, near syncope, and syncope, although some patients may be asymptomatic, depending on the sinus rate and consequent ventricular rate.

Approach to Management

Atropine and isoproterenol improve AV conduction if the level of block is in the AVN but may make it worse if the block is at the level of the His-Purkinje system. Therefore atropine is not recommended for suspected block in the His-Purkinje system. Depending on the level of block, approach to management follows recommendations and guidelines for Mobitz types I or II second-degree AVB. In the setting of acute MI with AVB, isoproterenol should be avoided because of the adverse effects of sinus tachycardia and ventricular ectopy (Table 2.4).

High-Degree Advanced Atrioventricular Block

Description

High-degree, or advanced, AVB occurs when two or more consecutive P waves are not conducted to the ventricles, but, because some P waves are conducted, CHB is not present. In the presence of atrial tachyarrhythmias, such as atrial fibrillation, long pauses (more than 5 seconds) can be considered to represent high-degree AVB. High-degree AVB may be associated with a narrow (Fig. 2.7) or wide (Fig. 2.8) QRS.

Associated Conditions

High-degree AVB can be benign (e.g., when due to an increase in vagal tone as may occur with vomiting, intubation, and suctioning, when it is referred to as "vagotonic" AVB), or it can be associated with serious and potentially life-threatening bradycardia-asystolic pauses. Causes include idiopathic degeneration of the conduction system, MI, surgery, trauma, myocarditis, infiltrative processes (e.g., amyloidosis), sarcoidosis, Lyme

2:1 ATRIOVENTRICULAR BLOCK MANAGEMENT

Setting	Therapy
AV nodal site of block suspected (usually narrow, normal-appearing QRS complex)	• If asymptomatic, evaluate (Holter monitor and exercise test for ventricular rates and diurnal variation) but no therapy.
	• Exercise testing may be required to help to elicit the site of block: if AV nodal, the AV conduction ratio will increase from 2:1 to 3:2 or higher.
	• If the AVB is intra-His or infra-Hisian, a higher degree of AV block will occur.
	• As AV nodal block may be due to a drug (e.g., digitalis, β-adrenergic blockers, calcium channel blockers, amiodarone), these drugs should be discontinued, if possible.
	• EP study with His bundle recording can help to determine the level of block, although this is rarely necessary in patients with AV nodal block.
	• In most cases, if observed over a period of time, 2:1 AV block will change to Mobitz type I or II second-degree AVB, allowing the site of block to be further characterized.
	• Atropine or isoproterenol can improve AV nodal conduction and may be useful as diagnostic maneuvers.
	• Block in the AV node is usually benign, but if it leads to asystole more than 3 seconds or complete heart block with escape rates of <40 per minute with symptoms in awake patients, permanent pacing is indicated.
	• Hemodynamic instability or symptomatic bradycardia with 2:1 AVB that is not reversible is an indication for permanent cardiac pacing.
Infranodal site of block suspected (usually wide QRS complex)	• If hemodynamically unstable, temporary pacing.
	• Infranodal block is suspected if bundle branch block is present, but even then the block can be in the AV node. May need EP study with His bundle recordings to clarify.
	• Observe long rhythm strips, including Holter monitoring, if feasible.
	• Attempt carotid massage and/or assess the effects of atropine or exercise to help determine level of block.
	• On rare occasions, it may be prudent to apply transcutaneous pacing electrodes.
	• If block is in the His-Purkinje system, a dual-chamber permanent pacemaker is indicated.
Inability to distinguish site of block by ECG or provocative maneuvers	• Electrophysiology study to evaluate the level of the block, although this rarely needs to be performed.
	• If block is intra-His or below, a permanent pacemaker is indicated.

Continued on following page

2:1 ATRIOVENTRICULAR BLOCK MANAGEMENT (Continued)

Setting	Therapy
MI	- If anterior infarction is evident, block is likely in the His-Purkinje system.
	- Temporary pacing should be performed; this is often accomplished at the time of percutaneous revascularization procedures.
	- Because more than 90% of patients recover with 1:1 AV conduction, generally within a few days, permanent pacing should be considered only if the block is persistent.
	- If inferior infarction is evident, the block is likely in the AVN.
	- Temporary pacing should be performed only if the patient is symptomatic or hemodynamically compromised and can be accomplished expeditiously, without delaying revascularization procedures.
	- Otherwise, intravenous atropine, together with rapid revascularization, is expected to resolve the block.
	- There is usually no need for a permanent pacemaker because the block almost always resolves.
Preoperative	- Perform provocative maneuvers or prolonged observation to define the site of the AVB.
	- If block is in the AVN, consider discontinuing drugs that may be initiating or maintaining the problem.
	- An exception might be the patient with coronary artery disease in whom perioperative β-blockade has morbidity and mortality advantages.
	- For cardiac surgery, epicardial pacing wires provide an opportunity for temporary AV sequential pacing if HR < 40 bpm or if there is:
	- Hemodynamic instability due to low heart rate
	- AV dyssynchrony
	- Symptoms
	- For noncardiac surgery and level of the block in the His-Purkinje system, temporary (if surgery emergent) or permanent (if surgery urgent or elective) pacing.
Postoperative	- Level of block needs to be determined.
	- Even if in the His-Purkinje system, in the first few days after cardiac surgery (e.g., CABG or valve surgery), it may resolve post-op.
	- AV block is often due to trauma to AV node or His bundle, and reversibility generally occurs; recovery, however, may not be robust if the block is in the His-Purkinje system.
	- If related to endocarditis or aortic valve surgery and block is in the His-Purkinje system, resolution is unlikely and permanent pacing will usually be required.

AV, Atrioventricular; *AVB*, atrioventricular block; *AVN*, atrioventricular node; *EP*, electrophysiology; *MI*, myocardial infarction.

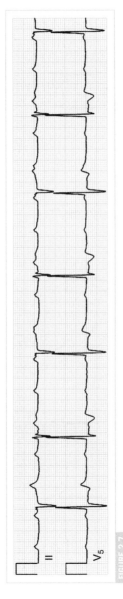

FIGURE 2.7

High-degree atrioventricular block with narrow QRS. This lead II and V$_5$ rhythm strip shows sinus tachycardia at approximately 105 bpm with high-degree AV block and alternating junctional escape and conducted beats. The conducted beats occur with a shorter R-R interval than the junctional escape interval.

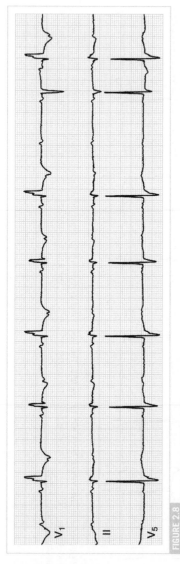

2:1 atrioventricular block followed by high-degree atrioventricular block. The first part shows 2:1 AV block with RBBB conduction. Every other QRS complex is slightly narrower with a shorter PR interval, indicating partial recovery of the right bundle during these beats. After the 5th QRS complex, there is high-degree AV block followed by a narrow QRS complex, suggesting conduction from the atrium or junctional escape with full right bundle recovery, followed by return of RBBB on the next beat. There is also ventriculophasic sinus arrhythmia; the P-P intervals without intervening QRS complexes are longer.

disease, neuromuscular diseases (e.g., myotonic muscular dystrophy, Erb limb-girdle muscular dystrophy, Kearns-Sayre syndrome, peroneal muscular atrophy), collagen vascular disease, or metastatic disease. When high-grade AVB is present due to block in the His-Purkinje system, the sinus rate tends to be normal to rapid, whereas if reduced, vagal tone is often the cause of the problem because the sinus rate will slow concomitantly. Sometimes, EP testing is needed to clarify the level of the block.

Clinical Symptoms and Presentation

Patients may be asymptomatic but often have significant symptoms, such as syncope, near syncope, lightheadedness, weakness, fatigue, palpitations, dyspnea, chest discomfort, or bradycardia-associated ventricular arrhythmias (specifically bradycardia- or pause-dependent polymorphic ventricular tachycardia [VT]) (Algorithm 2.3).

Approach to Management

Permanent pacemaker implantation is indicated for high-degree AVB with symptomatic bradycardia or ventricular arrhythmias related to the bradycardia, as long as an otherwise reversible cause cannot be eliminated, or drug therapy that produces the AVB is required (such as need for continued β-adrenergic blockers for CAD, heart failure, or arrhythmias). A pacemaker is also indicated in asymptomatic patients with advanced AVB and asystolic pauses of 3 or more seconds, escape rates of less than 40 bpm, or infranodal escape rhythms or conduction with BBB, both of which suggest His-Purkinje conduction system disease. However, most of the time, these patients are not truly asymptomatic, and a stressor (such as exercise testing) may be required to elicit symptoms (Table 2.5).

Third-Degree (Complete) Atrioventricular Block

Description

CHB, or third-degree AVB, occurs when there are no conducted impulses from the atria to the ventricles despite temporal opportunity for conduction. This can occur during sinus rhythm or any other atrial rhythm, such as atrial fibrillation or flutter. It may be persistent or transient. The QRS rhythm in CHB is regular and originates in the junction or ventricles. Although CHB is a form of AV dissociation, not all AV dissociation represents CHB. AV dissociation (Fig. 2.9) may occur from interference, isorhythmic competing rhythms between atria and ventricles, accelerated junctional or ventricular rhythms (including VTs with independent atrial rhythms), or SB with an escape rhythm. In these forms of AV dissociation, "capture" of the ventricles by atrial impulses is possible and will occur if there is temporal opportunity, unlike CHB.

In CHB, the atrial rate is faster than the ventricular rate. The escape rhythm can be junctional (with a narrow or wide QRS complex) (Fig. 2.10) or ventricular (with a wide QRS complex) (Fig. 2.11); in the latter case the focus of origin and therefore the rhythm is more unreliable, does not

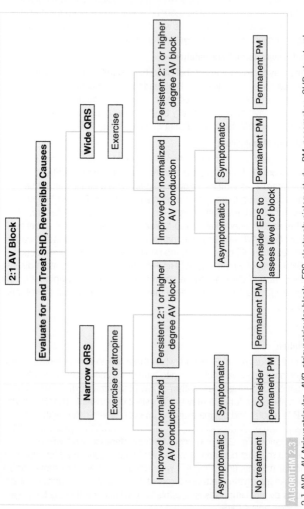

ALGORITHM 2.3

2:1 AVB. *AV,* Atrioventricular; *AVB,* atrioventricular block; *EPS,* electrophysiology study; *PM,* pacemaker; *SHD,* structural heart disease (no overt evidence of myocardial, valvular, congenital, or coronary heart disease).

TABLE 2.5

HIGH-DEGREE (ADVANCED) ATRIOVENTRICULAR BLOCK MANAGEMENT

Setting	Therapy
Asymptomatic	• High-grade AV block that is paroxysmal because of increases in vagal tone does not warrant a pacemaker, unless the episodes are the following:
	○ Highly symptomatic
	○ Recurrent
	○ Refractory to other therapies
	• A pacemaker is indicated in asymptomatic patients with the following:
	○ Advanced AVB and asystolic pauses of 3 seconds or more
	○ Escape rates of <40 bpm; pauses during atrial fibrillation of more than 5 seconds
	○ A level of block that is infranodal
	• Permanent pacing is indicated for advanced AVB associated with neuromuscular diseases.
Symptomatic	• A permanent pacemaker is indicated if high-degree AVB causes symptomatic bradycardia or bradycardia-dependent ventricular arrhythmias.
	• Permanent pacing is indicated if the block is not reversible or results from required drug therapy.
MI	• If symptomatic bradycardia occurs, a temporary pacemaker is indicated.
	○ High-degree AVB is relatively unusual during acute MI.
	• If advanced AVB occurs with an anterior infarction, permanent pacing is indicated if AVB persists for several days.
	• Advanced AVB in inferior MIs is generally in the AVN; because it is usually transient, there is no need for a permanent pacemaker.
	○ If it does not resolve over 1 to 2 weeks, a highly unusual circumstance in the current revascularization era, a permanent pacemaker may be indicated.
	○ Formal exercise testing prior to the decision to implant a permanent pacemaker can be considered, as the advanced AVB present at rest may improve considerably with an increase in sympathetic tone.
Preoperative	• Permanent pacemaker, unless the surgery is emergent.
	• Permanent pacemaker deferred after cardiovascular surgery due to risk of lead dislodgement.
	• If surgery is emergent, insert a temporary pacemaker preoperative with the plan for a permanent pacemaker after surgery.
Postoperative	• Temporary transvenous pacing or pacing via temporary epicardial wires placed at time of cardiac surgery.
	• A permanent pacemaker is indicated if there is damage to the AV conduction system (e.g., after aortic valve surgery) and the AVB does not resolve within 5-7 days.

AV, Atrioventricular; *AVB,* atrioventricular block; *AVN,* atrioventricular node; *MI,* myocardial infarction.

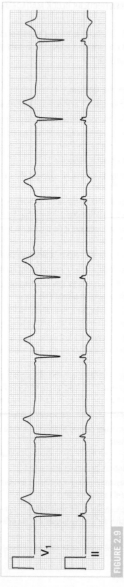

FIGURE 2.9

Isorhythmic atrioventricular dissociation (sinus bradycardia with junctional escape complexes and capture beats). This lead V₁ and II rhythm strip shows isorhythmic dissociation with junctional rhythm during an inferior MI. The sinus rhythm and the junctional rhythm rates are very close. The sinus rate is about 40 bpm and the junctional rhythm is about 41 bpm.

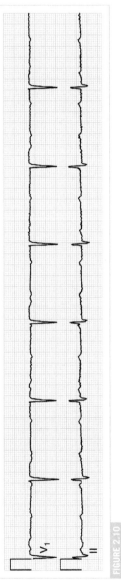

FIGURE 2.10

Congenital complete atrioventricular block with narrow QRS complex junctional escape rhythm. This lead II and V₁ rhythm strip shows sinus rhythm (rate: 103 bpm). There is a narrow QRS complex rhythm (rate: 43 bpm) that is independent of the sinus rhythm and that represents a junctional rhythm, probably escape, in a patient with known congenital complete AV block. AV dissociation, such as is shown here, does not necessarily imply AV block; however, in this case, failure to capture the ventricles despite temporal opportunity to do so indicates a diagnosis of AV block.

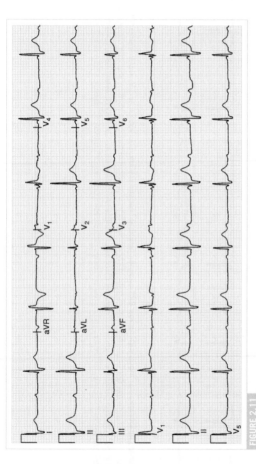

FIGURE 2.11

Acquired complete atrioventricular block with wide QRS ventricular escape rhythm. This 12-lead ECG shows complete AV block with P waves bearing no relationship to the QRS complexes, and with constant P-P and R-R intervals but variable PR intervals. Here the sinus rhythm (rate: 74 bpm) is completely dissociated from the escape rhythm (40 bpm). A ventricular origin of the QRS rhythm is indicated by the wide QRS complex and the slow rate. However, the QRS complexes have a typical right bundle branch block morphology, suggesting that this may be an escape rhythm coming from the junction, rather than the ventricle. There is also evidence of ventriculophasic sinus arrhythmia with some P-P intervals with intervening QRS complexes being slightly shorter than P-P intervals without QRS complexes.

respond to autonomic input, and is slower (<40 bpm). CHB during atrial fibrillation is characterized by narrow or wide QRS escape rhythms with a regular rate (Fig. 2.12); however, during atrial flutter, the ventricular rhythm may be regular, occurring at a fixed AV conduction ratio (e.g., 4:1). This does not represent CHB.

Associated Conditions

CHB may be congenital or more commonly acquired. Congenital CHB is generally associated with a narrow QRS complex (junctional) escape rhythm. Congenital CHB is associated with maternal lupus and maternal antibodies to SS-A (Ro) and SS-B (La). In acquired AVB the rhythm can be persistent or intermittent and may stop sometimes unpredictably and at other times after overdrive pacing or even premature ventricular contractions (PVCs). Aortic stenosis can be associated with CHB. Occasionally, acquired CHB is due to an antiarrhythmic drug (e.g., a class I antiarrhythmic or amiodarone), a calcium channel blocker, a β-adrenergic blocker, digoxin, or hyperkalemia. When it is due to a drug, there is likely an underlying conduction problem, or the drug doses were exceedingly high. CHB can occur after mitral and/or aortic valve repair or replacement. If after an aortic valve repair conduction is not likely to improve, it is due to conduction delay or block in the His-Purkinje system. CHB can follow ventricular septal defect (VSD) repair. A special circumstance is CHB after MI. In the case of an inferior MI the escape rhythm tends to be narrow (junctional) and relatively reliable. The CHB is usually transient and may be due to direct damage to the AVN or to the Bezold-Jarisch reflex. If CHB occurs during anterior wall MI, the CHB is associated with a wide QRS complex and is usually due to extensive infarction, with a high in-hospital and long-term mortality. Conduction is unlikely to resolve, and the patient will likely need a pacemaker or implantable cardioverter defibrillator (ICD). CHB can be due to a calcific or sclerodegenerative process in the conduction system, endocarditis with abscess in the conduction system, Lyme disease (in which case it is usually transient), and ablation of the AVN to control ventricular rates during atrial arrhythmias. CHB is also associated with cardiomyopathy, myocarditis, acute rheumatic fever, cardiac tumors of the conduction system, and high vagal tone and after radiation therapy for chest or breast malignancies (Algorithm 2.4).

Clinical Symptoms and Presentation

In congenital CHB with a narrow QRS complex escape rhythm, as long as the rate is more than 40 bpm, patients are usually asymptomatic; however, chronotropic incompetence may occur over time, which can cause symptoms of fatigue, lightheadedness, or weakness. Acquired CHB may also be asymptomatic, but more often is associated with symptoms such as syncope, near syncope, lightheadedness, weakness, fatigue, dyspnea, angina, or breathlessness. Ventricular arrhythmias may also be associated with the bradycardia. Sudden death is reported to occur with acquired CHB.

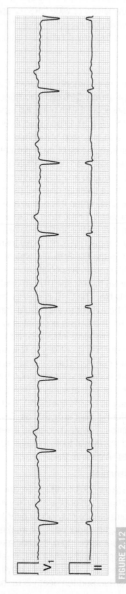

FIGURE 2.12

Complete atrioventricular block during atrial fibrillation. This rhythm strip of leads V₁ and II shows atrial fibrillation with CHB evident by the slow, regular, wide QRS ventricular rhythm. Supportive evidence for complete heart block is the complete regularity of the ventricular rhythm.

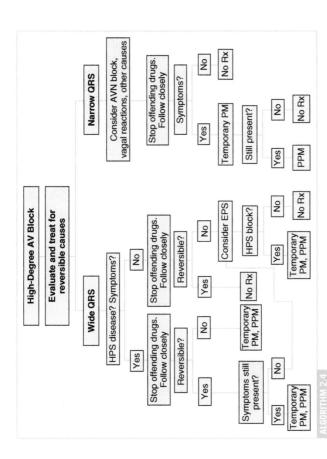

ALGORITHM 2.4

High-degree AVB. *AVN,* Atrioventricular node; *EPS,* electrophysiology study; *PM,* pacemaker; *PPM,* permanent pacemaker.

Approach to Management

In congenital CHB the risk of asystole is unknown, and some recent reports suggest that this condition is not always benign, especially when the ventricular rate is less than 40 bpm. Permanent pacemaker implantation is indicated in congenital heart block that causes symptoms, often due to chronotropic incompetence; pacemaker implantation is controversial in asymptomatic congenital CHB. In acquired CHB the escape rhythm is unreliable because of its origin in the ventricles; a permanent pacemaker is indicated to eliminate symptoms as well as to prevent cardiac arrest caused by asystole. Occasionally, acquired heart block is due to an antiarrhythmic drug effect or hyperkalemia. In cases associated with electrolyte abnormalities, antiarrhythmic or other drugs, or other reversible causes, correction of metabolic derangements or stopping the inciting cause can be curative without the need for a pacemaker. In CHB associated with inferior MI, a permanent pacemaker is not indicated unless the patient has a persistent CHB (more than 1 to 2 weeks) and/or symptoms. For anterior wall MI and CHB with a wide QRS complex, pacing (temporary or permanent) is often required for symptomatic bradycardia but may have little influence on long-term prognosis. Nevertheless, in this clinical scenario, permanent pacing is usually recommended for symptoms or persistent CHB (Table 2.6).

TABLE 2.6

COMPLETE HEART BLOCK MANAGEMENT

Setting	Therapy
Asymptomatic–Acquired	• Rule out reversible causes, including the following:
	Hyperkalemia
	Acute inferior MI
	Digoxin toxicity
	Excess calcium channel blocker therapy
	Lyme disease
	• If HR <40 bpm, first-line therapy is a permanent DDD pacemaker.
	• Temporary pacing is indicated if
	Heart rate <40 bpm.
	The patient has impaired hemodynamics and if permanent pacing cannot be accomplished expeditiously.
	The CHB has an identifiable and reversible cause, while awaiting recovery.
	• Temporary transvenous pacing must be used with caution in patients with any escape rhythm, particularly if wide QRS complex and slow.
	Overdrive suppression can occur rapidly.

TABLE 2.6

COMPLETE HEART BLOCK MANAGEMENT (Continued)

Setting	Therapy
	● If the rate of escape rhythm >40 bpm, permanent pacemaker insertion is controversial.
	○ Temporary pacing is to be avoided in asymptomatic patients whose ventricular rates are >40 bpm, especially if the QRS complex is narrow.
	● CHB due to radio frequency ablation of the AV junction to control ventricular response rate in atrial fibrillation requires permanent pacing.
	○ May occur even if the patient is asymptomatic from a slow ventricular rate (40 bpm) that may be quite stable over time.
	● Acquired CHB is associated with a poor short-term prognosis (>50% mortality in the first 6-12 months after diagnosis).
	○ If irreversible, pacing is indicated.
Symptomatic	● A permanent pacemaker is indicated.
	● Temporary pacing is indicated if permanent pacing cannot be done expeditiously or if CHB has an identifiable and reversible cause (e.g., drug overdose).
Congenital	● Usually associated with a narrow QRS complex with an escape rhythm arising in the AVN.
	○ Patients are usually asymptomatic.
	● In patients who are asymptomatic, the indications for a pacemaker are controversial.
	○ Patients will need close follow-up, at least annually, for evaluation of symptoms suggesting chronotropic incompetence.
	● If symptomatic bradycardia, a permanent pacemaker is indicated.
	● If rate is consistently <50 bpm and does not increase with exercise (chronotropic incompetence), a permanent pacemaker is indicated.
MI	● If symptomatic bradycardia, a temporary pacemaker is indicated.
	● If CHB block occurs in the setting of an anterior infarction, permanent pacing is indicated if AVB persists.
	● CHB in inferior MI is generally in the AVN.
	○ There is usually no need for a permanent pacemaker, as it usually resolves.
	○ If it does not resolve, a permanent pacemaker may be indicated in some cases.
Preoperative	● Permanent pacemaker first, unless the surgery is emergent.
	● If surgery is emergent, insert a temporary pacemaker pre-op with the plan for a permanent pacemaker after surgery.
Postoperative	● Transcutaneous or temporary transvenous pacing.
	● A permanent pacemaker is indicated if there is permanent damage to the AV conduction system (e.g., after aortic valve surgery or VSD repair).

AV, Atrioventricular; *AVB*, atrioventricular block; *AVN*, atrioventricular node; *CHB*, complete atrioventricular block; *MI*, myocardial infarction; *VSD*, ventricular septal defect.

Caveats

1. It is important to recognize whether the CHB is congenital or acquired.
2. If acquired, it is important to determine ventricular function and exclude the need for acute interventional therapy. If a patient requires bypass graft or other cardiovascular surgery, it should be performed prior to implanting a pacemaker because of the possibility of lead dislodgment occurring at the time of surgery. Temporary epicardial atrial and ventricular pacing wires can be placed at the time of surgery and can be relied on in most cases for several days.
3. If there is ventricular dysfunction, a pacemaker defibrillator may be a better option than a permanent pacemaker alone.
4. If there is ventricular dysfunction, a CRT-ICD or CRT pacing system is preferred. CRT-P is preferred over CRT-D if LVEF is ≥ 35%.
5. There are several indications for temporary pacing. These include episodic asystole, recurrent severe symptoms, hemodynamic collapse, and the reversible symptomatic problem that culminated in CHB.
6. External (transcutaneous) cardiac pacing is a poor substitute for an endocardial transvenous temporary pacemaker wire and should not be relied on in cases of symptomatic heart block or heart block associated with asystolic episodes.
7. If CHB is due to digoxin toxicity, digoxin-specific antibodies, although expensive, should be administered.
8. Patients with mild and moderate LV dysfunction and CHB may have progressive ventricular dysfunction with right ventricular apical pacing alone; upgrading to biventricular pacing systems is an option in these cases.
9. Dual-chamber pacing in patients with CHB is associated with reduced episodes of atrial fibrillation and is recommended, especially for younger individuals.

Atrioventricular Dissociation

AV dissociation is a condition in which atrial activation (usually from the sinus node) is independent from ventricular activation (originating from the AV junction, His-Purkinje system, or ventricles). The ventricular rate is usually more rapid than that of the atria in AV dissociation not related to CHB. When both atrial and ventricular rates are approximately the same, resulting in apparent association of the rhythms, the AV dissociation is termed *isorhythmic*. If the atrial rhythm is an ectopic tachycardia and the ventricular rhythm represents acceleration of a subsidiary pacemaker, *double tachycardia* is said to be present.

Emergence of ventricular activation can result from acceleration of a subsidiary ectopic focus due to enhanced automaticity from any cause (accelerated rhythm), reentry (e.g., VT due to structural heart disease), or as a result of slowing of the atrial rate below the intrinsic rate of an ectopic focus from the AV conduction system or the ventricles culminating in an escape rhythm. Causes of acceleration of the rate of subsidiary pacemakers include myocardial ischemia, high catecholamine state, digitalis toxicity, and atropine. Causes of slowing of atrial rate leading to emergence of an escape subsidiary pacemaker include SB, sinus arrhythmia, high vagal tone, and medications, such as β-adrenergic blockers and rate-sparing calcium channel blockers.

Although CHB is a form of AV dissociation, AV dissociation is not a form of CHB. In CHB, atrial impulses cannot be conducted to the ventricles despite a temporal opportunity for this to occur. In contrast, in AV dissociation, atrial impulses will capture (be conducted to and stimulate) the ventricles if temporal opportunity and nonrefractory tissue permit.

Capture beats, a hallmark of AV dissociation, are QRS complexes that occur prematurely relative to the rate of the subsidiary pacemaker. Capture beats often have morphologic features that are intermediate in configuration between QRS complexes that have been stimulated by atrial impulses and those that have been stimulated by ectopic foci (whether the focus is an accelerated one or an escape one). Such complexes are called fusion complexes. Because the occurrence of fusion implies capture of the ventricles from the supraventricular impulse, fusion complexes are also hallmarks of AV dissociation. Long rhythm strips must often be recorded to demonstrate their presence (Algorithm 2.5).

INTRAVENTRICULAR CONDUCTION ABNORMALITIES

Left Bundle Branch Block

Description
Left bundle branch (LBB) block (LBBB) (Fig. 2.13) is associated with a distinctive pattern on the ECG: wide (>0.12 seconds), predominantly negative QRS in lead V_1 and a prominent wide R or RR′ in I, aVL, and V_6. Secondary ST-T wave abnormalities accompany the pattern and consist of downsloping ST depression in the anterolateral leads and ST elevation in the right precordial leads. Because LV depolarization is abnormal, morphologic abnormalities, such as left ventricular hypertrophy (LVH), cannot be diagnosed from the ECG. The diagnosis of MI is also difficult, with concordant ST elevation of greater than or equal to 1 mm in any lead with positive QRS deflection and discordant ST depression greater than or equal to 1 mm in V_1, V_2, and V_3, having good specificity although lower sensitivity.

Associated Conditions
Although the overall incidence of LBBB in a normal population is 0.02% to 0.05%, LBBB almost always occurs in the presence of underlying structural heart disease, such as dilated cardiomyopathy, CAD, valvular heart disease, degenerative disease of the conduction system (Lev's disease, Lenegre's disease), and trauma. Lyme disease, sarcoidosis, or other infiltrative myocardial diseases may cause conduction disturbances,

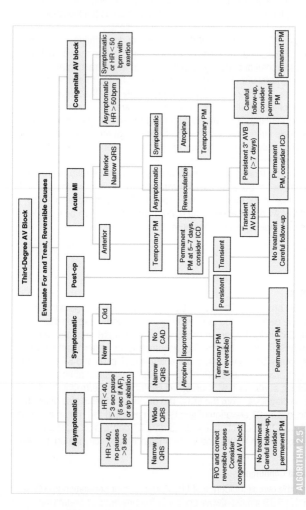

ALGORITHM 2.5

Third-degree AVB. *AVB*, Atrioventricular block; *CAD*, coronary artery disease; *ICD*, implantable cardioverter defibrillator; *MI*, myocardial infarction; *PM*, pacemaker.

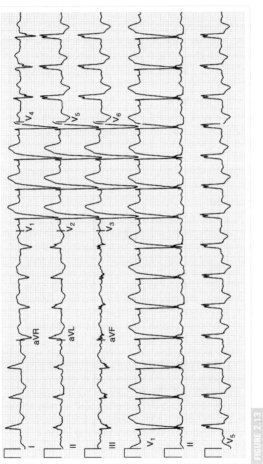

FIGURE 2.13

Left bundle branch block. This 12-lead ECG shows LBBB that is characterized by a wide (>0.12 seconds) QRS complex; broad monophasic R waves in leads V_5, V_6, and I that are commonly slurred or notched; rS or QS complexes in the right precordial leads; and secondary ST- and T-wave changes that are opposite in direction to the major QRS deflections. The mean frontal plane QRS axis is normal, but left-axis deviation may be present.

including LBBB. Rarely an LBBB pattern may be due to an atypical accessory (atriofascicular) conduction pathways (e.g., Mahaim fibers). If no other cardiac process is documented, the long-term prognosis is excellent; however, if heart disease is present, cumulative mortality is 50% at 10 years, five times the mortality of patients without LBBB. LBBB is associated with an increase in cardiac mortality as well, particularly sudden death due to ventricular fibrillation (VF). A causal relationship is not clear and may be due to the underlying heart disease. Progression to CHB is rare (approximately 1%); however, if left axis deviation is associated with LBBB, some reports indicate a higher mortality and up to a 6% long-term risk of CHB. Death in these cases is usually due to associated heart disease or rhythm abnormalities.

Clinical Symptoms and Presentation

Patients with LBBB are usually asymptomatic, unless there is bradycardia due to associated AVB, which may cause syncope, near syncope, lightheadedness, or dizziness; however, some patients with acquired LBBB may develop a cardiomyopathy and symptoms of heart failure caused by LV dyssynchrony with associated systolic dysfunction and mitral regurgitation. Some patients are symptomatic from LV dyssynchrony.

Approach to Management

No specific therapy is indicated for most patients, unless there is associated AVB or cardiomyopathy with congestive heart failure (CHF). If right heart catheterization (e.g., Swan-Ganz catheterization) is planned, catheter trauma to the right bundle may result in CHB and the need for temporary pacing. If there are symptoms associated with the LBBB, such as syncope, EP testing can demonstrate significant infra-Hisian conduction system disease that may indicate the need for a permanent pacemaker. His-Purkinje conduction (the histoventricular His to Ventricular [HV] interval) tends to be long in LBBB (60 to 80 ms), but this alone is insufficient reason to implant a pacemaker. However, if an HV interval exceeds 100 ms, pacemaker implantation is advised. If there is associated LV dysfunction with a left ventricular ejection fraction (LVEF) of 35% and New York Heart Association (NYHA) functional class II, III, or IV heart failure symptoms, implantation of a biventricular pacing-ICD system for cardiac resynchronization and defibrillation therapy (CRT-D) may not only improve symptoms and LV function and reduce hospitalizations for heart failure but may also even reduce sudden death mortality (Table 2.7).

Right Bundle Branch Block

Description

Right bundle branch (RBB) block (RBBB) (Fig. 2.14) is associated with a distinctive ECG pattern: a wide QRS complex duration (>0.12 seconds) and an RSR′ pattern in V_1, with terminal wide S waves in I, aVL, and V_5-V_6, indicating terminal rightward activation. Secondary ST-T waves occur in a

TABLE 2.7

LEFT BUNDLE BRANCH BLOCK MANAGEMENT

Setting	Therapy
Asymptomatic normal LV function	• No therapy—rule out structural heart disease, ischemic heart disease.
	• Requires long-term follow-up.
	• If instrumentation of the right ventricle is planned, be ready to temporarily pace (preferably externally or via a temporary pacemaker wire) if transient traumatic RBBB with resultant complete AVB is induced.
	◦ Trauma to the right bundle can last from minutes to more than 24 hours.
Symptomatic (syncope, lightheadedness)	• Admit, monitor, and evaluate for structural heart disease.
	• If syncope occurs, EP consultation and possible EP testing is indicated.
	• If HV interval is 100 ms or more or if infra-Hisian block is provoked with atrial pacing at rates of <160 bpm with or without procainamide challenge, implant a permanent pacemaker.
Symptomatic (CHF)	• LVEF is 35% or less, NYHA class II, III or IV heart failure symptoms are present with LBBB with QRS duration of more than 130 ms: CRT-D ICD implantation is indicated and may improve LV function and heart failure symptoms, and reduce the risk of sudden death.
MI	• New (or not known to be old) LBBB: revascularization with direct PTCA with or without stent.
	• Temporary pacemaker if second-degree or third-degree AVB is present.
	• New onset LBBB indicates extensive myocardial ischemia or infarction and can be associated with a poorer prognosis.
	• Have external (transcutaneous) pacing on standby if no AVB is present.
Preoperative	• No therapy is required if the patient is asymptomatic, whether or not coronary artery disease or systolic dysfunction is known to be present.
	• Cardiac workup (stress test, echocardiogram) to exclude structural heart disease if symptomatic.
	• LBBB is not per se an indication for treadmill testing. If stress testing is performed, imaging must accompany the test if the aim is to document the presence of obstructive coronary artery disease; imaging is not required if the aim of the stress test is the assessment of effort tolerance.
Postoperative	• No therapy if asymptomatic.
	• Common after aortic valve replacement (usually persistent) and after CABG (transient due to cardioplegia).
Alternating LBBB and RBBB	• Alternating BBB may be due to trifascicular disease (see trifascicular block).
	◦ Because of the high rate of progression to CHB, permanent pacemaker implantation is advised.
	• Alternating BBB may also be seen as a digitalis toxic rhythm, although in current practice this occurs only rarely.

AVB, Atrioventricular block; *BBB*, bundle branch block; *CABG*, coronary artery bypass graft; *CHB*, complete atrioventricular block; *CHF*, congestive heart failure; *CRT-D*, cardiac resynchronization and defibrillation therapy; *EP*, electrophysiology; *HV*, histoventricular; *ICD*, implantable cardioverter defibrillator; *LBBB*, left bundle branch block; *LV*, left ventricular; *LVEF*, left ventricular ejection fraction; *NYHA*, New York Heart Association; *RBBB*, right bundle branch block.

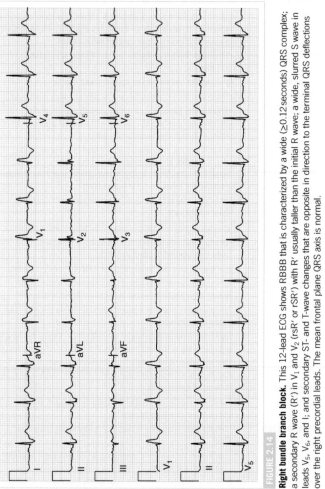

FIGURE 2.14

Right bundle branch block. This 12-lead ECG shows RBBB that is characterized by a wide (≥0.12 seconds) QRS complex; a secondary R wave (R') in V_1 and V_2 (rsR' or rSR') with R' usually taller than the initial R wave; a wide, slurred S wave in leads V_5, V_6, and I; and secondary ST- and T-wave changes that are opposite in direction to the terminal QRS deflections over the right precordial leads. The mean frontal plane QRS axis is normal.

direction opposite to the direction of the terminal part of the QRS. RBBB can be confused with Wolff-Parkinson-White syndrome with a left-sided accessory pathway, but the R wave in V_1 for a left-sided accessory pathway shows a slurred upstroke (delta wave) and does not have the typical RSR' pattern. RBBB does not per se cause tall R waves in V_1 or V_2, and if they are present, they are usually related to the depolarization abnormality and not necessarily to any associated conditions. Causes of tall R waves in V_1 and V_2 (without an RBBB pattern) include posterior wall MI, right ventricular hypertrophy, and myotonic dystrophy. The Brugada pattern can display a right-sided conduction delay in the right precordial leads, but the characteristic ST elevation with T inversion in these leads will clarify the diagnosis.

Associated Conditions

The incidence in a healthy population is approximately 0.16%, but the incidence increases with age and may be as high as 2.4% in an older population. RBBB is often associated with underlying structural heart disease and may be present after MI, cardiac surgery (especially involving the right ventricle), pulmonary embolism, myocarditis, or transient, direct trauma during right heart catheterization. It may also be present in pulmonary hypertension, congenital heart disease, or heart failure. Rate-related (usually tachycardia-dependent) RBBB is common and of no known clinical significance. RBBB in the Framingham study has been associated with (but not caused by) atrial fibrillation, atrial premature contractions, elevated cholesterol, diabetes, stroke, transient ischemic attacks, smoking, obesity, and hypertension. RBBB may be purposely induced with ablation to prevent bundle branch reentry VT. RBBB has been associated with an increased mortality, which may be related to its frequent association with underlying structural heart disease. The 10-year cumulative mortality is as high as 33% if cardiovascular disease is detected, but only 9% in the absence of organic heart disease (similar to that in patients without RBBB). In asymptomatic military recruits with RBBB (mean age of 42), only 1 of 37 (2.7%) had CAD documented by coronary angiography (Algorithm 2.6).

Symptoms and Clinical Presentation

RBBB does not per se cause symptoms. Symptoms would be those of underlying structural heart disease or syncope that may be related to other disorders (AVB, supraventricular tachycardia, and VT).

Approach to Management

Therapy is not required if asymptomatic, but patients with RBBB (especially those older than 65 years) should be carefully screened for cardiac disease. This includes evaluation for CAD, cardiomyopathy, RVH, and right ventricular dysfunction. If bifascicular block (RBBB plus left anterior fascicular block [LAFB] or left posterior fascicular block [LPFB]) develop during acute MI (usually extensive, involving the anterior wall and septum), temporary cardiac pacing may be indicated if there is associated second- or third-degree AVB (Table 2.8).

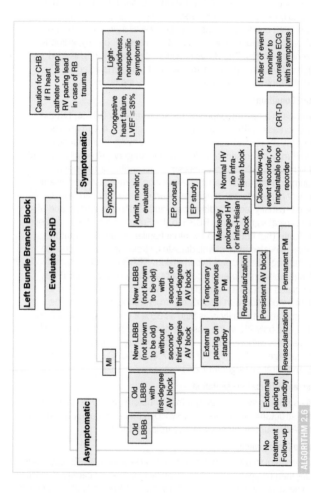

ALGORITHM 2.6

Left bundle branch block. *CHB,* Complete heart block; *LBBB,* left bundle branch block; *LVEF,* left ventricular ejection fraction; *MI,* myocardial infarction; *PM,* pacemaker; *SHD,* structural heart disease (no overt evidence of myocardial, valvular, congenital, or coronary heart disease).

RIGHT BUNDLE BRANCH BLOCK MANAGEMENT

Setting	Therapy
Outpatient asymptomatic	• No therapy.
	• May occur with instrumentation of the right ventricle (e.g., Swan-Ganz catheter) and trauma to the right bundle.
	• Can last up to 24 h.
Symptomatic (syncope)	• Admit the patient with RBBB who has syncope.
	• If symptoms of syncope occur (may be related to AVB or VT), attempt to correlate symptoms with rhythm by Holter or event monitoring.
	• Evaluate for underlying structural cardiac disease.
	• Consider EP testing to assess AV conduction and the presence of inducible VT (present in up to 30% of symptomatic RBBB patients) if the patient is syncopal.
MI	• Isolated RBBB: No therapy.
	• RBBB with LAFB or LPFB (that is new or not known to be old) or alternating BBB:
	• Temporary pacemaker
	• Alternatively, placement of a transcutaneous pacing system
	• RBBB occurs in 3% to 7% of MIs, often with LAFB, and usually because of anterior or anteroseptal infarction.
	• The combination is less common in the current era of early revascularization via percutaneous techniques.
Preoperative	• No therapy—temporary pacemaker not required.
	• Perform cardiac evaluation to exclude other cardiovascular disease.
Postoperative	• No treatment.
	• Most common conduction disturbance in this setting.
Alternating LBBB and RBBB	• Permanent pacemaker if not due to reversible cause.

AV, Atrioventricular; *AVB*, atrioventricular block; *EP*, electrophysiology; *LAFB*, left anterior fascicular block; *LBBB*, left bundle branch block; *LPFB*, left posterior fascicular block; *MI*, myocardial infarction; *RBBB*, right bundle branch block; *VT*, ventricular tachycardia.

Rate-Related Bundle Branch Block

Description

Rate-related BBB (Fig. 2.15) can have the morphology of either LBBB, RBBB, or both; fascicular block can also be rate dependent, although much more rarely.

Tachycardia-related (or dependent) ("phase 3") BBB most commonly involves the RBB. It may occur in patients with structurally normal hearts and is usually due to the physiologically longer refractory period of the RBB compared with that of the LBB. Thus IV aberration occurring after

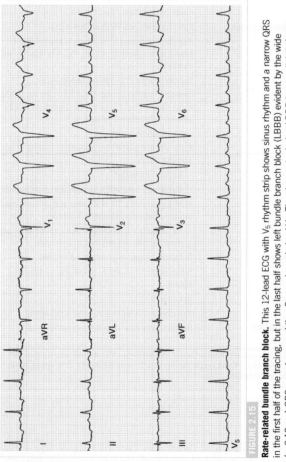

FIGURE 2.15

Rate-related bundle branch block. This 12-lead ECG with V₅ rhythm strip shows sinus rhythm and a narrow QRS in the first half of the tracing, but in the last half shows left bundle branch block (LBBB) evident by the wide (> 0.12 sec) QRS complexes and the rS complexes in lead V₁. The sinus rate during LBBB is very slightly faster.

atrial premature complexes or at rapid atrial rates usually involves the right bundle before the left bundle. The refractory period in the His-Purkinje system is proportional to the preceding coupling interval: after a short R-R interval or at a faster rate, the refractory period is shorter, but after a long R-R interval or slower rate, the refractory period is longer. Thus a premature atrial depolarization occurring at a short P-P interval after a longer P-P interval occurs at a time when the refractory period is longer in the His-Purkinje system. Because the RBB tends to have an even longer refractory period than the LBB, RBBB at the short interval is most likely. This phenomenon constitutes the basis for Ashman phenomenon during atrial fibrillation, where RBBB aberration occurs at a shorter R-R interval that follows a long R-R interval. After the initial aberrantly conducted QRS complex, the BBB may be continued for several complexes because of the phenomenon of "linking," in which concealed (not visible on the surface ECG) transseptal conduction penetrates the right bundle, propagating the RBBB pattern *(concealed perpetuated aberration)*. Although rate-related RBBB at rapid rates or with closely coupled atrial ectopy is usually considered normal physiology, rate-related LBBB typically is associated with structural heart disease and occurs at relatively slower rates compared with those associated with rate-related RBBB. It is possible for there to be RBBB and LBBB aberration in the same individual, and the aberrant morphologies can alternate. Rate-related BBB does not per se indicate trifascicular block (Algorithm 2.7).

Bradycardia-related *(phase 4)* aberrancy is much less common but occurs when there is apparent normal AV conduction and normal QRS duration at normal atrial rates, but with pauses or at slow rates, BBB patterns occur. This is usually due to damage in the His-Purkinje system that leads to *phase 4 depolarization* during bradycardia, causing chronic depolarization of one of the fascicles and allowing conduction to proceed only down to the other one. Bradycardia-related BBB is usually associated with advanced heart disease.

Associated Conditions

Rate-related RBBB is usually a normal, physiologic phenomenon; however, like LBBB, rate-related LBBB almost always occurs in the presence of underlying structural heart disease, such as dilated cardiomyopathy, CAD, valvular heart disease, degenerative disease of the conduction system (Lenegre's disease), calcification of the cardiac skeleton (Lev's disease), and trauma. Lyme disease, sarcoidosis, or other infiltrative myocardial diseases may cause conduction disturbances, including rate-dependent LBBB.

Clinical Symptoms and Presentation

Patients with rate-related BBB are usually asymptomatic, unless there is significant LV dyssynchrony during LBBB. The rate-related BBB may be detected during treadmill stress testing or Holter monitoring.

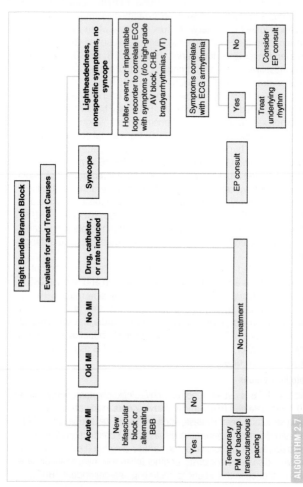

ALGORITHM 2.7

Right bundle branch block. *BBB,* Bundle branch block; *CHB,* complete heart block; *EP,* electrophysiology; *MI,* myocardial infarction; *PM,* pacemake; *VT,* ventricular tachycardia.

Approach to Management

No specific therapy is indicated for most patients, unless there is associated AVB or cardiomyopathy with heart failure. If there is associated LV dysfunction with LVEF of 35% or less and NYHA functional class III or IV heart failure symptoms, implantation of an ICD with biventricular pacing capabilities (CRT-D) may improve symptoms. If there is associated LV dysfunction with LVEF of 45% or less and NYHA functional class II-III heart failure symptoms, implantation of a biventricular pacer (CRT-P) may improve symptoms (Table 2.9).

Fascicular Block

Fascicular block refers to conduction delay or "block" in one of the three fascicles of the IV conduction system: the RBB and the left anterosuperior and inferoposterior fascicular radiation of the LBB. The QRS duration is usually slightly wide (≥100 ms but <120 ms). The RBB resembles a bundle rather than a fascicular radiation and is supplied mainly by the AV nodal (in 90% from the right coronary artery, in 10% from the circumflex artery) or LAD proximally and by the LAD distally. The anterosuperior division of the LBB is supplied by the left anterior descending coronary artery or AVN artery. The inferoposterior fascicular radiation of the left branch is composed of a wider spread or network of fascicular fibers and has a dual blood supply from the right and left circumflex coronary arteries.

Unifascicular Block

Description

Unifascicular block involving the right bundle does not produce a shift in the mean frontal plane QRS axis but does cause an RBBB pattern with a wide QRS complex. Fascicular block of the part of the LBB alone typically does not prolong the QRS duration longer than 0.12 seconds but does shift the mean frontal plane QRS axis. ECG characteristics of LAFB (Fig. 2.16) include QRS duration of 100 ms or more with left-axis deviation of more than –30 degrees, rS in leads II, III, and aVF, small Q wave in lead I and

---

TABLE 2.9

RATE-RELATED BUNDLE BRANCH BLOCK MANAGEMENT

Setting	Therapy
Asymptomatic normal LV function	• No therapy.
Symptomatic (CHF)	• If LVEF is 35% or less, NYHA Functional Class III or IV LBBB with QRS duration of more than 130 ms, cardiac resynchronization therapy with or without an ICD (CRT-P or CRT-D) may improve LV function and symptoms and reduce the risk of sudden death.

CHF, Congestive heart failure; *CRT-D,* cardiac resynchronization and defibrillation therapy; *ICD,* implantable cardioverter defibrillator; *LBBB,* left bundle branch block; *LV,* left ventricular; *LVEF,* left ventricular ejection fraction; *NYHA,* New York Heart Association.

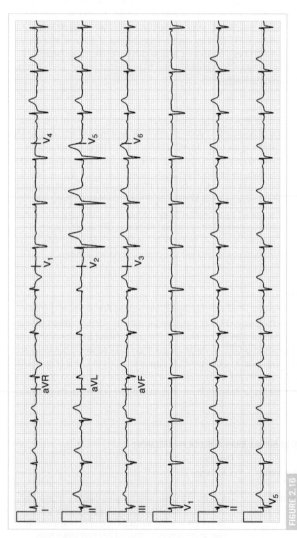

FIGURE 2.16

Left anterior fascicular block. This 12-lead ECG shows left anterior fascicular block, which is characterized by left-axis deviation (mean QRS axis between −45° and −90°); a qR complex in leads I and aVL; an rS complex in leads II, III, and aVF; QRS duration of 0.08–0.11 seconds; and poor R wave progression.

aVL, and a 40-ms delay between the onset of the QRS complex and the R-wave peak in leads I and aVL. Poor R-wave progression across the precordium (R-wave transition lead V_4 or later) and small (noninfarction) Q waves are common in V_2-V_6 in LAFB. This ECG pattern may also be seen with left-axis deviation due to LVH and may not indicate fascicular block. LAFB can be distinguished from left-axis deviation due to other causes by the timing of the R wave in aVL versus aVR. In LAFB the R wave in aVL precedes the late terminal R wave in aVR. The ECG characteristics of LPFB (Fig. 2.17) include duration of 100 ms or more and right-axis deviation with rS in lead I and small noninfarction Q waves in II, III, and aVF. Because isolated LPFB is rare, other causes of right-axis deviation should be sought in any ECG having this abnormality.

Associated Conditions

Unifascicular block is often an incidental finding on the ECG and may be unassociated with any clinically significant heart disease. The most common associated, but not necessarily causative, condition is CAD. Isolated fascicular block is often benign. The incidence of fascicular block is 2% to 5% in otherwise normal individuals; the incidence increases with age.

Clinical Symptoms and Presentation

Isolated unifascicular block does not produce symptoms. If symptoms occur, these are due to associated heart disease.

Approach to Management

No therapy is needed for isolated unifascicular block, and evaluation for underlying heart disease should not rest on this finding alone (Table 2.10).

Bifascicular Block

Description

Bifascicular block involves conduction delay or "block" below the AVN in two of the three fascicles (the RBB and left anterior and left posterior fascicles of the LBB). RBBB is typically combined with either LAFB (Fig. 2.18) or LPFB (Fig. 2.19). LBBB alone is not considered bifascicular block (LAFB plus LPFB), although anatomically this may be the case. Bifascicular block occurs in 1% to 2% of the adult population.

Associated Conditions

Bifascicular block is often associated with structural heart disease and may be associated with progression to high-grade block or CHB. The rate of progression to AVB is 1% to 4% per year and up to 17% per year for individuals with syncope. Bifascicular block in syncope patients is also associated with (but not causally related to) the presence of malignant ventricular arrhythmias. When first-degree AVB is associated with bifascicular block, there is the possibility (20% to 40% of cases in symptomatic patients) that there is *trifascicular* disease (i.e., the remaining

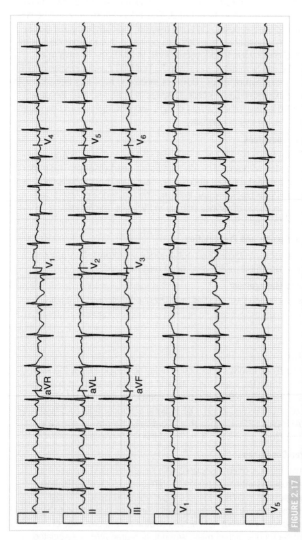

FIGURE 2.17

Left posterior fascicular block. This 12-lead ECG shows LPFB, which is characterized by right-axis deviation (mean QRS axis between +101 and +180 degrees); an S_1Q_3 pattern (deep S wave in lead I and Q wave in lead III); and normal or slightly prolonged QRS duration (0.08 to 0.10 seconds). Isolated LPFB is uncommon and an infrequent cause of right-axis deviation.

TABLE 2.10

FASCICULAR BLOCK MANAGEMENT

Setting	Therapy

Left anterior fascicular block	• No therapy.
	• Exclude other causes of left-axis deviation, including the following:
	  ◦ Emphysema
	  ◦ Left ventricular hypertrophy
	  ◦ Inferior MI
	  ◦ Congenital heart disease

Left posterior fascicular block	• Rare in normal individuals. • No therapy. • Rule out more common causes of right-axis deviation such as right ventricular hypertrophy of any etiology, lateral MI, and a vertical heart. • Usually occurs with RBBB (bifascicular block).
MI	• No specific therapy. • Monitoring for progression of unifascicular conduction delays to bifasicular and trifascicular block and also for AVB is indicated, as this may indicate a more extensive infarct and need for prophylactic temporary cardiac pacing.
Preoperative	• No therapy.
Postoperative	• No therapy. • If new onset, consider tachycardia dependency and acute ischemia as potential causes.

AVB, Atrioventricular block; *MI*, myocardial infarction; *RBBB*, right bundle branch block.

fascicle is also involved), although in most cases the prolonged PR interval is due to block in the AVN (and not the remaining fascicle). Bifascicular block involving the RBB and left anterior fascicle is more common than RBBB and LPFB. This is due to a single coronary artery blood supply (left anterior descending) to the anterior fascicle, as well as its relationship to the LV outflow tract, resulting in mechanotrauma to the fascicle. Bifascicular block involving the left posterior fascicle and the RBB is less common due to a dual blood supply (right and left circumflex coronary arteries), and this combination may be associated with more extensive underlying cardiac pathology. The risk for progression to CHB may be greater. The mortality may be as high as 15% in 2 years, with a 9% risk of sudden death.

Clinical Symptoms and Presentation

No symptoms will be present unless bradycardia caused by AVB exists.

Approach to Management

Treatment should be considered only if symptoms are present due to progression of AVB (e.g., to second-degree or higher AVB) (Table 2.11, Algorithm 2.8).

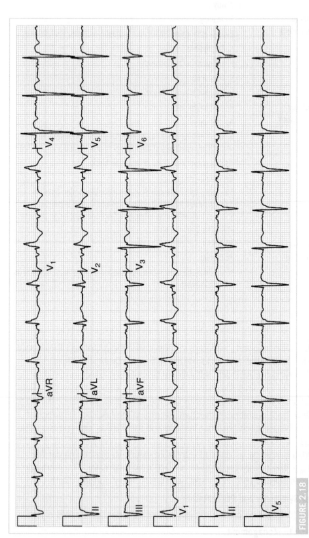

FIGURE 2.18

Right bundle branch block plus left anterior fascicular block–bifascicular block. This 12-lead ECG shows a sinus rhythm with RBBB and LAFB.

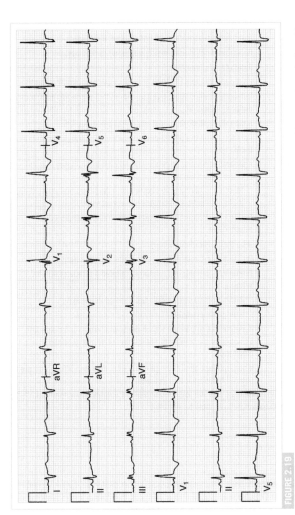

FIGURE 2.19

Right bundle branch block plus left posterior fascicular block–bifascicular block. This 12-lead ECG shows sinus rhythm with RBBB (wide rsR′ complex in lead V₁ with a deep and wide S wave in lead V₅ and V₆) and left anterior fascicular block (with axis> +100 degrees and no Q waves in I or aVL to suggest a lateral MI).

BIFASCICULAR BLOCK MANAGEMENT

Setting	Therapy
Asymptomatic	• No therapy.
	• Evaluate for structural heart disease if clinically warranted.
	• Assess when bifascicular block first occurred, if possible.
	• Recent onset may indicate rapidly progressive cardiac disease.
Symptomatic	• Assess cause of symptoms.
	• If not clear, may need EP testing or an EP consult to assess AV conduction.
MI	• Temporary pacing if Mobitz type II second- or third-degree AVB (CHB) occurs during an anterior MI.
	• Avoid antiarrhythmic drugs that may worsen preexisting AVB.
	• Does not constitute a contraindication to use of β-adrenergic blocker to treat the MI.
	• Associated with poorer prognosis, especially if it occurs in face of acute extensive anterior wall MI.
	– There is a higher mortality after MI even if the bifascicular block precedes the MI, although the exact cause of death not known.
Preoperative	• Evaluate for structural heart disease with an echocardiogram and treadmill test.
	• Not a contraindication to surgery.
Postoperative	• Persistent bifascicular block may occur after valvular surgery.
	• Permanent pacemaker implantation is indicated if associated with the following:
	– Recurring or persistent Mobitz type II second-degree AVB
	– High-grade or complete AV
	• If associated with transient second-degree or advanced or complete AVB, EP testing for site of AVB and measurement of HV interval should be considered.
	• If nonphysiologic block below the AVN or HV of more than 100 ms, permanent pacemaker implantation is indicated.

AV, Atrioventricular; *AVB*, atrioventricular block; *AVN*, atrioventricular node; *CHB*, complete atrioventricular block; *EP*, electrophysiology; *HV*, histoventricular; *MI*, myocardial infarction.

Trifascicular Block

Description

Trifascicular block implies that there is conduction delay or "block" in all three fascicles. One form of trifascicular block is the presence of alternating BBB or left fascicular block, with block alternating between the left anterosuperior and inferoposterior fascicles (LAFB and LPFB, respectively). In trifascicular block, complete block in all three fascicles simultaneously is not present, and the AV conduction ratio is 1:1; if trifascicular block is present simultaneously in all three fascicles, CHB would exist.

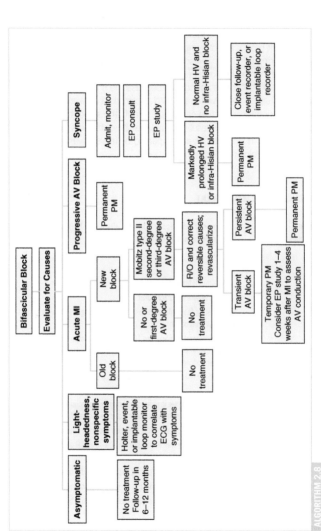

ALGORITHM 2.8

Bifascicular block. *EP,* Electrophysiology; *MI,* myocardial infarction; *PM,* pacemaker.

In trifascicular block the refractory period within a fascicle may be prolonged or conduction may simply be slowed. Another possibility to explain the QRS patterns is that there is concealed retrograde conduction through the fascicles; in this case there may not be trifascicular (antegrade) block at all, and therapy may not be indicated, especially if the fascicle block is intermittent, not productive of symptoms, and there is evidence of adequate conduction during EP study. Trifascicular block has also been considered to be present if there is first-degree AVB (prolonged PR) together with bifascicular block, but this is not correct because the first-degree AVB may represent conduction block within the AVN. IV atropine or exercise testing to facilitate AV nodal conduction can help to clarify the site of block in these cases: if the first-degree AVB resolves, then the site of block is in the AVN, but if the increase in sinus rate is accompanied by more advanced degrees of AVB, the site of block is likely infra-AV nodal.

TABLE 2.12

TRIFASCICULAR BLOCK MANAGEMENT

Setting	Therapy
Outpatient— Asymptomatic	• If evidence of trifascicular block with alternating BBB, intermittent high-grade, or complete heart block occurs:
	○ Admit.
	○ Monitor.
	○ Perform EP testing.
	○ Insert permanent pacemaker.
	• If alternating fascicular or BBB occurs, EP testing is indicated to assess AV conduction.
	• If the HV interval is more than 100 ms or infra-Hisian block is documented at baseline or with atrial pacing or procainamide, a permanent pacemaker is indicated.
Symptomatic	• If second- or third-degree AVB is present, a permanent pacemaker is indicated.
MI	• Temporary pacemaker is indicated if there is associated second- or third-degree AVB in the acute phase of anterior wall MI.
	• Permanent cardiac pacing has not been shown to improve survival.
	• AVB during inferior wall MI is usually intra-AV nodal and is expected to resolve.
	• Temporary transcutaneous pacing capability should be available.
Preoperative	• No acute change in condition and no symptoms: no therapy.
	• Temporary transcutaneous pacing capability should be immediately available.
Postoperative	• New onset suggests myocardial damage.
	• Rule out MI. Monitor continuously.
	• If no change from preoperative ECG, no specific therapy.

AV, Atrioventricular; *AVB,* atrioventricular block; *BBB,* bundle branch block; *ECG,* electrocardiogram; *EP,* electrophysiology; *HV,* histoventricular; *MI,* myocardial infarction.

Associated Conditions

Trifascicular block is often associated with underlying structural heart disease, such as CAD, including post-MI, degenerative disease of the conduction system (Lenegre's disease), calcification of the cardiac skeleton (Lev's disease), or other conditions that are associated with AVB. Trifascicular block can progress to high-grade and CHB.

Clinical Symptoms and Presentation

No symptoms may occur unless bradycardia caused by AVB is present.

Approach to Management

Treatment should be used if symptoms due to AVB are present or if the fascicular block occurs during or persists after the acute phase of an MI. If there are symptoms and alternating BBB, intermittent second-degree or high-grade or CHB, implantation of a permanent pacemaker is indicated. An EP test is indicated to assess AV conduction in symptomatic patients but no manifest AVB; in asymptomatic patients, close follow-up is necessary, and in selected cases, an EP study should be considered. At EP testing an HV interval of more than 100 ms is an indication for permanent pacemaker implantation (Table 2.12, Algorithm 2.9).

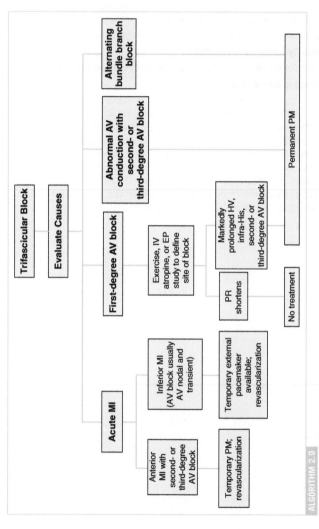

ALGORITHM 2.9

Trifascicular block. *AV,* Atrioventricular; *MI,* myocardial infarction; *PM,* pacemaker.

PREMATURE ATRIAL COMPLEXES

Description

Premature atrial complexes (PACs) are supraventricular ectopic depolarizations originating in or near the atria or in the pulmonary veins that supersede activation from the sinus node. The most common sites of origin appear to be in or around the pulmonary vein ostia, especially in patients who are at risk for atrial fibrillation (AF). They may be isolated and unifocal or multiform in a bigeminal (Fig. 3.1), trigeminal, or quadrigeminal fashion. PACs that are very early may not conduct to the ventricle due to block in the atrioventricular (AV) node or the His-Purkinje system; these blocked PACs (Fig. 3.2) are a common cause of brief pauses. At times, when the heart rhythm is more irregular, an early PAC following a longer R-R interval can conduct aberrantly; the resultant wide QRS (typically a right bundle branch block [RBBB] pattern) can resemble a premature ventricular complex (PVC) but is differentiated by the premature P wave preceding the QRS complex (Fig. 3.3).

PACs may also occur as couplets or as bursts of nonsustained atrial tachycardia. PACs are extremely common and probably occur in all people, whether or not structural heart disease is present. Most of the time they do not cause symptoms, but if they are not conducted to the ventricles and result in a low effective heart rate, symptoms can be present. Early-coupled PACs, in which atrial systole occurs in close temporal relationship to ventricular contraction and thus against closed AV valves, can produce symptoms because of an inability of the atria to empty, producing loss of stroke volume, as well as atrial stretch and increased atrial pressure (seen as cannon A waves), that can cause a sense of palpitations. Unlike many PVCs, most PACs do not encounter entrance block at the sinoatrial (SA) node and thus will reset the sinus node, resulting in a postextrasystolic pause that is less than fully compensatory; however, the type of postextrasystolic pause is not a good criterion of the origin of a premature depolarization. A PAC can occasionally initiate a sustained supraventricular tachycardia, such as AF. PACs can be confused with PVCs if the P wave is buried (hidden) in the preceding T wave, especially if intraventricular aberration of the conducted beat is present.

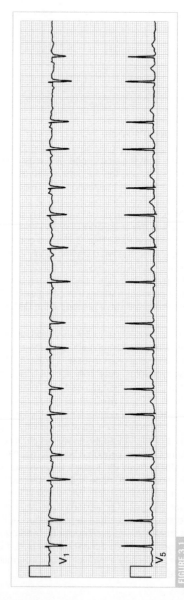

Premature atrial complexes. This rhythm strip of leads V_1 and V_5 shows sinus beats with frequent premature atrial complexes characterized by non-sinus (ectopic) P waves.

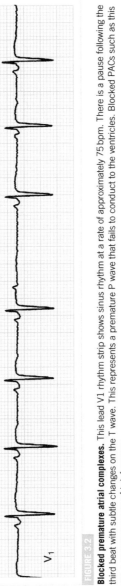

FIGURE 3.2

Blocked premature atrial complexes. This lead V1 rhythm strip shows sinus rhythm at a rate of approximately 75 bpm. There is a pause following the third beat with subtle changes on the T wave. This represents a premature P wave that fails to conduct to the ventricles. Blocked PACs such as this are a common cause of brief pauses.

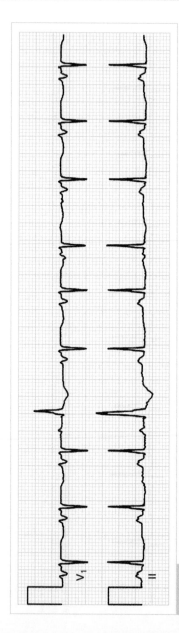

FIGURE 3.3

Premature atrial complex with aberrancy. This lead V1 and II rhythm strip shows sinus rhythm with two PACs. The second PAC conducts normally with a narrow QRS complex (seventh QRS complex), but the first PAC conducts aberrantly with a wide QRS complex (fourth QRS complex) that is due to right bundle branch block with left posterior fascicular block.

Associated Conditions

Atrial ectopy can be exacerbated by alcohol, caffeine, theobromine (chocolate), methylxanthines, catecholamines, smoking, stress, lack of sleep, fatigue, hypoxia, transient or chronic elevations in atrial pressure, or mechanical stimulation (e.g., from a Swan-Ganz catheter). Frequent PACs, especially if multiform, can mimic AF and may constitute a risk for its development. PACs are common after cardioversion of AF and may be a predictor of its early recurrence. They are rarely caused by an MI unless atrial infarction or pericarditis occurs. The underlying mechanism of PAC production during atrial infarction is unknown but may be due in some cases to focally discharging sites or microreentry located in or around the pulmonary vein ostia. PACs occurring in the presence of pericarditis may represent inflammatory irritation of specific foci.

Clinical Symptoms and Presentation

Occasional patients have palpitations, but only rarely are these intolerable. Frequent PACs are uncommon in the general population (<2% of healthy subjects have >100 PACs per 24-hour period), but their prevalence increases with age, especially when there is an associated atrial conduction abnormality, elevated atrial pressures, or atrial enlargement. PACs may be seen with lung disease and structural heart disease of any type; they may be a precursor to paroxysmal AF.

Approach to Management

Suppression is rarely indicated. The patient should be reassured and therapy discouraged unless severe or intolerable symptoms are present because the treatments to suppress these ectopic beats may be worse (e.g., side effects, proarrhythmia) than the rhythm itself. Patient education often helps in this regard. Suppression of PACs may be required early after DC cardioversion of AF because they may presage early AF recurrence. If PACs induce AF or are highly symptomatic, antiarrhythmic drug suppression or even ablation may be required (Table 3.1).

TABLE 3.1

PREMATURE ATRIAL COMPLEXES

Setting	Therapy
Mild or no symptoms	• No therapy.
	• Reassure the patient.
	• Assess risk for atrial fibrillation (e.g., enlarged atria, elevated atrial pressure), as PACs may trigger an episode.

Continued on following page

TABLE 3.1

PREMATURE ATRIAL COMPLEXES (Continued)

Setting	Therapy
Highly symptomatic	• Reassure the patient.
	• Eliminate potential triggers (e.g., caffeine, alcohol).
	• Explore cause for symptoms.
	• Consider an event monitor to correlate symptoms with the arrhythmia.
	• It is possible the two are not related and that treatment will not improve symptoms.
	• Rule out structural heart disease, especially mitral valve disease by history, physical examination, and echocardiogram.
	• First-line therapy: β-adrenergic blocker, which can be given on a PRN basis.
	• A calcium channel blocker may occasionally be effective.
	• Note: Data on the use of either of these drug classes are lacking.
	• In highly symptomatic patients who do not respond to β-adrenergic or calcium channel blockers, class IC antiarrhythmic drugs may be helpful if structural heart disease is not present.
	• Ablation is rarely indicated but may be considered in select cases in which the focus of origin is unifocal.
Triggers atrial fibrillation	• See also "Atrial Fibrillation."
	• Consider β-adrenergic blockers as the first-line therapy or treat as you would for atrial fibrillation (see "Atrial Fibrillation").
	• If symptomatic and refractory to β-adrenergic blockers, consider a class IC antiarrhythmic drug (no heart or coronary disease).
	• If structural heart disease or other specific risk factors for thromboembolism in atrial fibrillation, anticoagulation may be indicated.
	• PACs are common after DC cardioversion of atrial fibrillation but are expected to remit over minutes to hours to days.
	• Early use of antiarrhythmic drugs may be needed to prevent early recurrence of atrial fibrillation, after which the drugs can be stopped.
	• Ablation of the triggers of atrial fibrillation may prevent persistent or permanent atrial fibrillation.

TABLE 3.1

PREMATURE ATRIAL COMPLEXES (Continued)

Setting	Therapy
MI	• No therapy unless PACs:
	- Are frequent, highly symptomatic, or poorly tolerated hemodynamically
	- Trigger atrial fibrillation (in this case, a β-adrenergic blocker is first-line therapy)
Preoperative	• No therapy.
	• PACs may trigger atrial fibrillation, but prophylactic antiarrhythmic therapy is not indicated.
Postoperative	• If ectopic beats trigger paroxysmal atrial fibrillation, may need to suppress with β-adrenergic blockers as first-line therapy.
	• Short courses of antiarrhythmic drugs, including amiodarone for fibrillation, are occasionally necessary.
Nonconducted ("blocked") PACs	• No treatment.
	• Blocked PACs can cause brief pauses that may be confused with sinus pauses or second-degree AVB.
	• They are rarely symptomatic and rarely need treatment.
	• "Blocked bigeminy" can cause a low effective heart rate and produce symptoms of bradycardia; suppression may be helpful in such cases.

PREMATURE JUNCTIONAL COMPLEXES

Description

Premature junctional complexes (PJCs) originate in the AV junction. Postextrasystolic pauses may be fully compensatory or noncompensatory, depending on whether the junctional impulse encounters entrance block at the SA node (which does not disturb the rate of the sinus impulse, a fully compensatory pause) or penetrates it (depolarizing the sinus pacemaker cells and resetting the sinus rate). PJCs (Fig. 3.4) have a narrow QRS complex unless BBB is present. A PJC is often characterized as a premature beat with no P wave or with a retrograde P (inverted in leads II, III, and aVF) occurring just before, during, or after QRS complex. P waves may also be dissociated from the junctional complexes.

Associated Conditions

PJCs occur in structurally normal hearts, are usually of no clinical importance, and are self-limited. They may be seen in sinus node dysfunction. PJCs are rare during myocardial infarction (MI).

Clinical Symptoms and Presentation

PJCs may cause palpitations.

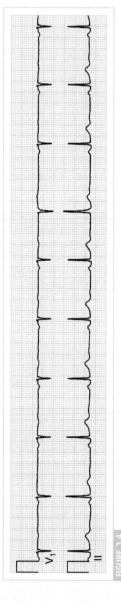

Premature junctional complex. This rhythm strip of leads V1 and II shows sinus rhythm. The seventh QRS complex is a PJC. It is premature, it is not preceded by a P wave, it has a very similar morphology as the sinus-stimulated QRS complexes, and it does not disrupt the sinus cycle length (the P-P intervals remain constant and the expected sinus P wave is seen in the ST segment of the PJC).

TABLE 3.2	
PREMATURE JUNCTIONAL COMPLEXES	
Setting	**Therapy**
Conducted	● No therapy.
	● If symptoms, treat the same as for PACs.
Nonconducted	● Same as conducted PACs and PJCs.
	● May mimic heart block.
MI	● No therapy.
Preoperative and Postoperative	● No therapy unless highly symptomatic.
	● If symptomatic, treat as PACs with β-adrenergic blockers as first-line therapy.

Approach to Management

Management is the same as for PACs. Treatment is generally not indicated unless the patient is symptomatic. PJCs may be difficult to suppress with an antiarrhythmic drug and are generally difficult or impossible to ablate without risk of complete heart block (Table 3.2).

PREMATURE VENTRICULAR COMPLEXES

Description

PVCs are premature ectopic beats arising from the right ventricle (RV) or left ventricle (LV) that can occur in a variety of patterns and can occasionally cause symptoms. PVCs can occur during sinus rhythm or any other prevailing cardiac rhythm. PVCs can cause a "compensatory pause" if no retrograde atrial activation is present or if retrograde atrial encounters entrance block at the sinus node, thereby producing no disturbance in the sinus firing rate; however, less than fully compensatory pauses will be produced if sinus node reset is produced by the retrograde atrial activation penetrating the node. The type of postextrasystolic pause may not distinguish PVCs from supraventricular complexes. "Interpolated" PVCs (Fig. 3.5) can occur in which the R-R interval enclosing the PVC is not disturbed, even though retrograde ("concealed") depolarization into the AV node often occurs producing "pseudo first-degree AV block" for one beat.

PVCs can occasionally be confused with other ectopic beats: PACs conducted to the ventricles aberrantly can mimic PVCs; however, a premature P wave is usually evident on close inspection of multiple simultaneously recorded ECG leads. A short burst of PACs can cause concealed conduction and result in perpetuated aberration that resembles multiple consecutive PVCs. PVCs can (1) occur as single unifocal complexes, (2) have multiple morphologies (multifocal or multiform) and fusion complexes (Fig. 3.6) in which the ventricles are depolarized via both the PVC and the antegrade conducted supraventricular impulse, (3) have multiple coupling intervals to the preceding sinus beats,

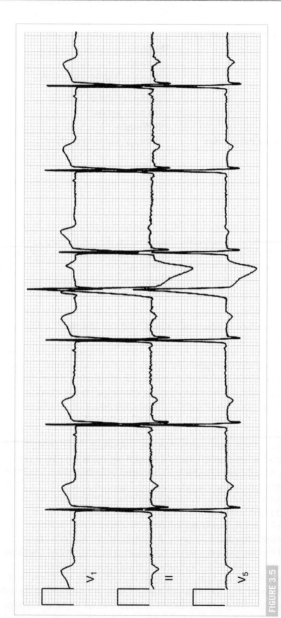

FIGURE 3.5

Interpolated premature ventricular complex. This lead V$_1$, II, and V$_5$ rhythm strip shows an interpolated premature ventricular contraction (PVC) (4th complex) in which the PVC occurs between two consecutive sinus beats with no compensatory pause.

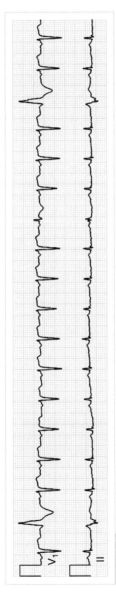

FIGURE 3.6

Premature ventricular complexes with fusion complexes. These simultaneously recorded leads V1 and II rhythm strips show normal sinus rhythm with PVCs. The second and sixteenth QRS complexes are PVCs. The 12th QRS complex is a PVC that follows a sinus P wave but is dissociated from it with a shorter PR interval and is a more narrow complex than the other PVCs; it is a fusion complex that represents simultaneous ventricular activation from two foci, in this case a sinus beat and a ventricular focus. The resultant QRS complex is intermediate in morphology between a sinus-stimulated QRS complex and the PVC. Fusion beats can have QRS durations less than 0.12 seconds.

(4) occur as couplets or triplets, or (5) initiate nonsustained or sustained ventricular tachycardia (VT). PVCs can alternate with every other beat (ventricular bigeminy) or every third beat (ventricular trigeminy) or occur every fourth beat (ventricular quadrigeminy) (Fig. 3.7). PVCs can also be a manifestation of a parasystolic focus, in which the focus fires at a constant rate that can be stable over years; the timing of its appearance on an ECG will reflect tissue refractoriness and varying degrees of exit (and entrance) block to depolarize surrounding ventricular tissue, and because it fires independently of surrounding depolarizations, it has no fixed coupled interval to preceding complexes. Ventricular parasystole is benign. Parasystolic tachycardia is extremely rare and difficult to diagnose.

Associated Conditions

PVCs are extremely common in patients with and without structural heart disease. The frequency of PVCs in normal healthy individuals ranges from 0.77% to 2.8% in a single ECG; on a Holter monitor the prevalence is 17% to 100%. In patients with normal hearts, PVCs (even if frequent) tend to be unifocal and often originate in the outflow tract, most commonly in the RV (Fig. 3.8) and less commonly in the LV outflow tract (Fig. 3.9), including the aortic cusp or other sites in the LV or RV. They may cause anxiety, which may increase their frequency. Complex ventricular ectopy (frequent, multiform complexes or bursts of VT) tends to occur in the older population and those with structural heart disease, with an incidence varying from 7% to 22% (up to 77% of elderly), depending on the population studied. They may occur in a variety of patterns and be exacerbated by exercise, emotional stress, alcohol, ischemia, heart failure, or mechanical stimulation (e.g., Swan-Ganz catheter).

"Frequent" PVCs (>10 PVCs per hour) may have prognostic significance for mortality in patients with ischemic heart disease, although arrhythmic mortality is not well predicted. In addition to causing symptoms, PVCs can occasionally have hemodynamic consequences acutely and over the long term can cause ventricular dysfunction. In some patients with very frequent PVCs, especially if a functional left bundle branch block (LBBB) is produced, cardiomyopathy may occur; suppression of the PVCs by medical or ablative approaches may improve the cardiomyopathy. PVCs appear to carry a benign prognosis in patients without structural heart disease and in patients with structural heart disease but normal ventricular function. The presence of frequent PVCs may be associated with a slightly increased risk of sudden cardiac death and total mortality, even in a population without structural heart disease, although this issue remains controversial. On the other hand, there are no data to indicate that treatment of PVCs in otherwise healthy individuals without structural heart disease will improve outcome. In contrast, frequent or complex PVCs are associated with increased total and cardiovascular mortality in patients with systolic ventricular dysfunction or after MI, with prognosis related to their frequency, complexity (couplets, triplets, nonsustained VT), and

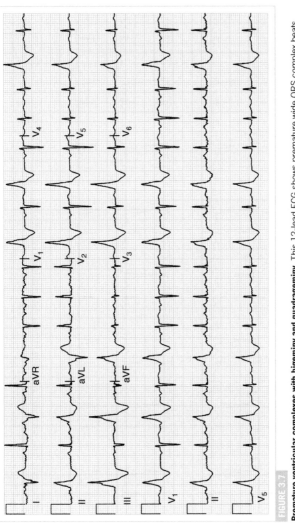

FIGURE 3.7

Premature ventricular complexes with bigeminy and quadrageminy. This 12-lead ECG shows premature wide QRS complex beats that are not preceded by P waves. These represent PVCs. For the first portion of the tracing, the PVCs appear in a bigeminal pattern (every other beat is a PVC), but in the fourth and sixth PVC are in a quadrigeminal pattern (every fourth beat is a PVC).

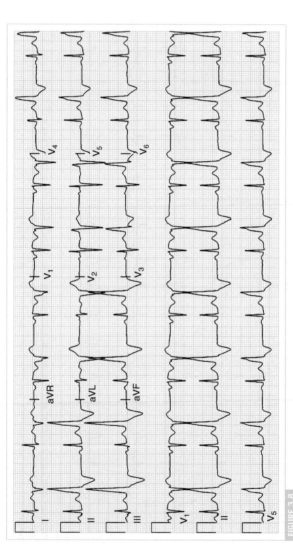

FIGURE 3.8

Premature ventricular complexes originating from the right ventricular outflow tract. This 12-lead ECG tracing with rhythm strips shows isolated premature ventricular complexes (PVCs) in a pattern of bigeminy in which the PVCs originate from either the right or the left ventricular outflow tract. The left bundle branch block pattern suggests a right ventricle origin, but the early R wave transition in V_3 suggests a left ventricular outflow tract origin could be possible. The outflow tract origin is evidenced by the mean frontal plane PVC axis, which is inferiorly directed, indicating a base-to-apex depolarization sequence.

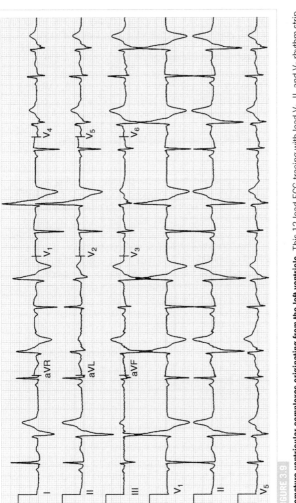

FIGURE 3.9

Premature ventricular complexes originating from the left ventricle. This 12-lead ECG tracing with lead V_1, II, and V_5 rhythm strip shows isolated premature ventricular complexes (PVCs) occurring in a bigeminal pattern in which the PVCs originate from the LV. This is evident from the right bundle branch block pattern. The superiorly directed mean frontal plane PVC axis indicates an apex-to-base depolarization sequence.

timing relative to acute clinical events. The incidence of PVCs peaks early after MI and then tapers gradually over time. The prognostic significance and mortality after MI increases if PVCs and complex ventricular ectopy occur 48 to 96 hours after MI, especially if the left ventricular ejection fraction (LVEF) is less than 0.40. PVCs therefore become a predictor of increased mortality similar to LVEF, multivessel coronary disease, abnormal signal-averaged ECG, abnormal heart rate variability, T-wave alternans, and a variety of other noninvasive parameters. The presence of isolated PVCs is not as highly predictive of mortality as some other risk factors, but patients with frequent PVCs (>10 per hour) occurring greater than 6 days after MI have been reported to have a 7% mortality after MI. The predictive value increases if the LVEF is less than 0.40 with an approximate doubling in mortality. However, much of this information was collected in the pre-percutaneous coronary intervention (pre-PCI) era and may not be applicable to aggressively managed acute MI patients nowadays.

Clinical Symptoms and Presentation

PVCs are usually asymptomatic, but in some patients, including those without structural heart disease, they may be associated with palpitations, dizziness, weakness, fatigue, shortness of breath, or chest discomfort. Most individuals feel the postextrasystolic beat after the PVC and do not feel the PVC itself because its early timing is associated with a lower stroke volume; however, the postextrasystolic (usually) compensatory pause allows a longer time for the ventricle to fill, and thus the sensation often can be described as a "skipped" beat followed by a forceful or strong beat. The sensation may also be due in part to postextrasystolic potentiation from the irregularity in pulse and from atrial contraction against closed AV valves. Pounding, slow palpitations are typical of bigeminal PVCs. In patients with symptoms consistent with PVCs, it is important to try to correlate the symptom with the arrhythmia. There are many symptoms that may mimic those from PVCs, but many PVCs still remain asymptomatic. New-onset PVCs in a patient at risk for or with known heart disease can be a red flag; such patients need to be evaluated carefully for the presence of developing or progressive heart disease.

Approach to Management

No Structural Heart Disease

In patients with no structural heart disease and PVCs, treatment to suppress PVCs has not been shown to improve survival (and mortality is low to begin with in these patients). In most cases no therapy is recommended, and reassuring the patient as to the benign nature of the rhythm is essential. Therapy is directed toward reduction or elimination in symptoms and may include β-adrenergic blockers, calcium channel blockers, or class I, II, or III antiarrhythmic drugs. Fish oil may be effective. Antiarrhythmic drugs should be used only if a patient has frequent and severe symptoms that cannot otherwise be controlled with a β-adrenergic blocker or a calcium channel blocker. There are few if any data to indicate that a β-adrenergic blocker or calcium channel blocker actually is effective in suppressing PVCs. Fish oil may suppress some symptomatic PVCs, but no other supplement is known to have any benefit. It is important to determine whether a patient has structural heart disease. It may be useful to follow the patient long term to determine whether new symptoms develop or whether there is a new onset of or progression in heart disease that was not present initially. For refractory symptoms or frequent PVCs leading to a PVC-associated cardiomyopathy or functional LBBB ventricular dyssynchrony, electrophysiology study with mapping and ablation of the PVC is helpful. This represents the distinct minority of patients without structural heart disease. PVCs can originate from the endocardium or epicardium of either ventricle (Algorithm 3.1).

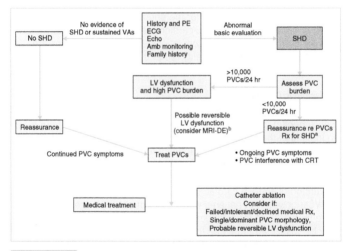

ALGORITHM 3.1

Management of PVCs. SHD = [a]Medical therapy + ICD; [b]Absence of high scar burden suggests reversibility. *CRT*, Cardiac resynchronization therapy; *ICD*, implantable cardioverter defibrillator; *LV*, left ventricular; *MRI-DE*, magnetic resonance imaging with delayed enhancement; *PE*, physical examination; *PVC*, premature ventricular complexes; *Rx*, therapy; *SHD*, structural heart disease; *VAs*, ventricular arrhythmias. (Modified from Pedersen CT, Kay GN, Kalman J, Borggrefe M, Della-Bella P, Dickfeld T, Dorian P, Huikuri H, Kim YH, Knight B, Marchlinski F, Ross D, Sacher F, Sapp J, Shivkumar K, Soejima K, Tada H, Alexander ME, Triedman JK, Yamada T, Kirchhof P, Lip GY, Kuck KH, Mont L, Haines D, Indik J, Dimarco J, Exner D, Iesaka Y, Savelieva I; EP-Europace,UK. Heart Rhythm. 2014 Oct;11(10):e166-e196. doi: 10.1016/j. hrthm.2014.07.024. Epub 2014 Aug 30.)

Post Myocardial Infarction

Early after MI, lidocaine had been used to suppress PVCs in hopes of avoiding progression to VT or ventricular fibrillation (VF); however, most studies show no benefit and possible harm (including death) from antiarrhythmic drug suppression of PVCs. As such, prophylactic lidocaine has little use. In the long term, class IC antiarrhythmic drugs have been shown to be associated with an increased mortality (almost triple) after MI despite suppression of PVCs. Similar data have been accumulated with class IA and III (d-sotalol and dl-sotalol) antiarrhythmic drugs. The only antiarrhythmic drugs that appear relatively neutral in this regard are amiodarone and dofetilide. Several studies have been performed with amiodarone after MI (e.g., EMIAT and CAMIAT); amiodarone has been found to reduce arrhythmic and sudden death, but overall mortality was not affected. There is currently no evidence that suppression of PVCs post-MI by an empiric antiarrhythmic drug is indicated. Implantation of an implantable cardioverter defibrillator (ICD) for the primary prevention of sudden death in patients with ischemic cardiomyopathy has been reported to improve mortality in selected populations, but these indications are intended for reduction of mortality rather than primarily for treatment of PVCs.

Nonischemic Cardiomyopathy

PVCs are common in other cardiac conditions, such as dilated (nonischemic) cardiomyopathy and valvular heart disease. There is no indication that empiric suppression of PVCs in these conditions will improve mortality. ICD implantation for patients with nonischemic cardiomyopathy has been shown to reduce mortality in patients with LVEF ≤ 35% (SCD-HeFT), but ICDs were studied for primary prevention of sudden cardiac death and not primarily for treatment of PVCs; however, in patients with very frequent PVCs (generally more than 10% of the total beats) in which the cardiomyopathy may be suspected to be due to the PVCs, pharmacologic or ablative suppression of PVCs may be beneficial in improving ventricular function.

Summary

PVCs may indicate a trend toward increased mortality, particularly if heart disease is present, although this increase is modest at best. The main indication to treat PVCs is for symptom reduction. However, empiric antiarrhythmic treatment may increase mortality, especially with structural heart disease, and the patient should be advised of this before treatment is instituted (Table 3.3).

TABLE 3.3

PREMATURE VENTRICULAR COMPLEX THERAPY AND SPECIFIC CLINICAL PRESENTATIONS

Setting	Therapy
Asymptomatic	• No treatment because treatment may increase mortality or have a neutral effect unless the PVCs are very frequent (typically > 10-20,000/day) and contributing to a tachycardia- or PVC-mediated cardiomyopathy.
	• Further clinical evaluation is indicated, especially if the PVCs are new onset and there are risk factors for heart disease.
	• PVCs may indicate proarrhythmic effects of antiarrhythmic drugs or other nonantiarrhythmic drugs, such as those that produce QT-interval prolongation.
	• Evaluation for the presence of structural heart disease is indicated.
	• The presence of PVCs that begin later in life (older than 40 years) should raise consideration that there may be a new or progressive cardiac process that is occurring, including ischemic heart disease.
	• However, in most of these patients, a diagnostic workup is unrevealing.
Symptomatic	• Heart disease
	◦ Avoid empiric treatment, unless required for symptom reduction.
	◦ Consider a β-adrenergic blocker.
	◦ Antiarrhythmic drugs, such as class IC antiarrhythmic drugs, can suppress PVCs, but risk of proarrhythmia exists and should be avoided.
	◦ Class III drugs (sotalol, amiodarone) may be considered for symptom reduction, although again risk of proarrhythmia or adverse effects exists.
	• No heart disease
	◦ Discuss goals of therapy with patient.
	◦ No therapy may be needed. Fish oil can be useful.
	◦ If patient remains highly symptomatic, a β-adrenergic blocker is usually the first-line drug.
	• In some patients, a second-line drug may be:
	◦ A class I, II, or III antiarrhythmic drug (IC: flecainide or propafenone).
	◦ Mexiletine, sotalol, or amiodarone (if no structural heart disease).
	• For refractory symptoms or tachycardia- or PVC-induced cardiomyopathy, an electrophysiology study with mapping and ablation can be considered.
	• If exercise or stress induced, the VT may be amenable to β-adrenergic blockers or radiofrequency ablation.
	• Exercise-induced PVCs or VT may indicate need for cardiac catheterization if there is an association with an ischemic response.
	• Exercise-induced right ventricular outflow tract VT is not uncommon in otherwise healthy individuals, and radiofrequency ablation can be curative.
	• Symptomatic PVCs may be seen associated with mitral valve prolapse (MVP).
	• There is little evidence that this increases mortality in typical MVP, but risk may be slightly increased.

Continued on following page

PREMATURE VENTRICULAR COMPLEX THERAPY AND SPECIFIC CLINICAL PRESENTATIONS (Continued)

Setting	Therapy
	• β-adrenergic blockers would be first-line therapy.
	• No other therapy has been shown to be useful.
	• In patients with LV dysfunction and CHF due to frequent PVCs (e.g., frequent or continuous bigeminy), catheter ablation may improve symptoms and cardiac function.
	• PVCs that begin later in life (older than 40 years) can suggest a new or progressive cardiac process, and a diagnostic workup can be considered.
MI	• Discussed previously.
	• No indication for empiric suppression or treatment unless needed for symptoms.
	• Up to 100% of individuals with MI will have PVCs, and up to 34% will have complex ectopy.
	• Frequent ectopy may indicate ongoing ischemia or LV dysfunction.
	• Frequently, PVCs represent a rhythm of reperfusion injury after fibrinolysis or PCI and generally resolve within hours to days.
Ischemic cardiomyopathy	• No indication for empiric suppression or treatment unless needed for symptoms.
	• A β-adrenergic blocker is first-line therapy but the goal is not necessarily elimination of PVCs.
	• For refractory symptoms, class III drugs (amiodarone, sotalol) are second-line choices.
Idiopathic dilated cardiomyopathy	• Common.
	• No indication for empiric suppression or treatment, unless needed for symptoms.
	• For symptoms, a β-adrenergic blocker would be first-line therapy.
	• For refractory symptoms, a class III drug (amiodarone, sotalol) is a second-line choice.
Hypertrophic cardiomyopathy	• No evidence that antiarrhythmic therapy will improve prognosis for patients with isolated PVCs and no other risk factors.
	• Nonsustained or sustained VT on Holter monitoring, syncope, or significant (>3 cm) ventricular hypertrophy are indications for ICD implantation.
	• The role of EP testing and empiric antiarrhythmic therapy, including the use of amiodarone, is controversial and is not routinely indicated.
Preoperative	• Before noncardiac surgery, consider the possibility that an untreated cardiac problem exists and treat appropriately.
	• No therapy for PVC suppression is indicated.
	• Expect that PVCs may increase in frequency postoperative.
	• This is likely due to increased adrenergic tone.
Postoperative	• Common after coronary artery bypass surgery.
	• The number of PVCs may increase by a factor of 10 but then diminish gradually over 4 to 6 weeks.
	• After noncardiac surgery, a modest increase in frequency of PVCs may be expected.
	• This usually does not warrant specific therapy.
	• β-adrenergic blockers are first-line therapy if patient is symptomatic.

Description

The hierarchy of the sources of electrical activation of the heart is the sinus node, AV node (or junction), and ventricle. Atrial myocardial tissue and His-Purkinje tissue, unless abnormal, do not commonly demonstrate automatic properties. The rate of the sinus node at rest is 50 to 100 bpm, but a slightly slower rate is not uncommon. The AV node or junction and the ventricle can provide an escape rhythm (i.e., a rhythm terminating pauses or slowing of rate) if the sinus node is not functioning (e.g., sinus arrest and/or SA block), if the sinus rate is slow, or if there is AV block. The typical junctional escape rate is 40 to 60 bpm. The typical ventricular escape rate is 20 to 40 bpm. Junctional or ventricular rhythms faster than these rates are termed accelerated rhythms. Accelerated rhythms may mask AV block and make it difficult to determine the level of the block. An accelerated junctional or ventricular rate occurring with an independent atrial rhythm can cause AV dissociation. AV dissociation is often confused with AV block, but it is *not* AV block, inasmuch as antegrade conduction of the atrial impulse will occur, given temporal opportunity to do so. Isorhythmic AV dissociation (Fig. 3.10) will be present when the atrial and the QRS rates are similar; long rhythm strips may be required to demonstrate the ability of the atrial impulse to conduct to the ventricles ("capture"); the captured QRS will be early relative to the cycle length of the accelerated junctional or ventricular rhythm.

Associated Conditions

Escape rhythms may exist concomitantly with sinus bradycardia (SB) or AV block. They may occur transiently with changes in autonomic tone and suppression of higher pacemakers. Patients with sinus node dysfunction often lack stable escape pacemakers.

Clinical Symptoms and Presentation

Escape and accelerated rhythms may cause palpitations or lightheadedness. AV dissociation may cause irregular neck or chest pounding (because of the variable and near simultaneity of atrial and ventricular contractions), weakness, or fatigue.

Approach to Management

Usually no therapy is required for accelerated rhythms, particularly if the patient is asymptomatic. If necessary, an increase in the atrial rate, either by pacing, drugs such as oral theophylline, or exercise, will eliminate the AV dissociation caused by accelerated rhythms. If AV block is present, causing escape rhythms that are slow and/or unstable, permanent cardiac

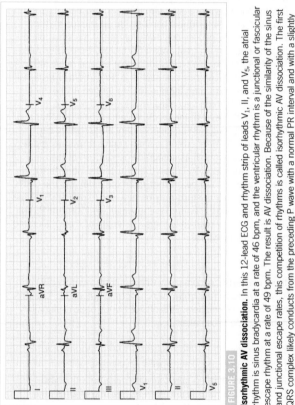

FIGURE 3.10

Isorhythmic AV dissociation. In this 12-lead ECG and rhythm strip of leads V_1, II, and V_5, the atrial rhythm is sinus bradycardia at a rate of 46 bpm, and the ventricular rhythm is a junctional or fascicular escape rhythm at a rate of 49 bpm. The result is AV dissociation. Because of the similarity of the sinus and junctional escape rates, this competition of rhythms is called isorhythmic AV dissociation. The first QRS complex likely conducts from the preceding P wave with a normal PR interval and with a slightly shorter interval than subsequent junctional escape beats that have short PR intervals. The escape rhythm has a narrow incomplete RBBB/LPFB QRS morphology, suggesting either a junctional escape with aberrancy or a fascicular escape from the left anterior fascicle. There are ST-T changes and inferior and anterior Q waves suggesting possible myocardial infarction of indeterminate age.

TABLE 3.4

ESCAPE BEATS AND RHYTHMS THERAPY

Setting	Therapy
Junctional	• No therapy, because the rate of the junctional escape rhythm is reasonable and the junction can respond to autonomic input, increasing its rate with exercise.
	• If there is symptomatic bradycardia due to sinus node disease or AV block, a pacemaker may be indicated.
	• Atropine accelerates the sinus node in symptomatic patients, but this is not a chronic therapy.
	• Atropine may also accelerate junctional pacemakers.
	• Consider atrial pacing if bothersome symptoms are presented.
	• Catecholamines can accelerate junctional pacemakers.
	• This is benign but may impair hemodynamics.
Ventricular	• Due to SB or AV block. If due to SB, AV dissociation may be present, which can be isorhythmic (see earlier); capture can occur.
	• AV dissociation is not synonymous with AV block and occurs when the atrial rate is slower than the ventricular rate.
	• Escape rhythms should not be suppressed because there may then be no QRS rhythm or an even slower one, which can be hemodynamically destabilizing.
	• A pacemaker may be needed if cause of the rhythm is not correctable.
	• Note: Temporary ventricular pacing can "overdrive suppress" the focus of an escape rhythm such that if pacing is stopped there may be no escape rhythm and prolonged asystolic pauses; this can occur despite the presence of what appears to be a stable escape rhythm for a long period of time.
MI	• May occur with transient AV block.
	• In some cases, temporary pacing may be required, depending on the origin, rate, and stability (junction more stable than ventricle) of the escape pacemaker.
	• Escape pacemakers and rhythms can be suppressed by antiarrhythmic drugs, including lidocaine; these should be avoided if possible.
Preoperative and Postoperative	• No specific treatment.
	• Assess underlying causes and treat.
	• If AV block or sinus node exists, treat these diseases as outlined.

pacing will be required. For congenital complete AV block with a junctional escape rhythm, demonstration of symptoms or chronotropic incompetence is an indication for permanent pacemaker implantation; there is evidence to suggest that permanent pacing is indicated even in the absence of symptoms (Table 3.4).

ECTOPIC ATRIAL RHYTHM

Description

Ectopic atrial rhythm (EAR) (Fig. 3.11) arises from pacemaker sites outside of the sinus node in the right or left atrium and results in a P-wave morphology different from that of sinus rhythm (e.g., P waves are not upright in leads II, III, and aVF or differ from sinus rhythm P wave morphology).

Associated Conditions

EAR is often seen as an escape rhythm in young adults, especially athletes with high vagal tone (transient and/or paroxysmal), or in patients with sinus node disease (in which case the EAR is often more persistent). EAR may also be an accelerated rhythm (rate exceeds sinus rate but <100 bpm) due to high catecholamine levels such as are induced by pain or anxiety. The ectopic focus is often in the low right atrium and may be associated with a short PR interval.

Clinical Symptoms and Presentation

EAR is not associated with increased risk for thromboembolism or adverse prognosis. Most patients are asymptomatic. Rarely, patients may experience palpitations, possibly related to short PR intervals (decreased diastolic filling time).

Approach to Management (Table 3.5)

TABLE 3.5

ECTOPIC ATRIAL RHYTHM APPROACH TO THERAPY

Setting	Therapy
Asymptomatic	• No therapy required.
Symptomatic	• Consider therapy with a β-adrenergic blocker, unless there is significant underlying SB.
MI	• Asymptomatic, rate < 90 bpm: no therapy.
	• Usually a transient problem and does not require long-term therapy.
Preoperative	• No therapy usually required.
Postoperative	• No therapy usually required.
	• EAR is often due to catecholamine elevation after surgery.

WANDERING ATRIAL PACEMAKER

Description

Wandering atrial pacemaker (WAP) (Fig. 3.12) is an atrial rhythm with multiple P-wave morphologies (three or more), often occurring in a repetitive pattern at a rate of less than 100 bpm. The pattern may be dependent on autonomic tone and the respiratory phase (with competing

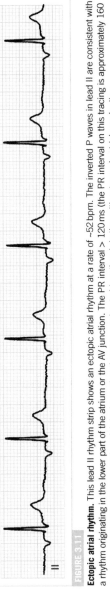

FIGURE 3.11

Ectopic atrial rhythm. This lead II rhythm strip shows an ectopic atrial rhythm at a rate of ~52 bpm. The inverted P waves in lead II are consistent with a rhythm originating in the lower part of the atrium or the AV junction. The PR interval on this tracing is approximately 160 msec) is consistent with an ectopic atrial rhythm rather than an accelerated junctional rhythm with retrograde atrial conduction.

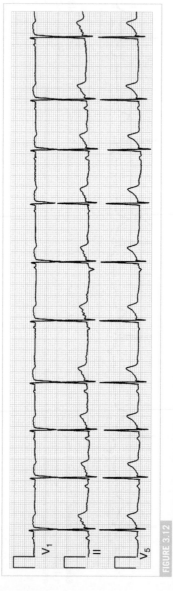

Wandering atrial pacemaker. This lead V_1, II, and V_5 rhythm strip shows wandering atrial pacemaker. There is an underlying sinus rhythm (first 4 beats, 8th and 9th beats) that slows and competes with an atrial rhythm arising from a nearby pacemaker (5th through 7th and 10th beats) from the low right atrium resulting in inverted P waves in lead II in a phasic manner. The ST-T fractionation is of uncertain significance.

activation from the sinus node, AV node, and other areas in the atria). WAP is distinguished from multifocal atrial tachycardia (MAT) on the basis of rate (WAP <100 bpm, MAT ≥100 bpm) and the repetitive nature of the changing P-wave morphology. It is generally due to multiple competing atrial pacemakers but may be related to competition between SA and AV nodal automaticity. It can be considered to be a different rhythm from multifocal atrial rhythm (Fig. 3.13), which is not a phasic rhythm and is unassociated with respiration.

WAP may be due to high vagal tone (it can occur in sinus node dysfunction). WAP tends to be stable, rather than progressive.

WAP is not typically associated with symptoms or hemodynamic compromise.

No therapy is indicated.

JUNCTIONAL RHYTHM

Junctional rhythm is a regular narrow QRS complex rhythm unless bundle branch block (BBB) is present. P waves may be absent, or retrograde P waves (inverted in leads II, III, and aVF) either precede the QRS with a PR of less than 0.12 seconds or follow the QRS complex. The junctional rate is usually 40 to 60 bpm. It can serve as an escape rhythm (Fig. 3.14) in cases of SB or AV block. Holter monitoring may be useful to document the presence of sinus node dysfunction and the cause of any symptoms that might result from the rhythm. Junctional rhythm can be an accelerated rhythm (Fig. 3.15), with its usual rate of 40 to 60 bpm being exceeded, particularly with adrenergic stimuli. Because the atrial and QRS rhythms are independent, AV dissociation will be present; capture beats will document the absence of AV block as the cause of the AV dissociation.

Junctional rhythm can be due to hypokalemia, MI (usually inferior), cardiac surgery, digitalis toxicity (rare today), sinus node dysfunction, or after ablation for AV node reentrant tachycardia. It can be caused by necessary medications (e.g., β-adrenergic blockers, verapamil, digitalis, sotalol, amiodarone). It can also be seen as part of tachy-brady syndrome. Junctional rhythm usually is associated with a benign course, but it can cause symptoms due to AV dyssynchrony (pseudo "pacemaker syndrome").

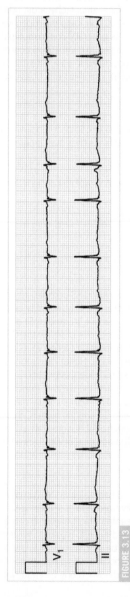

FIGURE 3.13

Multifocal atrial rhythm (or chaotic atrial mechanism). This rhythm strip of leads V$_1$ and II shows an atrial bradycardia with multiple (>3) P-wave morphologies arising from separate atrial foci. The atrial rate of less than 100 bpm and the varying P-P and PR intervals are all consistent with this rhythm diagnosis. This rhythm is distinguished from WAP by its lack of reproducibility or phasic nature. It is distinguished from MAT by its rate being less than 100 bpm.

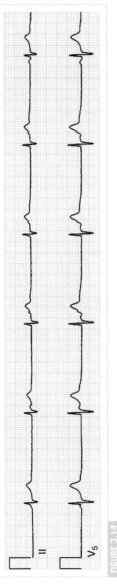

FIGURE 3.14

Junctional escape rhythm. This lead II and V$_5$ rhythm strip shows a regular narrow QRS complex rhythm (rate ~36 bpm). The first 2 QRS complexes compete with sinus P waves and then with further slowing of the sinus rate with junctional escape, retrograde atrial P waves are seen in the ST segments. Then on the final beat, the sinus P wave is faster and precedes the junctional escape complex.

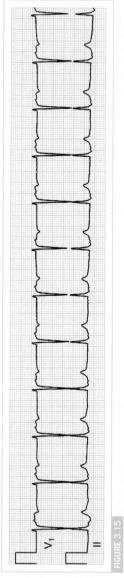

FIGURE 3.15

Accelerated junctional rhythm. This lead V₁ and II rhythm strip shows a narrow QRS complex rhythm (rate ~70 bpm) with no visible discrete preceding P waves and retrograde P waves evident in the ST segment, consistent with a junctional rhythm. However, since the rate exceeds that of normal junctional escape rhythms (40 bpm), this rhythm is considered an accelerated junctional rhythm.

Clinical Symptoms and Presentation

Junctional rhythm can cause symptoms due to bradycardia and/ or loss of AV synchrony. These symptoms (which can be vague and easily missed) include lightheadedness, palpitations, effort intolerance, chest heaviness, neck tightness or pounding, shortness of breath, and weakness.

Approach to Management

Treatment of the junctional rhythm is usually not necessary, but treatment of the underlying problem (e.g., underlying sinus or atrial bradycardia) may be needed. Discontinuation of medications that may slow the sinus rate may allow the atrial rate to increase and override a slower junctional rhythm ("capture"). Permanent pacemaker implantation can alleviate symptomatic junctional rhythm associated with sinus node dysfunction. For chronic symptomatic junctional rhythm not associated with sinus node dysfunction, ablation of the junctional focus may be considered but with risk of creating AV block (Table 3.6).

TABLE 3.6

JUNCTIONAL RHYTHM THERAPY AND SPECIFIC CLINICAL PRESENTATIONS

Setting	Therapy
Asymptomatic	• If heart rate is persistently < 40 bpm but responds to autonomic input (e.g., increased catecholamines with exercise), no therapy is required.
	• Assess the clinical situation that is responsible and consider if it needs to be treated.
	○ It may be an indication of high vagal tone that is common in healthy, young patients (especially if they are athletic).
	• May be difficult to assess symptoms in the elderly with this problem.
Symptomatic	• Discontinue potentially offending drugs (e.g., digoxin).
	• Theophylline and anticholinergics may be effective to increase sinus rate and override the slower junctional rhythm.
	• If the heart rate is slow, junctional rhythm may be an indication of sinus node dysfunction, and if symptomatic, the patient may need a permanent dual-chamber pacemaker.
	• Accelerated junctional rhythm (rate: 70-100 bpm) unrelated to drug toxicity or electrolyte problems:
	○ First line is β-adrenergic blocker.
	○ Second line is calcium channel blocker.
	• For chronic, symptomatic junctional rhythm, ablation of the focus of origin of the rhythm may be effective, although associated with risk for AV block.

Continued on following page

TABLE 3.6

JUNCTIONAL RHYTHM THERAPY AND SPECIFIC CLINICAL PRESENTATIONS (Continued)

Setting	Therapy
MI	• No therapy unless patient is hypotensive or symptomatic from the AV dyssynchrony or slow rate.
	• If symptomatic and hemodynamically compromised, consider atropine or atrial pacing just above junctional rate.
	• Usually transient.
	• Should not be confused with AV dissociation due to AV block.
Preoperative	• If symptomatic, first line is atropine, and second line is isoproterenol (if no coronary artery disease [CAD]); atrial pacing only if persistent and hemodynamically detrimental.
	• If asymptomatic, not a reason to delay or cancel surgery.
	• Common in young people and of no clinical significance.
	• Intubation and induction of anesthesia often enhance vagal tone and can worsen junctional rhythm and bradycardia (therapy: atropine or nothing; transcutaneous pacing may be used as a temporary measure if absolutely necessary).
Postoperative	• Stop offending drug (e.g., digoxin, β-adrenergic blocker, calcium channel blocker) if feasible.
	• Postoperative junctional rhythm tends to be accelerated and self-limited.

ACCELERATED IDIOVENTRICULAR RHYTHM

Description

Accelerated idioventricular rhythm (AIVR) (Fig. 3.16) is an automatic rhythm, independent of the sinus node, that originates in the ventricle and competes with sinus rhythm. AIVR is a regular rhythm with a wide QRS complex (>0.12 seconds). P waves may be absent, retrograde (following the QRS complex and negative in ECG leads II, III, and aVF), or independent of them (AV dissociation). Fusion complexes in which the ventricles are depolarized by both the sinus and ventricular impulses often occur. The ventricular rate is generally between 70 and 100 bpm (near the sinus rate) but should not be considered to be "slow VT." AIVR is distinguished from VT by its slower rate (<100 bpm). In contrast to AIVR, a ventricular escape rhythm can have a similar morphology, but its rates are 20 to 40 bpm.

Associated Conditions

AIVR is a generally benign rhythm. It is commonly seen during MI, occurring in 30% of inferior MIs and 5% of anterior MIs; it may or may not represent a reperfusion injury rhythm. Other conditions in which AIVR is observed include myocardial ischemia, digoxin toxicity, hypokalemia,

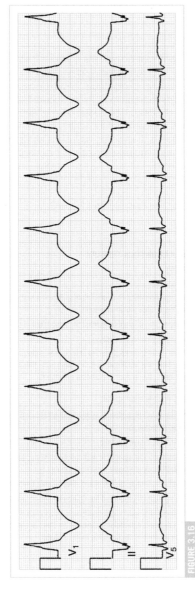

FIGURE 3.16

Accelerated idioventricular rhythm. This lead V₁, II, and V₅ rhythm strip shows a regular wide QRS complex rhythm (rate of ~62 bpm), representing accelerated ventricular rhythm. There appear to be retrograde P waves evident in the ST segments in lead II. The QRS is extremely wide and the QT very prolonged. The differential diagnosis includes ischemia, infarction, and electrolyte/metabolic abnormality.

and cardiac surgery, but these are not causative factors. AIVR may occasionally be seen in normal individuals and is generally an incidental finding.

Clinical Symptoms and Presentation

Patients are generally asymptomatic, and the rhythm is discovered only incidentally. Rarely, the loss of AV synchrony may produce a symptomatic reduction in cardiac output (lightheadedness, breathlessness), especially in patients with diastolic dysfunction (e.g., left ventricular hypertrophy [LVH]). AIVR is usually self-limited. The classic onset of AIVR is with mild slowing of sinus rate with emergence of the ventricular rhythm via fusion complexes; its classic offset is the reverse, via fusions with a mild increase in sinus rate. AIVR may also terminate abruptly. It is a benign rhythm and does not progress to VT or VF.

Approach to Management

None is indicated unless symptomatic (rare) (Table 3.7).

TABLE 3.7

ACCELERATED IDIOVENTRICULAR RHYTHM THERAPY

Setting	Therapy
Asymptomatic	• No therapy.
	• Exclude electrolyte abnormalities (e.g., hypokalemia) and digoxin toxicity, although these are rarely present.
Symptoms of low cardiac output, especially if chronic (rare) or recurrent	• Atropine may be used to increase the sinus rate and suppress the AIVR.
	• It cannot be used chronically.
	• Atrial (or AV sequential) pacing may be helpful because loss of AV synchrony and atrial contribution to ventricular filling ("atrial kick") may reduce cardiac output and produce symptoms.
	• It is virtually never needed.
MI	• No therapy usually required unless symptomatic (discussed previously).
	• Avoid isoproterenol.
Preoperative	• No therapy if asymptomatic.
	• If sustained and associated with hypotension, may need atropine, isoproterenol, or even AV sequential pacing.
	• Careful monitoring of rhythm and hemodynamic function is indicated.
Postoperative	• If persistent and sustained but stable rate and no symptoms, no therapy is indicated.
	• May be due to catecholamine excess, but consider that ischemia may have occurred in the operating room (unlikely).

Automaticity

The rate at which the sinus node discharges usually is faster than other latent or subsidiary automatic cardiac pacemakers. Subsidiary pacemakers can become dominant in the settings of acidosis, ischemia, sympathetic stimulation, and use of certain drugs. Normal automaticity can be suppressed by pacing but generally resumes after pacing stops.

Abnormal automaticity can be due to cell damage and abnormal depolarization. The partial depolarization and failure to reach or maintain the normal maximum diastolic potential may induce automatic discharge. Examples include accelerated junctional rhythm (i.e., nonparoxysmal junctional tachycardia), accelerated ventricular rhythms, certain atrial tachycardias, some ventricular tachycardias (VTs) in patients without structural heart disease, exercise-induced VT, and VT during the first several hours of acute myocardial infarction (MI).

Triggered Activity

Triggered activity is initiated by afterdepolarizations. If they occur before full repolarization, they are called early afterdepolarizations (EADs); if they occur after completion of repolarization, they are called delayed afterdepolarizations (DADs).

Early Afterdepolarizations

Occurring during phase 2 or 3 of the action potential, EADs are thought to be responsible for VTs associated with prolonged repolarization, such as long QT syndromes (acquired or congenital) and torsades de pointes (TdP) VT. Slower rates, including pauses after extrasystoles, augment EADs.

Delayed Afterdepolarizations

Occurring during phase 4, DADs have been recorded in Purkinje fibers and atrial and ventricular muscle. Faster rates may augment DADs. This type of triggered activity may underlie rhythms, such as those due to digitalis toxicity or catecholamine excess, acidosis, MI, and certain VTs (e.g., catecholaminergic polymorphic VT).

Reentry

Conduction delay or block can facilitate the development of reentry, the most common mechanism responsible for tachycardias.

Reentry requires the following:

- Alternate or separate pathways of conduction defined by anatomic barriers (e.g., myocardial scar, atrioventricular [AV] node, or an accessory pathway) or functional properties—contiguous fibers with different electrophysiologic properties (e.g., local differences in refractoriness, excitability, or anisotropic intercellular resistances)
- An area of unidirectional block in one pathway
- An area of conduction in the alternate pathway that is slow enough for the propagating and returning impulse to meet and excite tissue proximal to the block that has since recovered

Reentry is thought to be the mechanism underlying most pathologic tachycardias, including atrial flutter, AV nodal reentry, AV reentry involving accessory pathways (including Wolff-Parkinson-White [WPW] syndrome), and most VTs associated with ischemic heart disease and previous MI. Disordered reentry may cause atrial fibrillation or be passive due to triggered activity from the pulmonary veins.

NARROW QRS COMPLEX TACHYCARDIA

A narrow QRS complex tachycardia (QRS duration < 120 ms and rate > 100 bpm) indicates a supraventricular origin with ventricular activation occurring via the fast-conducting His-Purkinje system. The acute management of a regular narrow QRS complex tachycardia will depend on the hemodynamic state of the patient. In most but certainly not all instances the patient remains hemodynamically stable even if the rhythm is rapid; this is especially the case if the patient is younger and otherwise healthy; however, AV nodal and AV reentry tachycardias (Fig. 4.1) can cause severe symptoms of presyncope and frank syncope at any rate because of the retrograde atrial depolarization and atrial contraction against closed AV valves; this in turn produces not only loss of stroke volume but also, via atrial stretch receptor activation, reflex systemic hypotension, which can be refractory.

If the patient is stable, the first thing to try is a Valsalva maneuver (bearing down with closed mouth) or carotid sinus massage (if there is no carotid bruit or known vascular disease). If this is ineffective, it should be repeated with the patient in the Trendelenburg position or in combination. If this is ineffective, then adenosine between 6 mg or escalating doses of 12 mg or 18 mg given as an intravenous (IV) bolus followed by a saline "chaser" should be used; this will be expected to either terminate the tachycardia if it is dependent on the AV node for its maintenance or be diagnostic for what the atrial rhythm is during tachycardia, if the tachycardia is AV node independent. For example, sometimes a narrow QRS complex tachycardia, thought to be AV node or AV reentry, in fact turns out to be atrial flutter; adenosine, by producing AV block, thus allowing the atrial rhythm to be visible, will be diagnostic.

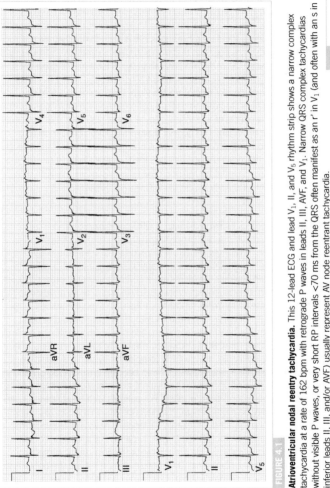

FIGURE 4.1

Atrioventricular nodal reentry tachycardia. This 12-lead ECG and lead V_1, II, and V_5 rhythm strip shows a narrow complex tachycardia at a rate of 162 bpm with retrograde P waves in leads II, III, AVF, and V_1. Narrow QRS complex tachycardias without visible P waves, or very short RP intervals <70 ms from the QRS often manifest as an r′ in V_1 (and often with an s in inferior leads II, III, and/or AVF) usually represent AV node reentrant tachycardia.

In some instances, adenosine is ineffective (sometimes due to the presence of theophylline or high levels of caffeine). If this is the case, a second option would be to give IV verapamil 5 to 15 mg; it is important to know that verapamil should *not* be given to the patient with a wide QRS complex tachycardia. If neither of these therapies is effective, a DC shock given with anesthesia may be effective; however, it should be recognized that adenosine and verapamil are indeed highly effective in terminating almost all supraventricular tachycardias (SVTs) and that if they do not work it is entirely possible that that the tachycardia is not an SVT but might be sinus tachycardia. IV digoxin is rarely given to terminate narrow QRS complex tachycardias because its action is not that of a direct AV nodal blocker but produces AV block through vagal mechanisms. Adenosine should not be given to heart transplant patients because prolonged asystole may follow; the effects of adenosine can be longer lasting in these patients than would be expected. The normal duration of action of adenosine is 10 to 20 seconds. Whereas theophylline and caffeine diminish the effects of adenosine, dipyridamole accentuates them. Adenosine can cause bronchospasm and atrial fibrillation; if the latter occurs in a patient with WPW syndrome, the atrial fibrillation can be potentially lethal.

WIDE QRS COMPLEX TACHYCARDIA

A regular wide QRS tachycardia (i.e., a QRS complex with a duration > 120 ms and a rate exceeding 100 bpm) is in most cases VT (Fig. 4.2), even in younger people. It is important to make the diagnosis before considering treatment, but in many instances it is not possible to know for certain whether the tachycardia is ventricular or supraventricular with aberration, bundle branch block (BBB) in origin, or an antidromic tachycardia caused by WPW syndrome. EP study is recommended if the diagnosis is not certain. In patients with underlying structural heart disease, MI, and/or heart failure, the chance of a wide complex tachycardia being VT is greater than 90%. However, even if the patient appears to be hemodynamically stable, a wide QRS complex tachycardia is not to be taken lightly because patients with VT can become unstable rapidly and may go on to develop ventricular fibrillation; this is particularly true if there is underlying structural heart disease. For patients with no structural heart disease, VT may be more benign, but nevertheless, in most cases urgent treatment will be required. Idiopathic VT tends to have one of two forms: left bundle branch block (LBBB) (Fig. 4.3) pattern with inferior frontal plane QRS axis or right bundle branch block (RBBB) (Fig. 4.4) pattern with superior frontal plane axis. These two tachycardias are the only VTs in which verapamil or β-adrenergic blockade may be useful; however, unless the diagnosis is known with certainty, neither β-adrenergic blockade nor verapamil are appropriate treatments.

To make the correct diagnosis of VT versus SVT with aberration, it is important to recognize that no criterion is 100% accurate to determine or distinguish SVT from VT. Various electrocardiographic criteria have

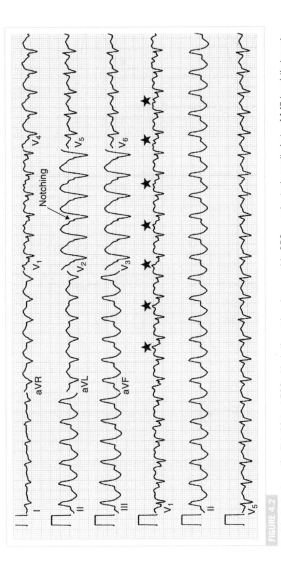

FIGURE 4.2

Ventricular tachycardia. This 12-lead ECG with rhythm strips shows a wide QRS complex tachycardia (rate of 143 bpm) that meets morphology criteria for ventricular tachycardia. It has LBBB-type morphology with notching on the downstroke of the QRS in V_2 and R<S in V_5 and V_6. There is also VA dissociation with P waves shown under the stars. The QRS width should be determined by viewing all leads, as it may appear to be narrow on certain leads or on rhythm strips. Here V_1 and V_5 look narrow, but inspection of other leads clearly has a wide QRS.

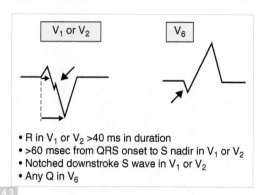

Morphology criteria for left bundle branch block pattern wide complex tachycardia.
(Adapted from Kindwall KE, Brown J, Josephson ME. Electrocardiographic criteria for ventricular tachycardia in wide complex left bundle branch block morphology tachycardias. Am J Cardiol 1988;61:1279–1283.)

FIGURE 4.3

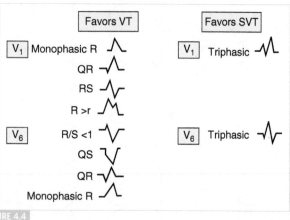

FIGURE 4.4

Morphology criteria for right bundle branch block pattern wide complex tachycardia.
(Adapted from Wellens HJJ, Bar FWHM, Lie KI. The value of the electrocardiogram in the differential diagnosis of a tachycardia with a widened QRS complex. Am J Med 1978;64:27–33.)

been applied, but the most potent predictor is the relationship between the P waves and the QRS complexes. If there is AV dissociation (e.g., more QRS complexes than P waves), then the rhythm is most likely VT. Other criteria have been used, including the QRS width and the frontal plane axis. The wider the QRS complex, the more likely the rhythm is VT;

however, because QRS duration is also related to left ventricle (LV) size and left ventricular ejection fraction (LVEF) (where it reflects prognosis), the rhythm may be supraventricular in origin. Unusual frontal plane axes are more consistent with VT. It is extremely important to recognize that if the tachycardia has similar QRS complex morphology to that seen during sinus rhythm, there is a high likelihood that it is a SVT, but even this criterion is not absolute. If the sinus-stimulated QRS complex is wide but is different from the observed wide QRS complex tachycardia, VT is likely. Other diagnostic clues include patient age and the presence of heart disease.

VTs are defined as three or more consecutive ventricular beats at rates exceeding 100 per minute. Nonsustained VT refers to a VT less than 30 seconds in duration; sustained VT has a more than 30-second duration, is immediately hemodynamically destabilizing, or requires an intervention (e.g., cardioversion) for termination. VTs are further described as being monomorphic or polymorphic and, if polymorphic and associated with a long QT interval, especially at tachycardia initiation, are termed "TdP" VT. Bursts of monomorphic VT can accelerate ("warm-up phenomenon") and thus may not be regular in rate. Hemodynamic tolerance of a tachycardia does not indicate its origin. Decompensation depends on tachycardia rate, on AV relationships (dissociation or association, as in 1:1 ventriculoatrial conduction), medications, and presence or absence of structural heart disease.

Other criteria that can help to determine whether the tachycardia is ventricular or supraventricular are the presence or absence of capture or fusion beats (Fig. 4.5), beat to beat QRS variation, and positive or negative concordance across the precordial leads. Physical findings that can be helpful to diagnose VT include a variable S_1, cannon A waves seen in the neck distinct from the pulse, or beat by beat fluctuations in blood pressure because these findings reflect AV dissociation and thus VT. The "Brugada" criteria are a four-step algorithm used to distinguish VT from SVT (Fig. 4.6). In step 1, if there is no RS in any precordial lead, VT is diagnosed. In step 2, if the onset of the R to the nadir of the S in any of the precordial leads is greater than 100 ms, then VT is diagnosed. In step 3, if AV dissociation is seen, VT is diagnosed. In step 4, if morphology criteria for VT are met in V_1 or V_2 and V_5 or V_6, VT is diagnosed. Otherwise, the diagnosis is SVT. Morphology criteria for LBBB morphology tachycardias (negative QRS in V_1) include: V_1 or V_2 width of R greater than 40 ms, greater than 60 ms from onset of QRS to nadir of S, or notch on the downstroke; V_5 or V_6 any Q wave. Morphology criteria for RBBB morphology, tachycardias (positive QRS in V_1) include: V_1 or V_2 R greater than r', monophasic R, QR, or RS; V_5 or V_6 R:S ratio less than 1, QS, QR, or monophasic R. Brugada criteria will not distinguish VT from antidromic SVT or SVT with antiarrhythmic drug-slowing IV conduction, unless AV dissociation is evident. The Vereckei algorithm is another approach to distinguish SVT from VT. It is based on the QRS complex morphology in aVR. An initial R wave, an initial R or Q wave greater than 40 ms, and a notch on the descending limb at the onset of a predominantly negative QRS imply VT.

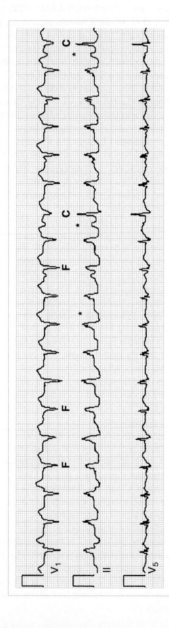

FIGURE 4.5

Fusion and capture beats. Fusion beats (F) are conducted supraventricular impulses that depolarize the ventricle coincident with ventricular depolarization from the ventricular tachycardia (VT). These may occur slightly early and the QRS is usually intermediate in width. Fusion beats are not pathognomonic for VT. For example, fusion can occur with a premature ventricular contraction during supraventricular tachycardia with bundle branch block aberrancy. Capture beats (C) represent conduction of a supraventricular impulse to the ventricle and depolarization before it is depolarized by the VT circuit. Capture beats are narrow complex beats with a shorter coupling interval than the tachycardia cycle length. Capture beats indicate the wide complex tachycardia is VT. Asterisks (*) indicate sinus rhythm P waves.

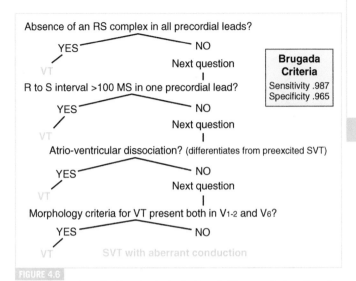

Absence of an RS complex in all precordial leads?

YES ——— NO

VT

Next question

R to S interval >100 MS in one precordial lead?

YES ——— NO

VT

Next question

Atrio-ventricular dissociation? (differentiates from preexcited SVT)

YES ——— NO

VT

Next question

Morphology criteria for VT present both in V1-2 and V6?

YES ——— NO

VT

SVT with aberrant conduction

Brugada Criteria
Sensitivity .987
Specificity .965

FIGURE 4.6

Wide complex tachycardia—Brugada criteria algorithm. *SVT,* Supraventricular tachycardia; *VT,* ventricular tachycardia. *(Adapted from Brugada P, Brugada J, Mont L, et al. A new approach to the differential diagnosis of a regular tachycardia with a wide QRS complex. Circulation 1991;83:1649–1659.)*

The approach to the patient with wide QRS complex tachycardia is to first determine hemodynamic stability. Then, determine whether it is VT. If the assessment cannot be made with any degree of certainty, treat as VT. Verapamil should not be administered. If the tachycardia is tolerated, carotid massage or IV adenosine is a possible diagnostic and therapeutic strategy, although the former is usually unproductive and the latter can cause significant hypotension with reflex increase in tachycardia rate (Fig. 4.7).

If the patient is hemodynamically stable, IV antiarrhythmic drugs could be tried: procainamide, 10 to 15 mg per kilogram over 30 to 60 minutes; lidocaine, 1.0 to 1.5 mg/kg as an initial bolus, reduced by half if elderly or heart failure or liver dysfunction present; or preferably, amiodarone, 150 mg over 10 minutes (or even slower). For individuals who have abnormal LVEFs (<40%), amiodarone is preferred over lidocaine. For patients with LVEFs greater than 40%, amiodarone or procainamide are the drugs of first choice, followed by lidocaine. If the rhythm is refractory, synchronized electrical (DC) cardioversion should be performed. If the tachycardia recurs, an antiarrhythmic drug can then be given with or without subsequent repeat DC cardioversion, or a temporary pacemaker wire can be placed in an attempt to pace-terminate (by overdrive techniques) the tachycardia. If the patient is unstable and hemodynamically compromised, a biphasic DC electrical shock (100 to 360 joules [J]) is recommended.

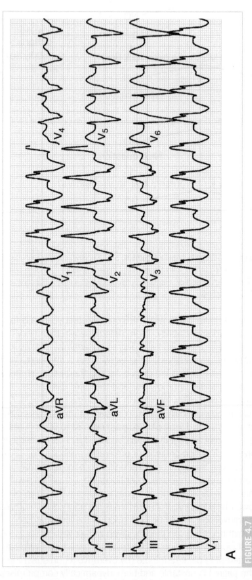

FIGURE 4.7

RBBB morphology ventricular tachycardia. A) This 12-lead ECG shows a wide complex tachycardia with RBBB morphology in V₁. There is an RS in V₄–V₆ (level 1 of the criteria). R to S interval is >100 ms in V₃ and V₄ (level 2), making a diagnosis of ventricular tachycardia. Incidentally, there is no evident AV dissociation (level 3), but the tachycardia also meets morphology criteria for RBBB morphology ventricular tachycardia in V₁ and V₂, as well as V₅ and V₆ (level 4; see Figure 4.5).

A

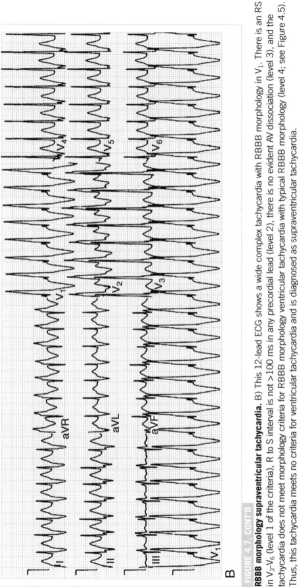

FIGURE 4.7. CONT'D

RBBB morphology supraventricular tachycardia. B) This 12-lead ECG shows a wide complex tachycardia with RBBB morphology in V_1. There is an RS in V_3–V_6 (level 1 of the criteria), R to S interval is not >100 ms in any precordial lead (level 2), there is no evident AV dissociation (level 3), and the tachycardia does not meet morphology criteria for RBBB morphology ventricular tachycardia with typical RBBB morphology (level 4; see Figure 4.5). Thus, this tachycardia meets no criteria for ventricular tachycardia and is diagnosed as supraventricular tachycardia.

After these maneuvers the patient will need to be admitted to the hospital and evaluated for the potential causes for the rhythm disturbance. EP study may be needed to secure a diagnosis and catheter ablation to treat the patient. In some patients with VT, implantable cardioverter defibrillators (ICDs) are already in place; the tachycardia can be below or above the programmed ICD rate cut-off. If the VT rate is above the rate cut-off and the patient is receiving appropriate shocks, start antiarrhythmic drugs. IV amiodarone is usually recommended. If the tachycardias are below the programmed detection criteria of the ICD, the device will not activate and treating the tachycardia and ICD reprogramming is necessary. If the tachycardia rate is sufficiently slow, antitachycardia pacing can be programmed; in this instance, it is probably best to avoid the use of rate-slowing drugs, due to the possibility of the tachycardia not being detected at all and the patient therefore not receiving the desired therapy. In these cases it may be useful to consider using an antiarrhythmic drug other than amiodarone, such as sotalol (if the LVEF greater than 35%) or mexiletine; these do not slow the tachycardia as much. The rationale for slowing the rate of the tachycardia is to avoid severe presyncope or syncope prior to ICD therapy delivery. If there are recurrent episodes despite medications, catheter ablation is recommended.

SUPRAVENTRICULAR TACHYCARDIA

Supraventricular tachycardia (SVT) is a rhythm disturbance with a rate greater than 100 that requires tissue from above the His-Purkinje system to perpetuate. SVT can be regular (e.g., atrioventricular [AV] node reentry), irregular (e.g., atrial flutter [AFL] with variable AV conduction), or irregularly irregular (e.g., multifocal atrial tachycardia [MAT], atrial fibrillation [AF]). SVT can be associated with a narrow QRS complex, a wide QRS complex, or both. When it is associated with a wide QRS complex, preexisting bundle branch block (BBB), tachycardia-dependent (phase 3) BBB (aberrancy), or an accessory pathway will be present. Intermittently wide QRS complexes caused by the Ashman phenomenon are commonly seen in AF and usually have a right bundle branch block (RBBB) pattern due to the long refractoriness of the right bundle branch that is present after long–short RR cycles. There can be a one-to-one atrial to ventricular relationship (such as is commonly seen in AV node reentry tachycardia or AV reentry tachycardia) or a two-to-one or greater relationship (commonly seen in AFL or atrial tachycardia [AT]). SVTs can be sustained, recurrent, and intermittent and/or paroxysmal.

The differential diagnosis for SVT includes sinus tachycardia (appropriate and inappropriate), AF, AFL, AV node reentry tachycardia, AV reentry tachycardia, AT (including multifocal), accelerated junctional tachycardia (JT) (junctional ectopic tachycardia), and sinoatrial (SA) reentry tachycardia. It is important to recognize the type of tachycardia because the need for and type of acute and chronic treatment vary depending on the specific rhythm (Algorithm 5.1).

Most SVTs are not life-threatening, but they can cause potential serious hemodynamic compromise, including presyncope and syncope, tachycardia-induced cardiomyopathy, congestive heart failure (CHF), and angina; palpitations and other rather nonspecific symptoms can have significant impact on quality of life. The aggressiveness of acute and long-term therapy depends on the perceived seriousness of the problem for the patient, based mainly on hemodynamic response to the arrhythmia. Before treatment, a precise rhythm diagnosis should be actively sought.

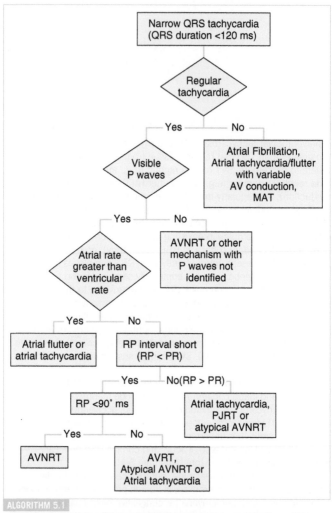

ALGORITHM 5.1

Differential diagnosis for adult narrow QRS tachycardia. Patients with JT may mimic the pattern of slow-fast AVNRT and may show AV dissociation and/or marked irregularity in the junctional rate. *RP refers to the interval from the onset of surface QRS to the onset of visible P wave (note that the 90-ms interval is defined from the surface ECG as opposed to the 70-ms ventriculoatrial interval that is used for intracardiac diagnosis. *AV,* Atrioventricular; *AVNRT,* atrioventricular nodal reentrant tachycardia; *AVRT,* atrioventricular reentrant tachycardia; *MAT,* multifocal atrial tachycardia; *PJRT,* permanent junctional reciprocating tachycardia. (*Reproduced with permission from Page RL et al. 2015 ACC/AHA/HRS Guideline for the Management of Adult Patients With Supraventricular Tachycardia. JACC 2016;67(13):e27-e115.*)

Description (Algorithm 5.2A and B**)**

AT (Fig. 5.1) is a less common type of SVT, responsible for 5% to 10% of cases of SVT. AT is suspected when there is a narrow QRS complex SVT with a long RP interval with variable coupling of the QRS to P wave interval or evidence for SVT with AV block. A long RP tachycardia can also occur

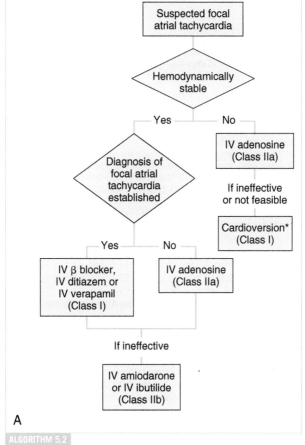

A

ALGORITHM 5.2

(A) Acute treatment of suspected focal atrial tachycardia. *For rhythms that break or recur spontaneously, synchronized cardioversion is not appropriate.

Continued on following page

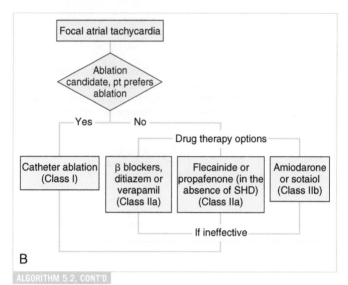

ALGORITHM 5.2, CONT'D

(B) Ongoing management of focal atrial tachycardia. *IV,* Intravenous; *Pt,* patient; *SHD,* structural heart disease (including ischemic heart disease). *(Reproduced with permission from Page RL et al. 2015 ACC/AHA/HRS Guideline for the Management of Adult Patients With Supraventricular Tachycardia. JACC 2016;67(13):e27-e115.)*

in an atrioventricular reentrant tachycardia (AVRT) mediated by a slow or decrementally conducting accessory pathway, or atypical atrioventricular nodal reentrant tachycardia (AVNRT).

P-wave morphology differs from sinus but can help to predict the origin of the tachycardia. Focal AT can be difficult to distinguish from atrial reentrant tachycardia (ART) on the surface ECG, and an electrophysiology (EP) study may be necessary to distinguish the two.

Several mechanisms can be responsible for AT; it can be difficult to differentiate one mechanism from the others. They can be macroreentrant or of focal origin.

Focal ATs may be triggered by autonomic activity (sympathetic activation), increased automaticity, or triggered automaticity or may be microreentrant. Focal tachycardias may be characterized by their location (e.g., sinus nodal or ectopic to the sinus node). Automatic AT (AAT) is a focal AT that is characterized by a gradual onset (speeding up, warm-up) and gradual offset (slowing), in contrast with ARTs that may have sudden onset after a premature beat, and sudden offset. Triggered ATs may have sudden onset and offset. If they are catecholamine dependent, they may occur with exercise.

Specific pulmonary vein ectopic-triggered tachycardias may be related to effects from the parasympathetic and sympathetic nervous system and from ganglionated plexuses to initiate AF.

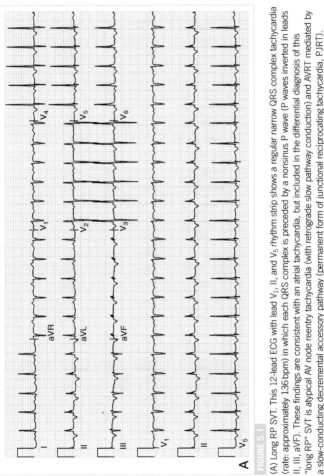

FIGURE 5.1

(A) Long RP SVT. This 12-lead ECG with lead V₁, II, and V₅ rhythm strip shows a regular narrow QRS complex tachycardia (rate: approximately 136bpm) in which each QRS complex is preceded by a nonsinus P wave (P waves inverted in leads II, III, and aVF). These findings are consistent with an atrial tachycardia, but included in the differential diagnosis of this "long RP" SVT is atypical AV node reentry tachycardia (with retrograde slow pathway conduction) and AVRT mediated by a slow-conducting decremental accessory pathway (permanent form of junctional reciprocating tachycardia, PJRT).

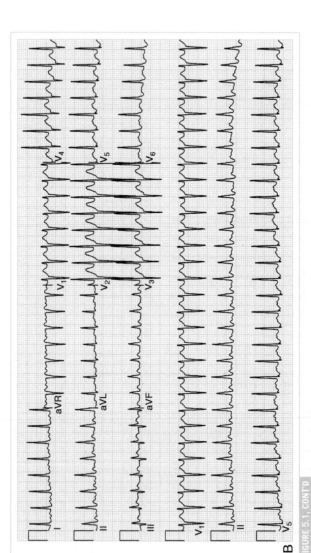

FIGURE 5.1, CONT'D

(B) AT. This ECG tracing shows an AT at a rate of approximately 185 bpm. The P waves are seen just after the QRS and are positive in leads II, III, and aVF, indicating a high-to-low activation pattern.

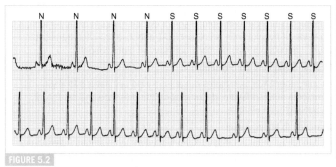

FIGURE 5.2

Sinoatrial node reentrant tachycardia. This rhythm strip shows sudden onset and offset of a regular narrow complex tachycardia with beats preceded by a P wave that is the same as that during sinus rhythm. The sudden onset and termination of this rhythm is not a feature of sinus tachycardia but is very consistent with SART (sinus P waves, sudden onset, and termination of tachycardia).

Whatever the mechanism of a focal AT, the approach to treatment is similar. If the tachycardia is focal, it can be ablated. Given the difficulty in mechanism differentiation, there is no specific approach to medical therapy should ablation not be first line for a specific patient and also for treatment in the acute phase of the tachycardia.

A unique and very rare form of AT is known as sinoatrial node reentrant tachycardia (SART) (Fig. 5.2). SART appears because of a reentry circuit involving the SA node. The P-wave morphology is the same as or similar to the sinus P wave. This tachycardia tends to be nonsustained and somewhat irregular with a relatively normal PR interval and a consistent P-wave morphology. The tachycardia can respond to autonomic maneuvers, as well as drugs, in particular verapamil, adenosine, digoxin, and less commonly β-adrenergic blockers and amiodarone. SART can be ablated; the ablation point may be in the inferior portion of the SA node as it exits into the crista terminalis.

Reentrant ATs may be due to "macro" reentry around structural or functional barriers in the right and/or left atria, or due to microreentrant circuits. AV block can be present during AT and may result in variable or 2:1 AV conduction. It is useful to look for this because it helps to differentiate this tachycardia from AVNRT and AVRT.

Associated Conditions

Although AT may occur in normal, healthy adults, it can be associated with acute myocardial infarction (MI), acute alcohol intoxication, exacerbation of chronic obstructive pulmonary disease (COPD), electrolyte abnormalities, and digoxin toxicity (especially if accompanied by AV block); this last one is now uncommon given the doses of digoxin in current use. AT due to digoxin can occur with normal serum digoxin levels in older persons, especially if hypokalemia is present. AAT episodes are often transient in young patients but may be more persistent in older patients.

Clinical Symptoms and Presentation

As with other SVTs, symptoms range from mild palpitations to angina or symptoms of heart failure, depending on the presence and severity of underlying heart disease.

Approach to Management

AT can occur as an isolated episode related to, for example, infection and acute alcohol ingestion and does not necessarily require chronic therapy, or it may be frequent and/or recurrent, causing disabling symptoms so that long-term treatment is necessary. Chronic persistent AT can cause tachycardia-induced cardiomyopathy, a reversible form of systolic heart failure caused by chronic rapid heart rates and similar symptoms to other SVTs. Acute therapy generally consists of treating any precipitating factors and terminating with antiarrhythmic drugs. Prevention of recurrences over the long term is typically addressed with drugs or catheter ablation (success rate: 50% to 80%). Asymptomatic or minimally symptomatic patients can usually be managed as outpatients unless tachy-brady syndrome is suspected. If the P wave can be seen and is similar to that in sinus rhythm, SART could be present; the patient may respond acutely to carotid massage, adenosine, a β-adrenergic blocker, calcium channel blocker, or digoxin (Table 5.1).

Automatic Atrial Tachycardia

Description

AAT is a rare type of SVT, responsible for less than 2% to 5% of cases. P-wave morphology differs from sinus but can help to predict the origin of the tachycardia. AAT can be difficult to distinguish from ART on the surface ECG, and an EP study may be necessary to distinguish the two. AAT is characterized by a gradual onset (speeding up) and offset (slowing), in contrast with reentrant tachycardias that may have sudden onset after a premature beat and sudden offset. AV block can be present during AAT and may result in variable or 2:1 AV conduction.

Associated Conditions

Although AAT may occur in normal, healthy adults, it is more often associated with acute MI, acute alcohol intoxication, exacerbation of COPD, electrolyte abnormalities, and digoxin toxicity (especially if accompanied by AV block); this last one is now uncommon given the lower doses of digoxin in current use. AAT can occur with normal serum digoxin levels in older patients, especially if hypokalemia is present. AAT episodes are often transient in young patients but may be more persistent in older patients.

ATRIAL TACHYCARDIA THERAPY

Acute therapy, unstable (hypotension, angina, heart failure symptoms)	• **First line:** Synchronized DCC (50-200 J with anesthesia); however, DCC may not convert AT to sinus rhythm, or if sinus rhythm is achieved, it may be transient. Using cardioversion, AT as a mechanism may be difficult to distinguish from other SVTs that respond to cardioversion (e.g., AV nodal reentrant, sinus nodal reentrant, or interatrial or intraatrial reentrant tachycardia). DCC should not be performed if digoxin toxicity is suspected because potentially lethal digoxin toxic rhythms, including VF, can be induced.
	• **Second line:** IV diltiazem or IV verapamil to control the ventricular response rate.
	• **Third line:** IV β-adrenergic blocker (e.g., esmolol or metoprolol). β-adrenergic blockers can produce some degree of AV block, thus slowing the ventricular rate, but they are not expected to terminate the atrial rhythm because the rhythm does not depend on the AV node for its maintenance.
	Similar responses occur in response to IV adenosine but use of adenosine may be useful diagnostically by demonstration of AV block during continued AT. In addition, some focal atrial tachycardias are adenosine dependent and will terminate with this drug.
Digoxin toxicity	• Digoxin antibody (Digibind) if the patient is unstable or the rhythm is associated with other more malignant arrhythmias such as PVCs or nonsustained or sustained VT.
	• Maintain serum K^+ >4.0 mEq/L.
Stable ventricular rate <120 bpm	• Ventricular rate control with IV or oral β-adrenergic blockers. Alternate: diltiazem.
	• Tachy-brady or unresponsive to rate control drugs: oral flecainide or propafenone (if normal LV function and no evidence of CAD, sotalol, dofetilide, or amiodarone); if tachy-brady syndrome, permanent cardiac pacing may be required.
	• Because the long-term goal is to achieve and maintain sinus rhythm, especially if symptoms are present, catheter ablation or drug therapy may be helpful.
Stable ventricular rate >120 bpm	• May require hospitalization.
	• IV β-adrenergic blocker or calcium channel blocker (diltiazem or verapamil) to control rate, followed by flecainide, propafenone, sotalol, dofetilide, or catheter ablation to terminate AT. If persistent, β-adrenergic blockers can occasionally terminate the arrhythmia, especially in young patients, where AT may be exercise induced.
	• Avoid digoxin if possible.
	• Treat precipitating factors (infection, CHF, digoxin toxicity) when present.
	• **Nonresponders:** Amiodarone (IV or oral) or catheter ablation (of the tachycardia [first line] or AV junctional ablation and pacemaker [last line]).

Continued on following page

ATRIAL TACHYCARDIA THERAPY (Continued)

Prevention (for patients with persistent risk for AT)	• Normal heart:
	1. β-adrenergic blocker.
	2. Catheter ablation.
	3. Drug therapy (preferred: class IC; alternate: class III, IA).
	• SHD, normal or near-normal LVEF (>40%):
	1. β-adrenergic blocker.
	2. Catheter ablation or drug therapy (preferred: sotalol; alternate: dofetilide, amiodarone, class IA).
	3. Catheter ablation.
	• SHD, poor LVEF (<40%):
	1. Catheter ablation or drug therapy (dofetilide, amiodarone).
	2. Catheter ablation. Avoid class IC drugs due to their proarrhythmic potential.
	• **Tachy-brady syndrome:** Catheter ablation or antiarrhythmic drug; pacemaker implantation if needed for symptomatic bradycardia or to facilitate use of antiarrhythmic drugs.
	• Catheter ablation of the atrial focus or foci is successful in 50% to 70% of ATs, which often originate in the crista terminalis, near the right atrial appendage, near the SA or AV nodes, or near the pulmonary veins; it is the preferred treatment. If unsuccessful and tachycardia-induced cardiomyopathy is present, consider catheter ablation of the AV junction and then placement of a mode-switching dual chamber pacemaker.
MI	• **First line:** β-adrenergic blocker if tolerated.
	• **Second line:** Sotalol or amiodarone.
	• If recurrent episodes, treat for several months as described for chronic prevention (above).
Preoperative/ postoperative	• Stable: Ventricular rate control (see Acute therapy, stable, above).
	• Unstable: Achieve sinus rhythm (see Acute therapy, unstable, above).
	• Transient postoperative: β-adrenergic blocker.

AV, Atrioventricular; *AT,* atrial tachycardia; *CAD,* coronary artery disease; *DCC,* direct current cardioversion; *IV,* intravenous; *LV,* left ventricle; *LVEF,* left ventricular ejection fraction; *MI,* myocardial infarction; *PVCs,* premature ventricular contraction; *SHD,* structural heart disease; *VF,* ventricular fibrillation.

Clinical Symptoms and Presentation

As with other SVTs, symptoms range from mild palpitations to angina or symptoms of heart failure, depending on the presence and severity of underlying heart disease.

Approach to Management

AAT can occur as an isolated episode related to, for example, infection and acute alcohol ingestion and does not require chronic therapy, or it may be frequent and/or recurrent, causing disabling symptoms. Chronic persistent AAT can cause tachycardia-induced cardiomyopathy, a reversible form of systolic heart failure caused by chronic rapid heart rates. Acute therapy generally consists of treating any precipitating factors and terminating with antiarrhythmic drugs. Prevention of recurrences over the long term is typically addressed with drugs or catheter ablation (a success rate of 50%). Asymptomatic or minimally symptomatic patients can be managed as outpatients unless severe tachy-brady syndrome is suspected (Table 5.2).

TABLE 5.2

AUTOMATIC ATRIAL TACHYCARDIA THERAPY

Acute therapy, unstable (hypotension, angina, heart failure symptoms)	• **First line:** Synchronized DCC (50-200 J with anesthesia). However, DCC may not convert AAT to sinus rhythm, or, if sinus rhythm is typically achieved, it may be transient. DCC should not be performed if digoxin toxicity is suspected, as potentially lethal digoxin toxic rhythms, including VF, can be induced.
	• **Second line:** IV diltiazem.
	• **Third line:** IV β-adrenergic blocker (e.g., esmolol or metoprolol). β-adrenergic blockers can produce some degree of AV block, thus slowing the ventricular rate, but they are not expected to terminate the atrial rhythm since the rhythm does not depend on the AV node for its maintenance.
	◦ Similar responses occur in response to IV adenosine, but response may be transient.
Digoxin toxicity	• Digoxin antibody (Digibind) if the patient is unstable or the rhythm is associated with other, more malignant arrhythmias such as PVCs or nonsustained or sustained VT.
	• Maintain serum K^+ >4.0 mEq/L.
Stable ventricular rate <120 bpm	• Ventricular rate control with IV or oral β-adrenergic blockers. Alternate: diltiazem.
	• If unresponsive to rate control drugs: oral flecainide or propafenone (if normal LV function and no evidence of CAD), sotalol, dofetilide, or amiodarone; if tachy-brady syndrome, permanent cardiac pacing will be required.
	• Because the long-term goal is to achieve and maintain sinus rhythm, especially if symptoms are present, catheter ablation (of the tachycardia itself) or drug therapy may be required.
Stable ventricular rate >120 bpm	• May require hospitalization.
	• IV β-adrenergic blocker or calcium channel blocker (diltiazem or verapamil) to control rate, followed by flecainide, propafenone, sotalol, dofetilide, or catheter ablation to terminate AAT. If persistent, β-adrenergic blockers can occasionally terminate the arrhythmia, especially in young patients, where AAT may be exercise induced.
	• Avoid digoxin, if possible.
	• Treat precipitating factors (infection, CHF, digoxin toxicity) when present.
	• **Nonresponders:** Amiodarone (IV or oral) or catheter ablation (of the tachycardia [first line] or AV junctional ablation and pacemaker [last line]).

Continued on following page

TABLE 5.2

AUTOMATIC ATRIAL TACHYCARDIA THERAPY (Continued)

Prevention (for patients with persistent risk for AAT)	• Normal heart:
	1. β-adrenergic blocker.
	2. Catheter ablation.
	3. Drug therapy (preferred: class IC; alternate: class III, IA).
	• SHD, normal or near-normal LVEF (>40%):
	1. β-adrenergic blocker.
	2. Catheter ablation or drug therapy (preferred: sotalol; alternate: dofetilide, amiodarone, class IA).
	3. Catheter ablation.
	• SHD, poor LVEF (<40%):
	1. Catheter ablation or drug therapy (dofetilide, amiodarone).
	2. Catheter ablation. Avoid class IC drugs due to their proarrhythmic potential.
	• **Tachy-brady syndrome:** Catheter ablation or antiarrhythmic drug; pacemaker implantation if needed for symptomatic bradycardia or to facilitate use of antiarrhythmic drugs.
	• Catheter ablation of the atrial focus or foci is successful in 50% to 70% of AATs, which often originate in the crista terminalis, near the SA or AV nodes, or near the pulmonary veins; it is the preferred treatment. If unsuccessful and tachycardia-induced cardiomyopathy is present, consider catheter ablation of the AV junction and then placement of a mode-switching dual chamber pacemaker.
MI	• **First line:** β-adrenergic blocker if tolerated.
	• **Second line:** Sotalol or amiodarone.
	• If recurrent episodes, treat for several months as described for chronic prevention (above).
Preoperative/postoperative	• **Stable:** Ventricular rate control (see Acute therapy, stable, above).
	• **Unstable:** Achieve sinus rhythm (see Acute therapy, unstable, above).
	• **Transient postoperative:** β-adrenergic blocker.

AAT, Automatic AT; *AV,* atrioventricular; *CAD,* coronary artery disease; *CHF,* congestive heart failure; *DCC,* direct current cardioversion; *IV,* intravenous; *LV,* left ventricle; *LVEF,* left ventricular ejection fraction; *MI,* myocardial infarction; *PVCs,* premature ventricular contraction; *SA,* sinoatrial; *SHD,* structural heart disease; *VF,* ventricular fibrillation.

Atrial Reentrant Tachycardia

Description

ART (Fig. 5.3) is an SVT that can be due to macroreentry (using large portions of the left or right atria) or microreentry. Macroreentrant ATs tend to occur around areas of scarring, including incisional scars from prior cardiac surgery, corrected congenital heart disease ("incisional or scar-related ART"), or trauma. ART causes 5% to 10% of SVTs. ART can be distinguished from AFL by discrete (nonsinus) P waves (which may be buried in the QRS complexes or T waves) and by their slower rate

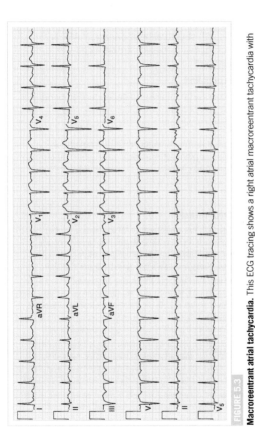

FIGURE 5.3

Macroreentrant atrial tachycardia. This ECG tracing shows a right atrial macroreentrant tachycardia with 2:1 AV conduction, proven by EP study, and ablation. Every other P wave is buried in the QRS. If one saw only the rhythm strips, this might mistakenly be diagnosed as a sinus tachycardia. However, the inferior leads III and aVF show negative P waves, indicating a low-to-high activation pattern that is not consistent with the typical sinus high-to-low atrial activation pattern that would inscribe a positive P wave. When this is seen, one should be prompted to look for 2:1 conduction and similar P waves buried in the QRS. In addition, the lack of discrete isoelectric baseline around the P waves suggests that this is a macroreentrant tachycardia rather than a focal tachycardia.

(170 to 220 bpm), but can be considered a slow atrial flutter. It can be distinguished from sinus tachycardia by its abrupt onset, persistence, and nonsinus P-wave morphology. Adenosine terminates ART in only approximately 15% of cases but can be used for diagnostic purposes because it causes transient AV block, uncovering the underlying P-wave rate and morphology. ART can be difficult to distinguish from AAT; an EP study may be needed.

Associated Conditions

ART is generally associated with structural heart disease. If ART is persistent, it can cause tachycardia-mediated cardiomyopathy or hemodynamic deterioration.

Clinical Symptoms and Presentation

Symptoms are similar to other SVTs but are also dependent on underlying heart disease.

Approach to Management

Terminating ART is the best first option, especially if the patient is symptomatic, unless ablation is planned, in which case mapping during tachycardia will be possible (Table 5.3).

TABLE 5.3	
ATRIAL REENTRANT TACHYCARDIA THERAPY	
Acute therapy in hemodynamically unstable patients	• **First line:** DCC. This may not work for AAT and therefore can be a diagnostic point. For AAT or ART unresponsive to cardioversion, use IV amiodarone, ibutilide, or procainamide to terminate ART or IV β-adrenergic blocker or diltiazem to increase the degree of AV block.
	• **Second line:** Atrial antitachycardia pacing (transvenous or transesophageal) to terminate ART; may attempt this as first line if pacing capability is in place (e.g., by use of temporary epicardial wires placed during cardiac surgery). A temporary intraatrial pacing lead can be placed to pace terminate frequent, recurrent, to poorly tolerated episodes.
	Subsequent therapy: Use oral antiarrhythmic drugs to prevent recurrence: Oral antiarrhythmic drugs are unlikely to cardiovert the rhythm to sinus (<20%) but may help to maintain sinus rhythm after it is achieved. Consider oral antiarrhythmic drugs after cardioversion or if recurrent ART paroxysms.
	• **First line:** Sotalol if preserved LVEF (>40%) with or without structural heart disease, amiodarone if structural heart disease and poor LVEF (<40%).
	• **Second line:** Dofetilide or class IA antiarrhythmic drugs.
	• **Third line:** Class IC drugs (propafenone, flecainide) if no structural heart disease is present; however, these drugs may stabilize the reentrant circuit by slowing atrial conduction, thus allowing 1:1 AV conduction and an increase in ventricular response. A concomitant AV nodal blocking drug may be needed.
	• Control ventricular response with β-adrenergic blocker, Ca^{2+} blocker, or digoxin (especially if low LVEF or CHF).
	• Evaluate and treat exacerbating cause(s) (e.g., pneumonia, CHF).

ATRIAL REENTRANT TACHYCARDIA THERAPY (Continued)

Chronic therapy	• Rate control alone is acceptable if the tachycardias are not rapid, are well tolerated, and are chronic.
	• **First line:** RF ablation; the success rate is 50% to 75%.
	• **Second line:** Antiarrhythmic drugs. If there is structural heart disease, consider class III antiarrhythmics. Sotalol is preferred if patient can tolerate the β-adrenergic blocker effect. Alternatively, dofetilide or class IA drugs are acceptable but have a higher incidence of side effects and proarrhythmic risk. Sotalol, dofetilide, and class IA drugs should be started in the hospital. Use amiodarone if poor LV function (LVEF <40%) or CHF.
	• **Third line:** ventricular rate control with β-adrenergic blockers or calcium blockers.
	• If drugs fail:
	• **First line:** Catheter ablation.
	• **Second line:** Catheter ablation of the AV node with placement of a dual-chamber mode-switching pacemaker. Modern pacemakers can sometimes allow for pace termination of atrial arrhythmias noninvasively.
MI	• See Acute therapy above; avoid class IC (flecainide, propafenone) antiarrhythmic drugs.
Preoperative	• Assess chronicity, hemodynamic tolerance, ventricular rate, and medical therapy. If well tolerated, no therapy is needed other than ventricular rate control (2:1 AV block or higher may be needed). However, even if rate is well controlled before surgery, increased catecholamine levels may increase ventricular rate and AV nodal blocking drugs may be required.
Postoperative	• See Acute therapy above.
Pregnancy	• Rare, control rate with β-adrenergic blocker.

AAT, Automatic AT; *ART,* atrial reentrant tachycardia; *AV,* atrioventricular; *CHF,* congestive heart failure; *DCC,* direct current cardioversion; *IV,* intravenous; *LV,* left ventricle; *LVEF,* left ventricular ejection fraction; *MI,* myocardial infarction; *RF,* radiofrequency.

Multifocal Atrial Tachycardia

Description

MAT (Fig. 5.4) is an SVT in which there are at least three distinct P-wave morphologies, indicating multifocality of the rhythm. The PP, PR, and RR intervals vary, and the ventricular rate is more than 100 bpm, usually ranging from 110 to 170 bpm. The multiple P-wave morphologies result from multiple depolarizing foci in the atria. The underlying mechanism may be enhanced automaticity or triggered activity. Whereas MAT is usually the predominant rhythm at a given time and does not occur in short bursts, on occasion other atrial arrhythmias (premature atrial complexes [PACs], AAT, sinus tachycardia, and even AFL and AF) may precede or follow a bout of MAT. The irregularly irregular ventricular rate can mimic AF. Differentiation from "coarse" AF can be made by the absence of isoelectric periods between P waves in AF. Distinction of MAT and AF is important because management strategies differ considerably.

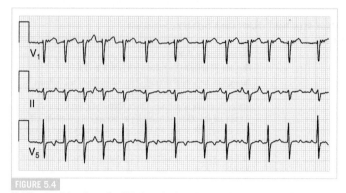

Multifocal atrial tachycardia. This three-lead rhythm strip (leads V_1, II, and V_5) shows an irregularly irregular narrow QRS complex rhythm. However, unlike AF, each QRS complex is preceded by discrete P waves. There are at least three different P wave morphologies and PR intervals, consistent with MAT.

Associated Conditions

The vast majority (approximately 60% to 85%) of cases occur in acutely ill older patients with severe COPD. However, in addition to COPD, MAT has been associated with severe coronary artery disease (CAD), cor pulmonale, pneumonia, sepsis, postoperative states, lung cancer, pulmonary embolism, congestive (usually systolic) heart failure, hypertensive heart disease, and other acute cardiac or pulmonary processes. Exacerbating factors include theophylline toxicity, catecholamine infusions, hypokalemia, hypomagnesemia, hypoxia, and acidosis. MAT usually lasts for days to weeks, especially in patients with exacerbations of COPD, and recurrences are common in acutely ill patients. Although MAT itself is rarely life-threatening (exception: rapid rate induces ischemia in those with severe coronary disease), acute mortality is approximately 30% to 40% because of the severity of the underlying disease, rather than the rhythm per se. MAT is rarely associated with acute MI.

Clinical Symptoms and Presentation

MAT is often asymptomatic but can be associated with rapid, irregular palpitations. Associated symptoms usually reflect the underlying illness (e.g., breathlessness in a COPD exacerbation).

Approach to Management

Primary treatment of MAT is extremely difficult and unrewarding because without effective treatment of the underlying disease the rhythm tends to persist; therapy should be directed at the acute illness. Electrolyte abnormalities should be corrected. Calcium channel blockers are preferable to β-adrenergic blockers, particularly if the underlying acute illness is COPD with bronchospasm (Table 5.4).

TABLE 5.4

MULTIFOCAL ATRIAL TACHYCARDIA THERAPY

Acute therapy, stable and unstable	• Treat underlying condition. Aggressive treatment of COPD exacerbation usually treats arrhythmia, but MAT may persist for hours to days after management of the underlying condition is effective. Treatment of the MAT itself does not affect the course or prognosis of the medical illness. Avoid digoxin as AV block and slowing of ventricular rate is unlikely to occur. DCC is ineffective in terminating the rhythm.
	• Cardioversion is of no benefit for MAT. However, AF may be confused with MAT; if the diagnosis is uncertain and the patient is hemodynamically unstable, cardioversion can be considered in selected cases. Hemodynamic instability generally results from the underlying medical condition and not from the rhythm or rapid rate per se.
	• Lower the dose of sympathomimetics and methylxanthines, as tolerated, if applicable.
	• Maintain K^+ and Mg^{2+} within normal limits.
	• Drugs to control ventricular rate (data on effectiveness are inconclusive): Preferred: calcium blocker (IV or oral diltiazem). Verapamil can cause substantial hypotension in patients with COPD but may be effective. Ventricular rate control is difficult due to excess catecholamines for most of these patients. β-adrenergic blockers rarely can be given due to concurrent bronchospastic pulmonary disease.
	• IV magnesium 2- to 4-g bolus of magnesium sulfate may terminate the episodes and help to control the ventricular rate, but success is limited and unpredictable.
	• Digoxin may worsen MAT and is unlikely to control the ventricular response.
	• Amiodarone can be considered to control ventricular rate and suppress the arrhythmia, but there are no data to support its use.
Chronic prevention	• Options include calcium channel blockers (e.g., oral diltiazem) for ventricular rate control or possibly amiodarone to prevent recurrences; drug therapy without aggressive treatment of the underlying condition is often futile.
	• Treat pulmonary disease; maintain $K^+ >4.0$ and $Mg^{2+} >2.0$, if possible.
MI	• See Acute therapy above. Rapid rate and ineffective atrial kick (PR interval <0.14 s) can worsen ischemia and CHF. Rate control is often required. A calcium channel blocker such as diltiazem is the first-line therapy, unless β-adrenergic blockers can be tolerated.

AV, Atrioventricular; *AF,* atrial fibrillation; *DCC,* direct current cardioversion; *COPD,* chronic obstructive pulmonary disease; *IV,* intravenous; *MAT,* multifocal atrial tachycardia.

ATRIAL FIBRILLATION

Description

AF is the most common SVT that requires long-term therapy. Depolarization of the atria occurs in rapid, multiple waves, with continuously changing pathways. Intraatrial activation can be recorded as irregular, rapid depolarizations, often at rates greater than 300 to 400 bpm. These depolarizations result in loss of coordinated atrial contraction and in irregular conduction to the ventricle due to irregular arrival and decremental conduction of impulses in the AV node. On the surface ECG, discrete P waves are absent and irregular fibrillatory waves are seen; the ventricular response is irregularly irregular and can be fast (>100 bpm; Fig. 5.5), moderate (60 to 100 bpm; Fig. 5.6), or slow (<60 bpm; Fig. 5.7), unless complete AV block is present, in which case the QRS rhythm results from a regularly firing escape focus (Fig. 5.8). At times, the irregular fibrillatory waves are accompanied by more regular, but still varying, flutter-like waves (Fig. 5.9); this still represents AF rather than AFL. MAT (see Fig. 5.4) and sinus with frequent PACs (Fig. 5.10) can mimic AF with its irregularly irregular rhythm but are distinguished from AF by the presence of P waves preceding each QRS complex.

In the presence of an underlying BBB (or intraventricular conduction delay), AF can present as a wide QRS complex rhythm (Fig. 5.11) that could mimic ventricular tachycardia (VT) (except that AF remains irregularly irregular). Intraventricular aberrancy with a BBB pattern can result in wide QRS complexes and occasionally mimic VT if the BBB pattern is not classic. Aberration is usually initiated by a long-short sequence (Ashman phenomenon) (Fig. 5.12); RBBB aberration is more common than left bundle branch block (LBBB) aberration in the absence of structural heart disease. AF at extremely high ventricular rates (e.g., 200 to 300 bpm) should suggest the presence of a bypass tract (Fig. 5.13), and the wide QRS complex is typically due to conduction down the bypass tract. Another instance of an irregularly irregular wide QRS complex tachycardia is AF in the setting of a dual-chamber pacemaker, in which the pacemaker tracks atrial activations at or near its upper rate limit.

Triggering sites, typically arising from the ostia of the pulmonary veins, have been recognized to initiate AF, particularly in lone AF (AF without structural heart disease). These triggers can potentially be ablated or isolated from atrial tissue using catheter-based or surgical pulmonary vein isolation, aiming for long-term cure.

Associated Conditions

AF occurs in normal, healthy adults ("lone" AF) but is often associated with structural heart disease (ischemic, valvular [especially mitral], rheumatic, cardiomyopathic, congenital). Other associated conditions include advancing age, hypertension, diabetes mellitus, postoperative

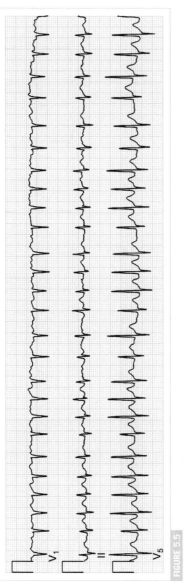

FIGURE 5.5

Atrial fibrillation with rapid ventricular response. This lead V_1, II, and V_5 rhythm strip shows AF with rapid (>100 bpm) ventricular response. Rapid ventricular rates are the most common finding when AF first presents (usually in the absence of any AV nodal blocking drugs).

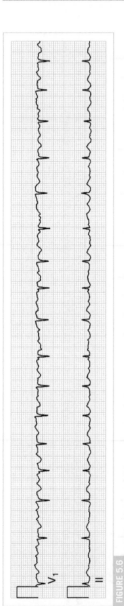

FIGURE 5.6

Atrial fibrillation with moderate ventricular response. This lead V$_1$ and II rhythm strip shows AF with moderate (60 to 100 bpm) ventricular response, reflecting a more controlled ventricular response, most often due to the use of drugs that block the AV node.

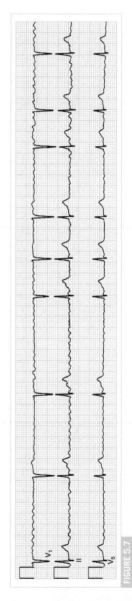

FIGURE 5.7

Atrial fibrillation with slow ventricular response. This lead V$_1$, II, and V$_5$ rhythm strip shows AF with slow (<60 bpm) ventricular response (in this case as slow as 33 bpm) that can reflect excessive nodal blocking effects by drugs, drug toxicity (e.g., digitalis toxicity), or the presence of underlying conduction system disease.

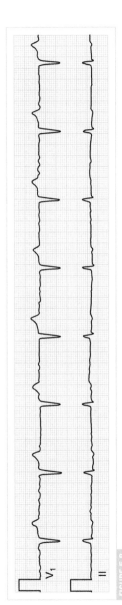

FIGURE 5.8

Atrial fibrillation with regular (slow) ventricular response. This lead V_1 and II rhythm strip shows AF with a very very regular ventricular response. In this case the regular response is due to CHB with an idioventricular rhythm.

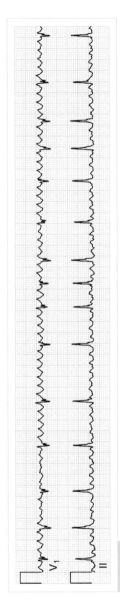

FIGURE 5.9

Atrial fibrillation with atypical flutter. This lead V_1 and II rhythm strip shows an irregularly irregular narrow QRS complex rhythm. At times it looks like coarse AF, and then at times it looks like atypical AFL (although not always regular and sometimes faster than typical AFL). This is called AF-flutter and is considered a form of AF.

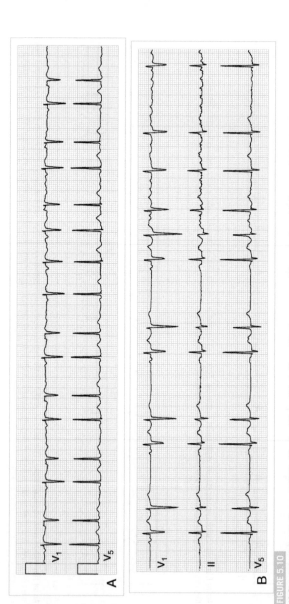

FIGURE 5.10

(A) Sinus rhythm with frequent PACs. The lead V₁ and V₅ rhythm strip shows normal sinus rhythm with frequent PACs in a bigeminal pattern for the first eight complexes, then an irregular rhythm for the last half of the tracing. Although the last half is irregular, there is a discrete P wave preceding each and every QRS complex. There is an underlying sinus rhythm, and the early QRS complexes have a nonsinus P wave preceding them.

(B) Frequent PACs initiating AF. The first half of this lead V₁, II, and V₅ rhythm strip shows atrial bigeminy. The last half of the tracing shows a premature atrial complex initiating AF, as shown by the fibrillatory baseline and absence of discrete P waves.

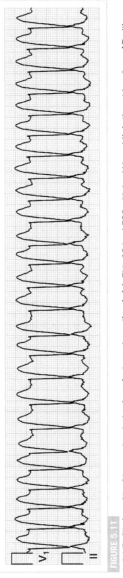

FIGURE 5.11

Atrial fibrillation with wide complex rhythm (ventricular tachycardia mimic). This 12-lead ECG with lead V_1 and II rhythm strips shows AF with a rapid response with an LBBB pattern. The result is a wide complex tachycardia that could be confused with VT. However, closer examination reveals an irregularly irregular rhythm characteristic of AF, and the QRS morphology shows a typical LBBB pattern.

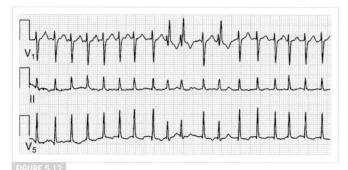

FIGURE 5.12

Atrial fibrillation with aberrancy. This lead V_1, II, and V_5 rhythm strip shows AF with the 9th, 10th, and 12th beats showing a wide QRS complex in a RBBB pattern. Although premature wide QRS complex beats can be premature ventricular contractions (PVCs), they may also arise from aberrant conduction (i.e., rate-related changes in conduction), as is the case here. The basic property involved is that the refractoriness of the bundle branches are related to the RR interval of the preceding beat. In this case there is a typical long–short sequence in which a late-coupled beat with long RR (which prolongs the refractoriness of the bundles for the subsequent beat) is followed by an early beat that exhibits an increased QRS duration due to incomplete recovery of excitability down one of the bundle branches. The right bundle branch typically has a longer refractory period than the left bundle. As such, the typical features of Ashman phenomenon are seen with (a) a long–short interval and (b) a wide QRS that is typically with an RBBB morphology. Of note, Ashman phenomenon explains the aberrancy of the 9th and 12th beat of the tracing, but not the aberrancy of the 10th beat. In this case a phenomenon called concealed perpetuated aberration, or linking, is involved. In this case the 9th (aberrantly conducted) beat activated down the left bundle branch, then the interventricular septum, and then retrogradely up the right bundle. Because the surface ECG does not show activation in the bundles, this retrograde activation is "concealed" but becomes evident with the next early-coupled beat that propagates down the bundle of His but finds the right bundle refractory (and thus conducts with a RBBB pattern). The next conducted beat proceeds down both bundles and does not show aberrancy.

states (especially after cardiac surgery with incidences after aortocoronary bypass procedures ranging from 15% to 40%, and after valve surgery, 40% to 60%), pericarditis, pulmonary embolism, chronic lung disease, thyrotoxicosis, acute alcohol ingestion ("holiday heart"), excessive caffeine, drugs (especially sympathomimetic drugs), autonomic fluctuation (vagal or sympathetic), hypokalemia or other metabolic derangements, systemic infection, sinus node dysfunction (tachy-brady syndrome), degenerative conduction system disease, and Wolff-Parkinson-White (WPW) syndrome. Long-term consequences include the risk of embolic stroke or transient ischemic attack (TIA) (with incidences in rheumatic

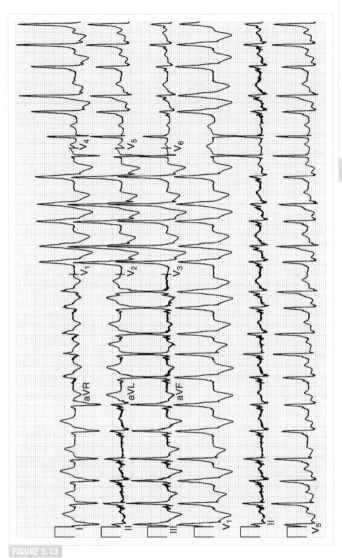

FIGURE 5.13

Atrial fibrillation with bypass tract. This 12-lead ECG with lead V_1 rhythm strip shows a rapid irregularly irregular wide complex tachycardia, consistent with AF in a patient with WPW syndrome. Note marked variability in QRS morphology due to variable degrees of preexcitation. WPW should be suspected when there is AF with very rapid rates (>200 bpm) and/or irregularly irregular rhythms with varying QRS morphologies. The combination of an irregularly irregular rhythm with a rapid wide QRS complex and varying QRS widths indicating varying degrees of fusion should always bring to mind AF with WPW syndrome and rapid conduction over an accessory AV pathway.

AF of 10% to 12% per year; nonvalvular AF of 1% to 7% per year) and reduced exercise capacity due to reduction in stroke volume caused by loss of atrial kick and to left ventricular (LV) dysfunction (impaired diastolic filling during rapid ventricular response, tachycardia-mediated cardiomyopathy). There is a twofold increase in mortality in AF patients, possibly related to underlying heart disease and proarrhythmia rather than AF per se.

Clinical Symptoms and Presentation

Depending on the presence and severity of underlying heart disease, patients may be asymptomatic and have mild palpitations or significant symptoms, such as angina, CHF, syncope, or hemodynamic collapse. Symptoms may occur due to rapid rates, irregularity of the rhythm, and loss of AV synchrony and the atrial kick. AF is strongly associated with TIA, stroke, or other thromboembolic complications, which are not infrequently the initial manifestation of AF that has not been previously known to exist. AF is the most common cause of cardioembolic stroke and is a common cause of cryptogenic stroke.

AF may be categorized by its presentation into several types. *Newly diagnosed AF* characterizes patients presenting with AF for the first time, regardless of duration. *Paroxysmal AF* is AF that self terminates, usually within 48 hours after its onset (but sometimes up to 7 days). *Persistent AF* lasts more than 7 days or requires an intervention (pharmacologic or electrical) for cardioversion. *Long-standing persistent AF* is AF that has persisted continuously for more than 1 year. *Permanent AF* is AF that has been accepted to remain with either failure of rhythm control efforts and/or no additional efforts planned to restore sinus rhythm.

Approach to Management

The management of AF can be focused into three main aspects: (1) control of the ventricular rate (rate control), (2) control of the atrial rhythm (rhythm control), and (3) antithrombotic therapy to reduce the risk of stroke and other thromboembolic complications. For any patient with AF, all three aspects of management should be considered, but all are not necessarily required for a given patient.

Acute management of symptomatic AF with rapid ventricular rates includes consideration of urgent electrical cardioversion if there is evidence of hemodynamic instability, significant myocardial ischemia, or pulmonary edema. Electrical or pharmacologic cardioversion is also reasonable therapy for new-onset symptomatic AF. Ventricular rate control can usually be attempted while preparing for cardioversion, using intravenous (IV) or oral β-adrenergic blockers, diltiazem or verapamil, or digoxin (see Table 5.5). Rhythm control with intent to

TABLE 5.5

PHARMACOLOGIC AND NONPHARMACOLOGIC OPTIONS FOR MANAGEMENT OF ATRIAL FIBRILLATION

	Rate Control	Achievement and Maintenance of Sinus Rhythm	Antithrombotic Therapy
Pharmacologic	β-adrenergic blockers	Antiarrhythmic drugs	Warfarin, heparin, LMWH
	Ca²⁺-channel blockers	Class IA	NOAC
	Digoxin	quinidine	Apixaban
		procainamide	Dabigatran
		disopyramide	Edoxaban
		Class IC	Rivaroxaban
		flecainide	
		propafenone	
		Class III	
		sotalol	
		dofetilide	
		dronedarone	
		amiodarone	
		ibutilide	
Nonpharmacologic	AV junction ablation and pacing	Catheter ablation/PVI	LAA ligation, removal, or occlusion
		Surgical maze/PVI	

LAA, Left atrial appendage; *NOAC,* non-vitamin K oral anticoagulants; *PVI,* pulmonary vein isolation.

convert the AF to sinus rhythm can be begun with pharmacologic or electrical cardioversion. Anticoagulation strategies should be addressed before conversion. If the AF duration is more than 24-48 hours, anticoagulation with warfarin with international normalized ratios (INRs) therapeutic (between 2 and 3) or NOACs (e.g., dabigatran, rivaroxaban, apixaban, or edoxaban) for at least 3 weeks is needed and should be documented. Alternatively, if left atrial thrombus is not demonstrated by transesophageal echocardiography (TEE) and the patient is therapeutically anticoagulated (with heparin, warfarin with INR ≥2.0, or NOACs), cardioversion can be done and anticoagulation with warfarin or an NOAC initiated or continued for at least 3 to 6 weeks and indefinitely for many patients with risk factors. For AF duration of less than 48 hours, anticoagulation should still be considered, particularly if the patient has structural heart disease or risk factors for stroke or thromboembolism. Anticoagulation should be strongly considered for the postcardioversion period. Cardioversion can be attempted by electrical means or by antiarrhythmic drugs. The latter may include oral class I or class III antiarrhythmic drugs, such as IV ibutilide, procainamide, or amiodarone. A new drug, vernakalant, not yet approved, appears to also be highly effective to convert AF to sinus rhythm.

Long-term management should include all three aspects of management listed previously here, as well as evaluation for underlying structural heart disease, risk factors for stroke or thromboembolism, or other associated conditions associated with AF. However, appropriate management of associated conditions does not guarantee that AF will not recur. Evaluation includes an echocardiogram to assess for ventricular dysfunction, valve disease, and atrial size. Treadmill exercise testing and/or cardiac catheterization to assess coronary anatomy may be indicated in selected patients and/or patients considered for class IC (flecainide or propafenone) antiarrhythmic drugs. Patients with structural heart disease or CAD should not be treated with class IC drugs. Thyroid function tests should be checked at least once because hyperthyroidism can initiate AF. Anticoagulation using warfarin, a NOAC, aspirin, or aspirin plus clopidogrel should be considered in all patients. Ventricular rate control can be generally achieved with β-adrenergic blockers, diltiazem, or verapamil; digoxin can be used but is not a direct AV nodal blocker, and its AV nodal blocking effect will generally be lost with the vagolysis of activity. Rhythm control, with restoration and maintenance of sinus rhythm using cardioversion and/or antiarrhythmic therapy, should be considered; even though no significant overall survival benefit has been demonstrated for either approach, rhythm control is important in selected highly symptomatic patients (often with lone AF) in whom better survival in sinus rhythm and improved functional status and quality of life can be demonstrated. Because AF can be clinically silent, it is important that anticoagulation not be discontinued in patients at risk for thromboembolic complications, even if sinus rhythm appears during clinical follow-up to be maintained. Those patients who remain anticoagulated with warfarin or a NOAC have a lower risk of stroke. For new-onset AF or for those with continued symptoms despite rate control, a rhythm control strategy is still beneficial and is recommended (Table 5.5).

Rate-Control Strategies

The mainstays of ventricular rate control are the β-adrenergic blockers, diltiazem or verapamil, and digoxin. IV AV nodal blocking drugs may be most efficacious and easily titrated during acute management of rapid ventricular rates. Digoxin is less effective, although it can be used in patients with CHF, but has a delayed onset, narrow therapeutic window, and less effect in hyperadrenergic states (e.g., in postoperative states, intensive care units). For patients in whom sinus rhythm cannot be maintained and who have continued difficulty with rapid ventricular rates despite medical therapies, AV junction ablation with implantation of a rate-responsive permanent ventricular pacemaker can improve symptoms and ventricular function. This approach can also be used in patients with paroxysmal AF (in whom dual-chamber pacing is recommended). AV junction ablation results in complete heart block (CHB) with a QRS rhythm originating in ventricular tissue, usually at rates in the 30s; the functional LBBB induced by RV apical pacing can lead to intraventricular dyssynchrony and reduced left ventricular ejection fraction (LVEF). In these cases, upgrading the pacing system to a biventricular one (cardiac resynchronization therapy) may be of benefit.

Rhythm-Control Strategies

Electrical cardioversion is the most effective way to terminate AF. One method to control AF is to perform cardioversion whenever AF episodes occur. This is appropriate if the AF episodes are not too closely spaced in time. Those patients who are most likely to have recurrence of AF after cardioversion include those who have large left atria, who are older, and who have had episodes of long duration.

Control of blood pressure and avoidance or treatment of any identified precipitating conditions or clinical triggers, such as stimulant use or hyperthyroidism, may be potentially helpful in reducing the risk of AF.

Pharmacologic cardioversion is less effective when there is long-standing AF. In some instances, after cardioversion, there is immediate or early return of AF; in these cases IV verapamil or IV ibutilide can help to maintain sinus rhythm after cardioversion. In addition, atropine IV may be useful in patients who have slow rates with their AF and may have high vagal tone that reinitiates the arrhythmia. Slow ventricular rates in AF (see Fig. 5.7) do not necessarily portend slow rates in sinus rhythm after cardioversion, but caution must be used, especially in patients who have been taking digoxin because they are at risk for malignant ventricular arrhythmias after cardioversion.

Antiarrhythmic drugs that can help to maintain sinus rhythm (and even help to stop AF in some instances) include class IA (quinidine, procainamide, disopyramide), class IC (flecainide, propafenone), and class III (sotalol, dofetilide, amiodarone, dronedarone) drugs.

The success rate of maintaining sinus rhythm is approximately 50% to 70%, depending on the drug and the definition of success; however, the goal of medical therapy to control the rhythm is to decrease the incidence of symptomatic AF, not necessarily to suppress the AF completely, which might require higher doses of antiarrhythmic drugs with their attendant side effects or toxicity. Thus recurrences are expected, and occasional recurrences do not necessarily constitute failure of this approach. Antiarrhythmic drug selection is individualized, based on the presence of structural heart disease or other individual factors, such as patient compliance with the regimen. In patients with no or minimal structural heart disease, flecainide, propafenone, sotalol, or dronedarone are first-line choices, followed by dofetilide and amiodarone. For these patients, flecainide or propafenone can be given intermittently on a pro rata nata (PRN) basis during episodes of AF ("pill in the pocket"). Dofetilide must be started in the hospital. For patients with hypertension and significant LV hypertrophy, amiodarone or dronedarone is recommended. For patients with CAD, IC drugs (flecainide, propafenone) must be avoided. First-line therapy for these patients includes sotalol, dronedarone, and dofetilide, followed by amiodarone. For patients with heart failure, amiodarone or dofetilide are first-line therapies and dronedarone should be avoided. Class IA antiarrhythmic drugs are rarely used because of high risk of toxicity and side effects.

The reason to use antiarrhythmic drug therapy is to reduce the risk of recurrent AF and in most cases to prevent symptoms. It is not clear how many patients have AF that remains undetectable or undetected, although implanted device interrogation suggests that up to 50% of AF episodes are unassociated with symptoms and therefore not detected clinically. Although symptom reduction is the main reason to treat AF, other reasons also are important to recognize, including the progression of ventricular dysfunction caused by tachycardia and symptomatic heart failure.

Another nonpharmacologic adjunctive therapy includes permanent pacemaker implantation for tachy-brady syndrome when long pauses and/or symptomatic bradycardia is present. Permanent pacemakers can be indicated in patients with symptomatic post-AF conversion pauses or other symptomatic bradyarrhythmias (including those due to ventricular rate control medications). Dual-chamber (DDD) pacing in which AV synchrony is preserved and the atria may be paced to avoid atrial bradycardia is associated with less AF recurrences than single chamber ventricular (VVI) pacing systems. Some pacemakers have an option of allowing atrial overdrive pacing just above the continuously sensed sinus rate to prevent irregularities of rate and pauses that may be related to the initiation or reinitiation of AF.

Potential curative catheter ablation directed toward electrical isolation of the pulmonary vein ostia and other arrhythmogenic atrial substrates can be considered for patients with symptomatic AF who have not responded to an antiarrhythmic drug. Radiofrequency (RF) or other energy or freezing (e.g., cryoablation) is applied segmentally or circumferentially to the antra of the pulmonary vein ostia to isolate the ostia. Fractionated electrical potentials, sites of vagal attachments, or ganglionated plexes or connecting areas between ostia may be targeted. The surgical maze or surgical pulmonary vein isolation procedure can be performed with minimally invasive or open cardiac surgical approaches. The maze procedure is performed by making incisions and resuturing the atria or by applying RF, cryo ablation, or other energy to create lines of conduction block. Much of the success of this approach has likely been due to the surgically created pulmonary vein antral isolation, and modifications of the maze procedure, including pulmonary vein isolation approaches, have been developed. Currently, surgical ablation is most commonly performed as a concomitant procedure during other cardiac operations.

Anticoagulation

Because stroke is one of the most important clinical consequences of and a source of major morbidity associated with AF, addressing anticoagulation is critical with each step in the management of AF. Multiple risk stratification schemes have been published. Two useful scoring systems for assessing thromboembolic risk are the CHADS$_2$ score (Table 5.6A), and the CHA$_2$DS$_2$-VASc score (Table 5.6B), which are two schemes for identifying patients at high and low risk for stroke. Recommended guidelines for long-term antithrombotic therapy are listed in Table 5.7. Studies also suggest that for patients with AF who are at risk for stroke but who have contraindications to warfarin, aspirin plus clopidogrel may be beneficial. The magnitude of benefit is not as great as warfarin, and the magnitude of benefit over aspirin is relatively small. This combination therapy is associated with a higher risk of bleeding than with aspirin alone. Dabigatran, a direct thrombin inhibitor, and several factor Xa inhibitors, rivaroxaban, edoxaban, and apixaban (commonly, the group is known as non-vitamin K oral anticoagulants [i.e., "NOACs"]) were approved for reduction of the risk of stroke and systemic embolism in patients with nonvalvular AF. See Chapter 12 for further anticoagulation information. Left atrial appendage occlusion or resection is also an approach for reducing thromboembolic complications for those patients who cannot take an anticoagulant or refuse to take one but are at high risk of thromboembolic events (Algorithm 5.3).

There are several advantages of NOACs over warfarin: (1) anticoagulation is rapid, (2) bleeding risks are equal to of superior to warfarin, (3) outcomes regarding thromboembolic events are equal to or superior to warfarin, (4) there is no need to monitor INRs, (5) anticoagulation is immediate, and (6) stopping a NOAC leads to rapid reversal of the anticoagulation. There is a downside to NOACs: (1) NOACs are excreted renally, and this may be a problem in patients with renal insufficiency; (2) NOACs are not approved for patients with valvular disease because outcomes are better in those taking warfarin; (3) costs are higher; (4) one of the NOACs cannot be given for those with creatinine clearance greater than 95; (5) fluctuating renal function may be an issue about anticoagulation; (6) many of the NOACS have no reversing agent; and (7) noncompliance is an issue, and it can be impossible to know if a patient is actually taking the drug.

TABLE 5.6A

CHADS₂ SCORE FOR PATIENTS WITH NONVALVULAR ATRIAL FIBRILLATION NOT TREATED WITH ANTICOAGULATION

Risk Factor	Score	$CHADS_2$ Score	Adjusted Stroke Rate (95% CI)[a]
CHF	1	0	1.9 (1.2-3.0)
Hypertension	1	1	2.8 (2.0-3.8)
Age ≥75 years	1	2	4.0 (3.1-5.1)
Diabetes	1	3	5.9 (4.6-7.3)
Stroke or TIA, prior	2	4	8.5 (6.3-11.1)
Maximum score	6	5	12.5 (8.2-17.5)
—		6	18.2 (10.5-27.4)

CHF, Congestive heart failure; *TIA,* transient ischemic attack.

[a] Expected stroke rate/100 patient-years, assuming aspirin was not taken, based on data from the National Registry of Atrial Fibrillation (NRAF) Participants.

TABLE 5.6B

CHA₂DS₂-VASc SCORE

Risk Factor	Score	CHA_2DS_2-VASc Score	Thromboembolism Rate Adjusted for Aspirin, %/year[a]	Thromboembolism Rate Adjusted for Warfarin, %/year[b]
CHF failure/LV dysfunction	1	0	0	0
Hypertension	1	1	0.7	1.3
Age ≥75 years	2	2	1.9	2.2
Diabetes mellitus	1	3	4.7	3.2
Stroke, TIA, or TE	2	4	2.3	4.0
Vascular disease (prior MI, PAD or aortic plaque)	1	5	3.9	6.7
Age 65-74 years	1	6	4.5	9.8
Sex, female	1	7	10.1	9.6
Maximum score	9	8	14.2	6.7
—		9	100	15.2

CHF, Congestive heart failure; *LV,* left ventricle; *MI,* myocardial infarction; *PAD,* peripheral artery disease; *TE,* thromboembolism, *TIA,* transient ischemic attack.

[a] Theoretical TE rates without therapy, adjusted for aspirin use, assuming aspirin provides 22% reduction in TE risk. Modified from Lip GYH, Nieuwlaat R, Pisters R, Lane DA, Crijns HJGM. *Chest* 2010;137:263-272.

[b] Theoretical TE rates without therapy, adjusted for warfarin use, assuming warfarin provides 64% reduction in TE risk. Modified from Lip GYH, Frison L, Halperin JL, Lane DA. *Stroke.* 2010;41:2731-2738.

Modified from European Heart Rhythm Association; European Association for Cardio-Thoracic Surgery, Camm AJ, et al. Guidelines for the management of atrial fibrillation. Eur Heart J. 2010;31:2369-2429.

TABLE 5.7

SUMMARY OF RECOMMENDATIONS FOR RISK-BASED ANTITHROMBOTIC THERAPY

Recommendations	COR	LOE
Antithrombotic therapy based on shared decision making, discussion of risks of stroke and bleeding, and patient's preferences	I	C
Selection of antithrombotic therapy based on risk of thromboembolism	I	B
CHA$_2$DS$_2$-VASc score recommended to assess stroke risk	I	B
Warfarin recommended for mechanical heart valves and target INR intensity based on type and location of prosthesis	I	B
With prior stroke, TIA, or CHA$_2$DS$_2$-VASc score ≥ 2, oral anticoagulants recommended. Options include:		
Warfarin	I	A
Dabigatran, rivaroxaban, or apixaban	I	B
With warfarin, determine INR at least weekly during initiation of therapy and monthly when stable	I	A
Direct thrombin or factor Xa inhibitor recommended if unable to maintain therapeutic INR	I	C
Reevaluate the need for anticoagulation at periodic intervals	I	C
Bridging therapy with UFH or LMWH recommended with a mechanical heart valve if warfarin is interrupted. Bridging therapy should balance risks of stroke and bleeding	I	C
For patients without mechanical heart valves, bridging therapy decisions should balance stroke and bleeding risks against duration of time patient will not be anticoagulated	I	C
Evaluate renal function before initiation of direct thrombin or factor Xa inhibitors, and reevaluate when clinically indicated and at least annually	I	B
For atrial flutter, antithrombotic therapy is recommended as for AF	I	C
With nonvalvular AF and CHA$_2$DS$_2$-VASc score of 0, it is reasonable to omit antithrombotic therapy	IIa	B
With CHA$_2$DS$_2$-VASc score ≥ 2 and end-stage CKD (CrCl < 15mL/min) or on hemodialysis, it is reasonable to prescribe warfarin for oral anticoagulation	IIa	B
With nonvalvular AF and a CHA$_2$DS$_2$-VASc score of 1, no antithrombotic therapy or treatment with oral anticoagulant or aspirin may be considered	IIb	C
With moderate-to-severe CKD and CHA$_2$DS$_2$-VASc scores ≥ 2, reduced doses of direct thrombin or factor Xa inhibitors may be considered	IIb	C
For PCI, BMS may be considered to minimize duration of DAPT	IIb	C
After coronary revascularization in patients with CHA$_2$DS$_2$-VASc score ≥ 2, it may be reasonable to use clopidogrel concurrently with oral anticoagulants but without aspirin	IIb	B
Direct thrombin dabigatran and factor Xa inhibitor rivaroxaban are not recommended in patients with AF and end-stage CKD or on dialysis because of a lack of evidence from clinical trials regarding the balance of risks and benefits	III: No Benefit	C
Direct thrombin inhibitor dabigatran should not be used with a mechanical heart valve	III: Harm	B

AF indicates atrial fibrillation; *BMS*, bare-metal stent; *CHA$_2$DS$_2$-VASc*, Congestive heart failure, Hypertension, Age $\geq$ 75 years (doubled), Diabetes mellitus, Prior Stroke or TIA or thromboembolism (doubled), Vascular disease, Age 65 to 74 years, Sex category; *CKD*, chronic kidney disease; *COR*, Class of Recommendation; *CrCl*, creatinine clearance; *DAPT*, dual antiplatelet therapy; *INR*, international normalized ratio; *LMWH*, low-molecular-weight heparin; *LOE*, Level of Evidence; *N/A*, not applicable; *PCI*, percutaneous coronary intervention; *TIA*, transient ischemic attack; and *UFH*, unfractionated heparin.
From January CT, Wann LS, Alpert JS, et al. 2014 AHA/ACC/HRS guideline for the management of patients with atrial fibrillation: a report of the American College of Cardiology/American Heart Association Task Force on Practice Guidelines and the Heart Rhythm Society. J Am Coll Cardiol 2014;64:e1–76.

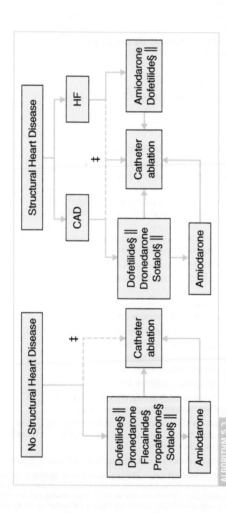

ALGORITHM 5.3
Rhythm control strategies for atrial fibrillation. *CAD,* Coronary artery disease; *HF,* heart failure. *(Reproduced with permission from January CT, Wann LS, Alpert JS, et al. 2014 AHA/ACC/HRS guideline for the management of patients with atrial fibrillation. J Am Coll Cardiol. 2014;64:2246-2280.)*

Anticoagulation Around the Time of Electrical or Pharmacologic Cardioversion

For AF of 48 hours in duration or more, or when duration is unknown, anticoagulation with warfarin (e.g., warfarin, INR ≥2.0, target 2.0 to 3.0) or a NOAC is recommended for at least 3 weeks before and 4 weeks after cardioversion. If the patient appears to be at risk for recurrence of AF and the CHADS$_2$-VASc score is at least 2, long-term anticoagulation is recommended. For AF of more than a 48-hour duration requiring immediate cardioversion due to hemodynamic instability, heparin should be administered concurrently (unless contraindicated) by an initial IV bolus followed by a continuous infusion (activated partial thromboplastin time [aPTT] 1.5 to 2 times control). Thereafter therapeutic oral anticoagulation should be provided for at least 4 weeks, as it is for patients undergoing elective cardioversion. Some data support subcutaneous administration of low-molecular-weight heparin for heparin. Another option is to initiate a NOAC to achieve immediate anticoagulation. For AF of less than 48 hours in duration associated with hemodynamic instability (shock, pulmonary edema), angina, or MI, cardioversion should be performed immediately without delaying for initiation of anticoagulation. As an alternative to 3 weeks of anticoagulation before cardioversion of AF, it is reasonable to perform TEE to exclude left atrial thrombus. For patients with no identifiable thrombus, cardioversion may be performed immediately if achievement of therapeutic anticoagulation with heparin, warfarin, or a NOAC has been achieved. For patients with an identified thrombus, oral anticoagulation (if warfarin, INR 2.0 to 3.0) should be administered for at least 4 to 6 weeks before and 4 weeks, often longer or indefinitely, after restoration of sinus rhythm. Another TEE may be considered prior to cardioversion to determine if the thrombus has resolved. For all patients undergoing cardioversion, long-term anticoagulation beyond the 4 weeks after cardioversion should be considered if other indications for long-term anticoagulation also exist, often based on the CHA2DS2-VASc score (Table 5.8, Algorithms 5.4 to 5.9).

ATRIAL FLUTTER

Description

AFL (Fig. 5.14) is a common, macroreentrant AT that occurs frequently in patients who also have AF; AFL may be the precursor of AF in up to approximately 5% to 10% of cases. The incidence of AFL is lower than that of AF.

Text continued on p. 179

TABLE 5.8

ATRIAL FIBRILLATION APPROACH TO THERAPY

Outpatient management versus inpatient management	• Inpatient management is indicated for patients with moderate and severe symptoms (angina, syncope, CHF); impaired LV function; hypotension; uncontrolled ventricular rate; initiation of antiarrhythmic drugs sotalol, dofetilide, quinidine, procainamide, disopyramide, or high-dose amiodarone; initiation of antiarrhythmic drugs when AF has been permanent or persistent for a long period of time (e.g., months), as pharmacologic conversion may be associated with long postconversion pauses and symptomatic SB. See Acute therapy below.
	• Anticoagulation: Warfarin, low-molecular-weight heparin or a NOAC can be started as an inpatient or outpatient (heparin as an inpatient). All episodes of AF lasting longer than 24–48 h should be anticoagulated if cardioversion is being considered and anticoagulation should be continued during and after cardioversion for at least 1 month or longer depending on the CHA2DS2VASc score.
	• Outpatient management may be acceptable for patients with absent or mild symptoms; no heart failure; controlled ventricular rate; paroxysmal AF; and patients with no cardiac disease and normal LV function.
	• Outpatient treatment: Flecainide and propafenone can be used and initiated in the outpatient setting in patients with paroxysmal AF and no structural heart disease. Amiodarone can be started at doses of 200–600 mg/day in stable patients with structural heart disease. DCC can be accomplished in an anticoagulated patient on or off antiarrhythmic drugs.
Acute therapy, symptomatic with rapid rates	• Ventricular rate control. Cardiac monitoring may be helpful.
	• If good LV function (>0.40 LVEF), β-adrenergic blockers (IV esmolol or metoprolol or oral metoprolol, propranolol, or atenolol), or Ca²⁺ channel blockers (IV or oral diltiazem, verapamil) to keep ventricular rate <110 bpm at rest. LV function should be assessed, as additional or stricter rate control, especially with exercise, may be required if there is LV dysfunction. Digoxin is a second-line drug because better rate control can be achieved with β-adrenergic blockers and Ca²⁺ blockers than with digoxin. May combine drugs if rate not controlled, but extreme caution should be used when using both β-adrenergic blockers and calcium channel blockers together. If LV dysfunction (LVEF <0.40) or CHF is present, digoxin may be used as adjunctive therapy. Because the goal is to lower ventricular rate, there is no absolute contraindication to use of β-adrenergic blockers or calcium channel blockers in patients with LV dysfunction; caution and monitoring are required.
	• DCC—Emergent if hypotensive, ischemic, pulmonary edema (only after and with necessary anticoagulation as indicated).
	• Digoxin has a longer onset of action and may increase risk of DCC to sinus rhythm if levels are high; it may also cause irreversible VF. Checking digoxin levels if time permits is advised. If cardioversion is nonemergent, holding digoxin on the day of the procedure is advised.

Chronic therapy	○ Rate-control drug therapy—poor LV function: digoxin, β-adrenergic blocker as tolerated; good LV function—diltiazem, verapamil, β-adrenergic blocker.
	○ Rhythm-control drug therapy: Sinus rhythm may be preferable if the patient has symptoms or CHF despite adequate rate control. LV function may improve with rate or rhythm control if prior rates have been rapid. There is no evidence that longevity is increased with a rhythm control approach.
	○ Risk of recurrent AF after cardioversion is approximately 50%, perhaps slightly less when amiodarone is used. However, the goal of medical therapy to control the rhythm is to decrease symptoms of AF, not necessarily complete suppression of AF, which might require higher doses of antiarrhythmic drugs that might risk side effects or toxicity.
Conversion to sinus rhythm	○ Pharmacologic conversion: IV ibutilide (1 mg over 10 min and give another 1 mg over 10 min if the rhythm does not convert to sinus and the QT <500 ms), procainamide, or amiodarone may convert AF; amiodarone may not convert the rhythm until several hours have passed. Oral regimens may be effective in approximately 30% to 70% of patients, particularly if given early after onset of the AF. Vernakalant is still investigational. N.B. Make sure the patient is properly anticoagulated.
	○ **First line:** Electrical cardioversion of AF.
	1. Proper patch or paddle placement is essential: Anterior–posterior patch positioning may be more effective in converting AF, but repositioning or pressure application to patches may be required if initial attempts are unsuccessful.
	2. Always synchronize the shock to the QRS to avoid ventricular fibrillation; check the cardioverter ECG to assess the displayed point of shock delivery.
	3. Always use general anesthesia if the patient is awake.
	4. Start with 100-200 J (biphasic shock), and increase the output to 200-360 J if needed. Biphasic shocks require lower energies and have been associated with higher efficacy.
	5. May give two to five shocks at one sitting, if necessary, particularly if starting at lower energies. If ineffective in one vector, change patch location. Make sure there is adequate contact and pressure of the patches with the patient.
	6. Sometimes intracardiac shocks in the right atrium will convert a patient if external shocks are ineffective.
	○ If cardioversion is not successful, there are possible sequelae:
	1. No return of sinus rhythm. Consider patch placement, contact, and vector of energy delivery; may need to try biphasic or higher energy shocks. Consider use of drugs associated with lower atrial defibrillation thresholds (e.g., sotalol, ibutilide) prior to a repeat attempt.
	2. Immediate recurrence of AF. Consider use of or alternative antiarrhythmic drugs (including IV verapamil and ibutilide) and repeat cardioversion, or consider ablation.

Continued on following page

TABLE 5.8

ATRIAL FIBRILLATION APPROACH TO THERAPY (Continued)

Maintenance of sinus rhythm	• Conversion to and maintenance of sinus rhythm may be preferable in new-onset AF, younger patients, and patients with symptoms despite ventricular rate control.
	• Maintenance of sinus rhythm has not been associated with reduced thromboembolic risk in patients in whom anticoagulation has been discontinued; consider long-term anticoagulation with warfarin or a NOAC as indicated or aspirin plus clopidogrel therapy.
	• It is acceptable to cardiovert a patient either electrically or pharmacologically; for a patient with one episode or rare episodes of AF, drugs may not need to be continued.
	• The duration of episodes of AF inversely correlates with success in maintaining sinus rhythm.
	• Patients with recurrences often require long-term oral antiarrhythmic drug therapy.
	• Repeat DC shocks on drug therapy may be needed, but if AF is infrequent, there may be no need to change drugs.
	• Nonpharmacologic therapies: Catheter ablation directed toward pulmonary vein ostial sources/isolation, surgical pulmonary vein isolation, or the Maze procedure and variants.
	• "Pill in the pocket" approach—Can be useful in some patients with lone AF and rare episodes. AF may be shortened or converted using PRN doses of flecainide or propafenone. AV nodal blocking drugs may also be required.
Recurrent episodes after cardioversion	• Antiarrhythmic drugs used for AF include class IC drugs used in the absence of LV dysfunction or CAD (flecainide, propafenone), class IA drugs (procainamide, disopyramide, quinidine), and class III drugs (sotalol, dronedarone, dofetilide, amiodarone). Selection of drugs is based on the presence or absence of structural heart disease, age, and proarrhythmia risk.
	• Recurrent episodes do not necessarily mean the drug is not useful. If a drug has prevented frequent recurrences but there is an occasional recurrence (e.g., one to two times per year), it is reasonable to continue the drug and cardiovert the patient intermittently as long as the patient is fully anticoagulated.
	• Frequent, symptomatic recurrent episodes mean the drug therapy may not be successful. Another drug or changing to a rate-control drug alone or nonpharmacologic approaches (AF ablation/pulmonary vein isolation, AV junction ablation with adjunctive pacing) should be considered.

Nonresponders to cardioversion or antiarrhythmic drugs

- Rate control with digoxin, Ca²⁺ channel blockers (verapamil, diltiazem), β-adrenergic blockers may be used. If necessary as a second-line drug, amiodarone can help to control the rate.

- Catheter ablation or isolation of sites initiating AF, typically at the pulmonary vein ostia, may be curative. Risks include a small but improving (with improved techniques) risk of pulmonary vein stenosis and risk of stroke during the procedure. The first few months after catheter ablation can be associated with frequent recurrences of AF or AFL, which are generally short lived. Catheter ablation may be performed as adjunctive therapy to antiarrhythmic drug therapy for AF associated with AFL.

- Surgical pulmonary vein isolation or the surgical maze procedure has been performed for primary cure of AF or as a concomitant procedure with other cardiac surgery, such as mitral valve procedures.

- If rate control cannot be achieved, AV nodal ablation can be performed with implantation of a permanent rate-responsive pacemaker: VVI(R) if permanent AF, DDD(R) if paroxysmal AF. These patients may have a wide QRS rate of 35 to 40/min (originating in fascicular of ventricular tissue). Functional LBBB caused by right ventricular pacing can induce LV dyssynchrony and a fall in LVEF. When a permanent pacemaker is placed after AV junctional ablation, the rate should be programmed initially at 90/min to avoid relative bradycardia-dependent ventricular arrhythmias; the pacing rate can be reduced to optimal levels after 2 to 3 months.

Drug interactions to consider

- Amiodarone will increase the INR and prothrombin time in patients taking coumarin derivatives and increase the time that the prothrombin time remains elevated.

- Amiodarone will increase (nearly double) digoxin levels and will have a synergistic effect with digoxin on AV node blockade.

- Quinidine, rarely used today, will increase digoxin levels.

- A class IA drug used without an AV nodal blocking drug can cause exceedingly rapid ventricular rates in AF.

- Class IC drug (flecainide, propafenone) and other antiarrhythmic drugs may reduce AF recurrences, but a recurrence may manifest as AFL with 1:1 AV conduction. Thus AV node-blocking drugs are usually used concomitantly with IC drugs.

- Approximately 7% of patients taking propafenone are slow metabolizers and may manifest significant β-adrenergic blocker effects. In this situation additional AV node blockers must be used with caution.

Continued on following page

TABLE 5.8

ATRIAL FIBRILLATION APPROACH TO THERAPY (Continued)

Slow ventricular response (<60, independent of drug therapy)	• Avoid drugs that may slow ventricular response, unless necessary to treat another condition (e.g., heart failure); consider permanent pacing for ventricular rate support in these cases.
	• If symptomatic, may attempt cardioversion, but postconversion resulting rhythm may be an escape rhythm and may be slow.
	• If AF with long pauses (more than 3 s in sinus rhythm, or 5 s in AF, or escape rate <40 bpm): permanent VVI(R) pacemaker if paroxysmal, DDD(R) pacing system.
	• Usually reflects underlying AV node or sinus node disease.
	• Be prepared to pace temporarily at the time of cardioversion; up to 15% of DCC for AF can be associated with postconversion pauses or bradycardia. Have atropine, isoproterenol, a secure IV, and an external (transcutaneous) pacemaker immediately available.
	• Do not cardiovert if there is a possibility of digoxin toxicity (check digoxin level, hold dose the morning of the procedure).
Regular ventricular response (no possibility of digoxin toxicity)	• Indicates high-grade or CHB, make sure that the atrial rhythm is not AFL with fixed AV conduction ratio.
	• If CHB with a slow ventricular rate, permanent pacing is usually indicated.
Digoxin toxicity possible	• Usually presents with high-degree or complete AV block with either an accelerated junctional rhythm or a slow QRS rhythm originating in ventricular tissue.
	• Electrical DCC is contraindicated due to the risk of life-threatening VF.
	• Check digoxin level.
	• Correct electrolyte imbalances, consider FAb fragment therapy; watchful waiting is often the best approach.
	• Do not give digoxin or verapamil. May give IV procainamide to slow conduction in the accessory pathway, or ibutilide.
Wide QRS complexes (WPW suspected)	• IV β-adrenergic blocker (esmolol or metoprolol) can be used with caution, as hypotension may result.
	• Cardiovert if not tolerated.
Wide QRS Due to BBB	• May be due to preexisting or rate-dependent BBB; check a prior ECG if available.
	• May treat with AV nodal blockers.

Preoperative

- For cardiac surgery, convert to NSR if adequate anticoagulation has been achieved or ensure that ventricular response is well controlled.

- If surgery is elective and AF is chronic, antiarrhythmic drugs or catheter ablation may be considered. However, anticoagulation should be continued at least 3 weeks after conversion of longer-term (>48 h) AFL prior to elective surgery. Anticoagulation should be stopped for surgery, and this depends on which one is being used. For NOACs, only a few days are needed. For warfarin, it is 3-7 days.

- If the AF is well tolerated and asymptomatic and/or longstanding and if there is adequate rate control, anticoagulation can be stopped for surgery, and surgery can proceed with adequate monitoring during surgery if possible at time of surgery.

- For more urgent surgery in which anticoagulation cannot be used, consider rate control without cardioversion or start a NOAC postoperatively when risk of bleeding is low.

- For short-duration (<48 h) AF, DCC can be performed (may consider heparin/NOAC before DCC).

Postoperative

- AF occurs in 10% to 30% of all patients after cardiac surgery or major thoracic surgery (50% if there is valve surgery). The incidence peaks at days 2 to 3. It is more common in older patients. It rarely occurs after other types of surgery but management is similar. AF may resolve spontaneously; however, the rhythm can increase the length of hospital stay, exacerbate heart failure, slow the recovery process, and cause symptoms.

- In patients undergoing major cardiac or thoracic surgeries with high risk for postoperative AF, prophylactic amiodarone or β-blockers can be considered.

- Control rate with β-adrenergic blocker if no CHF or bronchospastic disease and good LVEF (>40%). Diltiazem is often successful as a second-line drug, but use with caution in patients with poor LVEF. Digoxin for rate control is less effective but may be considered particularly in patients with poor LV function.

- IV then oral amiodarone may be useful for persistent, poorly tolerated and/or recurrent AF; it may be continued 4-6 weeks after surgery in a tapering dose.

- DCC is often successful though AF may recur and may be best used if highly symptomatic or impossible to control rate and BP. Anticoagulation recommendations for DCC should be followed, especially if AF duration is >48 h.

- Discontinue inotropic drugs, if possible.

AFL, Atrial flutter; *AF* atrial fibrillation; *CHF,* congestive heart failure; *CHB,* complete heart block; *DCC,* direct current cardioversion; *ECG,* electrocardiogram; *IV,* intravenous; *LV,* left ventricle; *LVEF,* left ventricular ejection fraction; *NOAC,* non-vitamin K oral anticoagulants; *NSR,* normal sinus rhythm; *PRN,* pro rata nata; *SB,* sinus bradycardia; *VF,* ventricular fibrillation *WPW,* Wolff-Parkinson-White.

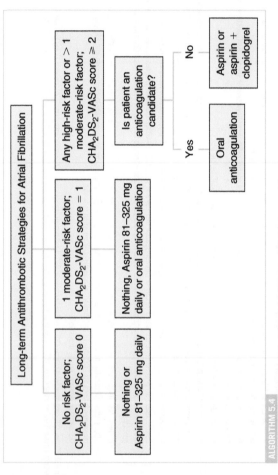

ALGORITHM 5.4

Long-term antithrombotic therapy for atrial fibrillation. See Table 5.6 for CHA$_2$DS$_2$-VASc and CHADS$_2$ scoring and Table 5.7 for risk factor categorization. Aspirin dosage 81 to 325 mg daily. Oral anticoagulation = warfarin (INR 2.0 to 3.0, target 2.5) or an NOAC 150 mg BID.

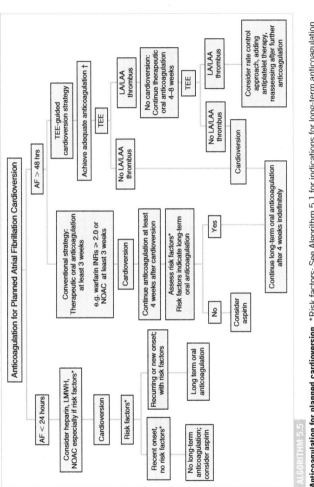

Anticoagulation for planned cardioversion. *Risk factors: See Algorithm 5.1 for indications for long-term anticoagulation by risk factors. †Oral anticoagulation=warfarin (INR 2.0 to 3.0, target 2.5) or dabigatran 75 to 150 mg BID. *AF,* Atrial fibrillation; *NOACs,* non-vitamin K oral anticoagulants; *TEE,* transesophageal echocardiography.

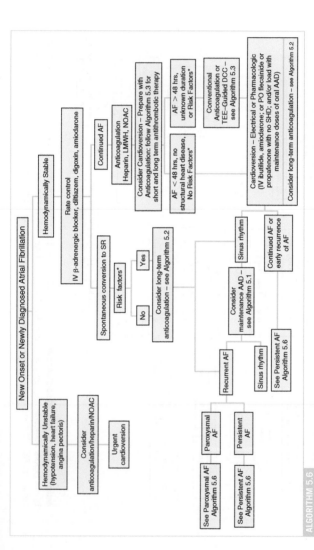

ALGORITHM 5.6

New onset or newly diagnosed atrial fibrillation. *Risk factors = risk factors for thromboembolism/stroke: see Tables 5.6 and 5.7. *AAD,* Antiarrhythmic drug; *AF,* atrial fibrillation; *IV,* intravenous; *NOACs,* non-vitamin K oral anticoagulants; *SHD,* structural heart disease (no overt evidence of myocardial, valvular, congenital, or coronary heart disease); *SR,* sinus rhythm; *TEE,* transesophageal echocardiography.

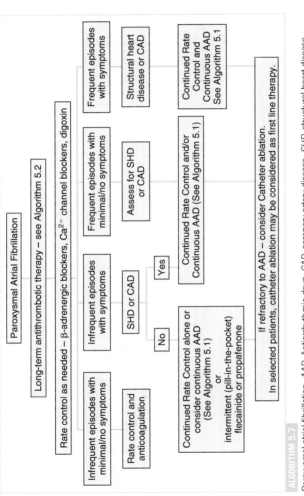

ALGORITHM 5.7

Paroxysmal atrial fibrillation. *AAD,* Antiarrhythmic drug; *CAD,* coronary artery disease; *SHD,* structural heart disease (no overt evidence of myocardial, valvular, congenital, or coronary heart disease).

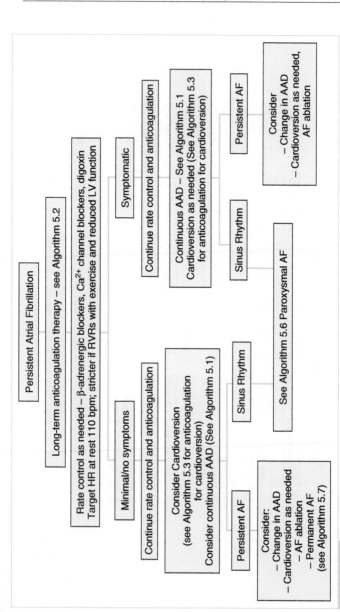

ALGORITHM 5.8

Persistent atrial fibrillation. *AAD,* Antiarrhythmic drug; *AF,* atrial fibrillation; *HR,* heart rate; *LV,* left ventricle; *RVR,* rapid ventricular rates.

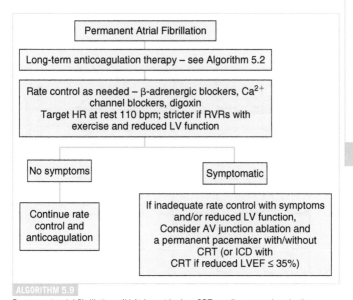

ALGORITHM 5.9

Permanent atrial fibrillation. *AV,* Atrioventricular; *CRT,* cardiac resynchronization therapy; *HR,* heart rate; *ICD,* implantable cardioverter-defibrillator; *LV,* left ventricular; *RVR,* rapid ventricular rate.

There are several types of AFL. Typical AFL (type I or isthmus-dependent AFL) is due to macroreentry within the right atrium, typically occurring in a counterclockwise direction (Fig. 5.15), proceeding craniocaudally down the free wall, through the cavotricuspid isthmus between the tricuspid valve and inferior vena cava, and caudalcranially up the atrial septum. Looking at the tricuspid valve from below, electrical activation around the valve occurs in a counterclockwise direction. Activation of the left atrium is passive. This depolarization sequence results in the inscription of the typical sawtooth flutter waves that are usually or mainly negative in the inferior leads (II, III, aVF); they often deform the ST segments, causing pseudo-ST elevation and pseudo-ST depression patterns. In lead V_1, because this is an anteroposterior lead, flutter waves are inscribed as discrete upright P waves. Clockwise reentry can also occur around the tricuspid valve (Fig. 5.16), inscribing positive flutter waves in the inferior leads. In this form of AFL, discrete upright P waves will also be recorded in lead V_1. Type I AFL can be terminated with atrial overdrive pacing in some patients and can be cured (with success rates of 75% to 90%) by catheter ablation, which creates a line of conduction block across the cavotricuspid isthmus. The isthmus is present between the tricuspid valve and the inferior vena cava.

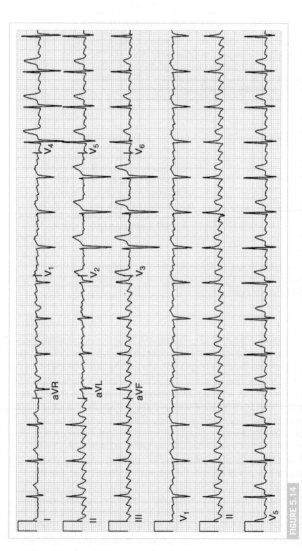

FIGURE 5.14

Typical atrial flutter. This 12-lead ECG and leads V₁, II, and V₅ rhythm strip shows AFL with 4:1 AV conduction and an overall ventricular rate of approximately 80 bpm. The sawtooth flutter wave pattern in the inferior leads is characteristic of typical, or type I, AFL. Typical AFL usually represents counterclockwise activation around the right atrium through the cavotricuspid isthmus.

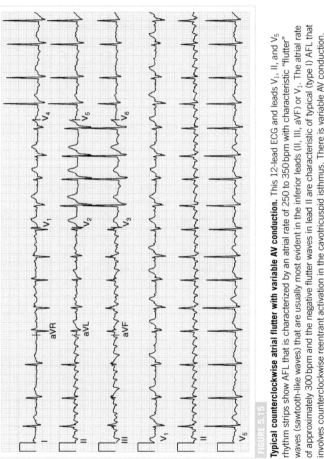

FIGURE 5.15

Typical counterclockwise atrial flutter with variable AV conduction. This 12-lead ECG and leads V_1, II, and V_5 rhythm strips show AFL that is characterized by an atrial rate of 250 to 350 bpm with characteristic "flutter" waves (sawtooth-like waves) that are usually most evident in the inferior leads (II, III, aVF) or V_1. The atrial rate of approximately 300 bpm and the negative flutter waves in lead II are characteristic of typical (type I) AFL that involves counterclockwise reentrant activation in the cavotricuspid isthmus. There is variable AV conduction.

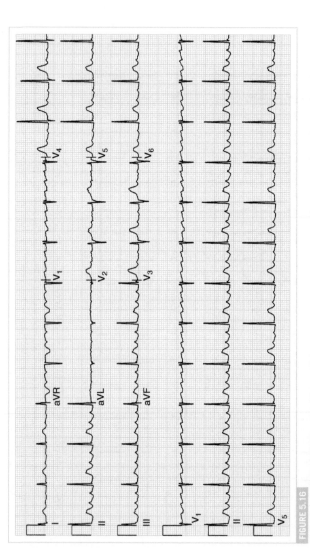

FIGURE 5.16

Typical clockwise atrial flutter. This 12-lead ECG tracing with rhythm strips shows AFL with 4:1 AV conduction. However, in contrast to Fig. 5.15, the flutter waves in lead II, III, and aVF are upright, consistent with reentry around the cavotricuspid isthmus in a clockwise direction, although other forms of AFL cannot be excluded.

It is just lateral to the os of the coronary sinus and the right atrial septum. Conduction block created within a reentry circuit will disallow perpetuation of the arrhythmia.

Type II AFL may be functionally determined without a necessary area of anatomic block. Atrial pacing may or may not terminate this type of AFL. This is a less common form of flutter and is associated with a relatively rapid atrial rate (Fig. 5.17).

There are other forms of right AFLs. These are non–isthmus-dependent right AFLs, including "upper loop reentry" and "lower loop reentry" tachycardias. These are macroreentrant tachycardias that use other circuits within the right atrium. Although these AFLs are also ablatable, they are more challenging than typical isthmus-dependent right AFLs.

Other forms of AFL include non–isthmus-dependent macroreentrant ATs originating from the left atrium. This type of flutter is often associated with AF; it is also associated with ablation of AF in which new anatomic pathways are created, determined by the ablation lesions themselves. Left AFLs also tend to occur in patients who have had cardiac surgery, in particular mitral valve surgery. Although these types of flutters can be ablatable, they are more challenging than isthmus-dependent right AFLs.

AFL may be due to reentry around areas of right or left atrial scars, including those caused by prior surgical incisions. For example, in patients who have had an atrial septal defect repair, reentry may occur around that repair area. The atrial rate is determined by atrial conduction time and the size of the macroreentrant pathway. The cavotricuspid isthmus is usually not a critical part of this type of circuit.

In the absence of antiarrhythmic medications that slow intraatrial or interatrial conduction, the atrial rate of typical (type I) AFL is 250 to 300 bpm, often associated with 2:1 AV conduction (Fig. 5.18), resulting in a regular ventricular rate of 150 bpm. Slower ventricular rates with higher AV conduction ratios (including Wenckebach conduction) can occur with AV nodal blocking drugs or in the setting of AV node system disease. The ventricular response often occurs with 2:1, 4:1 (see Fig. 5.15), or alternating 2:1/4:1 AV ratios; variable conduction patterns can be present as well. Thus the ventricular rhythm may be regular, or variable and irregular, or grouped, suggesting Wenckebach periodicity. A 1:1 AV conduction may be occasionally seen in hyperadrenergic states (Fig. 5.19) or preexcitation syndromes (WPW syndrome). IV adenosine can be used to elucidate the atrial rhythm in AFL with rapid ventricular rate.

Ventricular rate control is more difficult to achieve in AFL than in AF, as there is less decremental conduction in the AV node from atrial impulses in AFL compared with AF. Although the rate can be controlled at rest in many instances, minimal activity can lead to rapid rates, which are often highly symptomatic. In some instances, rate control is achieved but is very slow; termination of the flutter in these cases does not predict slow rates in sinus rhythm.

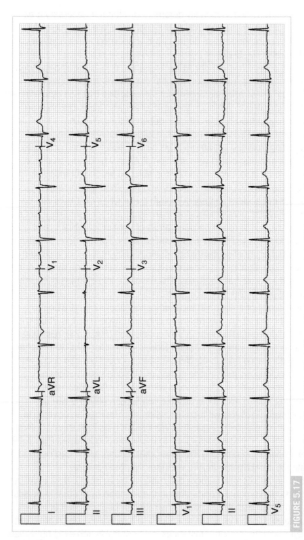

FIGURE 5.17

Atypical atrial flutter. This 12-lead ECG with rhythm strips shows atypical AFL/tachycardia that does not involve the cavotricuspid isthmus. The flutter waves lack the sawtooth morphology seen in typical AFL. There is 4:1 AV conduction.

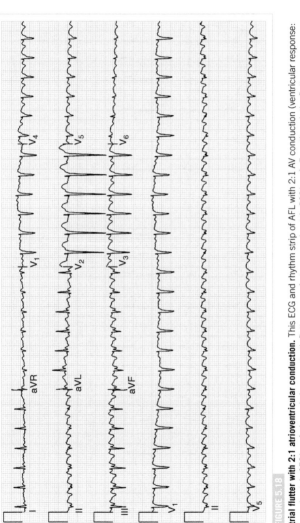

FIGURE 5.18

Atrial flutter with 2:1 atrioventricular conduction. This ECG and rhythm strip of AFL with 2:1 AV conduction (ventricular response: approximately 150 bpm) show obvious sawtooth flutter waves (rate: approximately 300 bpm). Even though the flutter waves are often superimposed on the ST segment, their prominence in lead II make the diagnosis relatively straightforward.

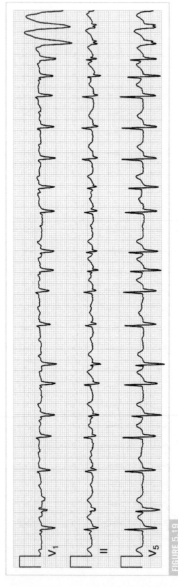

FIGURE 5.19

Atrial flutter/tachycardia with variable and then 1:1 atrioventricular conduction. This lead V_1, II, and V_5 rhythm strip shows AFL/tachycardia, which is most apparent in the first portion of the lead V_1 and II rhythm strips. Variable AV conduction is noted, at times resulting in a rapid (1:1) ventricular response (end of the strip). At the end of the tracing there is 1:1 ventricular response associated with aberrant conduction (that resembles ventricular tachycardia), and earlier in the tracing there are beats with aberrancy occurring after long–short coupling intervals. At the far right, when there are wide complex beats, the RR cycle lengths are similar to the atrial cycle lengths, supporting 1:1 AV conduction.

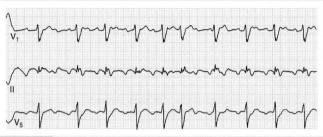

FIGURE 5.20

Slow atrial flutter. This lead V_1, II, and V_5 rhythm strip shows flutter-like waves in lead II, as well as lead V_1. Here the flutter rate is on the order of approximately 175 bpm. Although this is much slower than the typical AFL rate of 250 to 350 bpm, it represents a slow form of typical AFL with typical sawtooth flutter waves that are inverted in lead II and upright in V_1. In this case the patient was on a number of antiarrhythmic drugs that slowed the flutter rate below the normal range.

Atrial conduction can be slowed by class IA, IC, and III antiarrhythmic drugs (Fig. 5.20), leading to sufficient slowing of the atrial rate that 1:1 AV conduction occurs (e.g., the atrial rate may slow from 300 to 200 bpm, a rate at which the AV node may be able to conduct 1:1). Vagal maneuvers or IV adenosine may help to establish the diagnosis of AFL by enhancing AV block and slowing the ventricular rate enough to show flutter waves. Intracardiac atrial electrograms or esophageal electrograms may also be diagnostic. AFL is considered "the great pretender." It can mimic sinus rhythm, ectopic atrial rhythm, tachycardia, and/or RBBB (in lead V_1) and can produce ST abnormalities suggesting MI or QRS alternans by superposition of the flutter waves on the QRST complexes. Mimics of AFL include AF and sinus tachycardia.

Associated Conditions

AFL is often associated with underlying structural heart disease but may occur in structurally normal hearts. AFL often coexists with AF. Conditions associated with AFL are similar to those associated with AF and include CAD, rheumatic and nonrheumatic valve disease (especially mitral), cardiomyopathy, hypertension, pulmonary disease, hyperthyroidism, alcohol or caffeine use, pericarditis, acute MI (rare), pulmonary embolism, and congenital heart disease or its repair. A form of slow AFL is due to drug treatment of AF. If AFL is present in a young, healthy person, evaluation to rule out underlying structural heart disease should be undertaken.

Clinical Symptoms and Presentation

AFL may be paroxysmal or persistent. AFL commonly coexists with AF, and recurrences on antiarrhythmic drugs may present as AFL rather than AF. AFL may also occur in the postoperative state. AFL is usually symptomatic. Symptoms include palpitations, neck pounding (due to flutter waves occurring in proximity to the QRS complexes, like cannon waves), lightheadedness, shortness of breath, chest discomfort, fatigue, and effort intolerance.

Approach to Management (Algorithm 5.10)

The use of drugs to slow ventricular rate and to maintain sinus rhythm can be occasionally effective; however, there are few long-term controlled trials showing efficacy of drug therapy for AFL alone, and efficacy of antiarrhythmic drugs may be less than that for AF. Control of the ventricular rate often requires larger doses of AV nodal blocking drugs than for AF; these drugs include β-adrenergic blockers, verapamil, diltiazem, or digoxin. Digoxin is least effective because its AV nodal blocking effect is not direct but depends on vagal mechanisms; thus the vagolysis occurring during activity will reduce any benefit present at rest. Direct current cardioversion (DCC) is effective and requires lower energies (e.g., 25 to 100 J biphasic) than AF, but low-energy shocks may also initiate AF. Rapid atrial overdrive pacing may terminate type I AFL and may be useful, particularly after cardiac surgery in which temporary atrial pacing wires have been placed or if a permanent pacemaker with this capability has been implanted. Class IA, IC, or III antiarrhythmic drugs have been successfully used for control of atrial rate in AFL; however, use of drugs that slow atrial conduction may slow the AFL rate, allowing 1:1 AV conduction, occasionally with a wide QRS resembling VT. The use of concomitant AV nodal block drugs is generally required to prevent 1:1 AV conduction. Long-term treatment of AFL is often difficult with medications alone. Nonpharmacologic therapy, such as ablation, can cure typical or classic AFL in more than 90% of cases. Atypical or non–isthmus-dependent AFL may also be mapped and ablated, although with a lower success rate. Ablation of AFL has also been used successfully as adjunctive therapy in patients requiring antiarrhythmic therapy for AF but whose recurrences are in the form of AFL. If AFL requires urgent cardioversion, strategies for anticoagulation similar to AF should be used; if elective cardioversion is planned, TEE to rule out left atrial thrombus is recommended unless the patient has been anticoagulated for at least 3 to 4 weeks and, if anticoagulation is with warfarin, has had INR levels in the therapeutic range. Management of anticoagulation of AFL is the same as AF (Table 5.9).

ATRIOVENTRICULAR NODAL REENTRY TACHYCARDIA

Description

AVNRT (Fig. 5.21) is responsible for 60% to 70% of all paroxysmal regular SVTs. AVNRT uses the AV node and perinodal tissue. At least two functional and anatomic pathways of conduction are present in patients with AVNRT. In typical AVNRT a fast pathway conducts retrograde rapidly and a slow

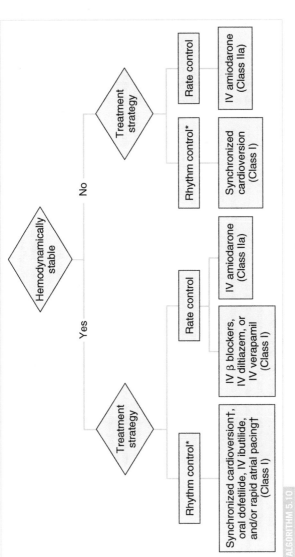

ALGORITHM 5.10

Acute treatment of atrial flutter. *Anticoagulation as per guideline is mandatory. †For rhythms that break or recur spontaneously, synchronized cardioversion, or rapid atrial pacing is not appropriate. *IV,* Intravenous. *(Reproduced with permission from Page RL et al. 2015 ACC/AHA/HRS Guideline for the Management of Adult Patients With Supraventricular Tachycardia. JACC 2016;67(13):e27-e115.)*

TABLE 5.9

ATRIAL FLUTTER THERAPY

| Acute therapy for poorly tolerated AFL or continuous rapid ventricular rate | <ul><li>If prolonged (i.e., >48 to 72 h), anticoagulation with heparin followed by therapeutic warfarin or a NOAC as cardioversion may be associated with thromboembolic risk. Anticoagulation guidelines for cardioversion are the same as for atrial fibrillation and may indicate need for a TEE for prolonged episodes. Adenosine and carotid massage can be used to help to diagnose AFL masquerading as sinus rhythm.</li><li>**First line:** DCC under anesthesia with anticoagulation as necessary. Consider the length of the episode.</li><li>**Second line:** Ibutilide or procainamide may be attempted for conversion prior to DCC attempts. Ibutilide may be 70% effective if AFL has been present for <48 h, although how often this is not known with certainty. Procainamide may help to maintain sinus rhythm.</li><li>**Alternate:** Rapid atrial pacing (esophageal, epicardial, or endocardial, depending on the situation). To pace terminate, pace for 10 to 15 s at a rate of 10% to 20% faster than rate of flutter. If ineffective, burst pace 10 bpm faster at a time for 10 to 15 s at a time until conversion to AF or sinus rhythm. Adding procainamide may help to pace termination efficacy; however, it may speed AV conduction if the ventricular response is not adequately controlled with AV nodal blocker drugs (see Chronic prevention, below); 20% to 30% will pace to AF and 10% to 20% will have no effect from pacing, depending on patient selection for the procedure. When AF occurs, it is usually short-lived and terminates spontaneously within 24 h. If persistent, DCC can be attempted with or without antiarrhythmic drugs. Rapid AFL (atrial rate >350) and atrial fib/flutter usually cannot be pace terminated. However, slower AFL (rate <350) of any flutter wave morphology can often be pace terminated.</li><li>Oral drug loading alone to terminate AFL is rarely useful.</li><li>If recurrent episodes, use class IC or III antiarrhythmic drugs until steady state achieved, then attempt cardioversion. These drugs (particularly 1C drugs) may stabilize the flutter circuit. It may also create another form of AFL—"1C" AFL—from AF. Ablation remains first-line therapy, especially if AFL is isthmus dependent.</li><li>Consider ablation for all persistent, refractory, or symptomatic AFL. However, despite AFL ablation, AF may occur, especially in individuals with underlying structural heart disease.</li><li>AV nodal ablation, although not preferable, could be considered when ventricular rate control cannot be achieved and flutter cannot be ablated, or if symptomatic, refractory, and/or if associated with tachycardia-induced cardiomyopathy. This option may be considered in cases where individuals have multiple forms of nonablatable AFL or AF and especially for those who do have non-isthmus-dependent AFL.</li></ul> |

Chronic prevention
- If structural heart disease without CHF: sotalol (initiate in the hospital), dofetilide, amiodarone.
- If structural heart disease with CHF: amiodarone, dofetilide.
- If no structural heart disease: propafenone, flecainide, sotalol, dofetilide, or amiodarone, but propafenone or flecainide may need concomitant AV nodal blocking drugs to prevent 1:1 conduction.
- If class I or III drugs are used, first control the ventricular response rate with an AV nodal blocking drug. Otherwise, the vagolytic effects of class IA drugs can enhance AV nodal conduction, and both 1A and 1C drugs can lead to AFL with 1:1 AV conduction.
- Drug therapy alone for pure AFL flutter is usually not effective.
- Consider radiofrequency catheter ablation early; it has become first-line therapy.

Nonresponders with severe symptoms
- If type I AFL, radiofrequency ablation of the right atrial isthmus.
- Atypical AFL is more difficult to ablate, and depends on the location of reentrant circuit. Success rates are lower than that for typical AFL. It is more difficult when there is congenital heart disease, valve disease, or prior surgery in which significant areas of scar are present.
- Ventricular rate control, antiarrhythmic drugs, or AV node ablation (less preferable) can be performed for atypical, nonablatable AFL.
- If AV node ablation and pacing is performed and AFL is intermittent, mode-switching function should be programmed "ON."

MI
- If hemodynamic intolerance or ongoing refractory myocardial ischemia, emergent cardioversion. AFL may increase MVO2 due to rapid ventricular rate, causing further ischemia, diastolic dysfunction, and pulmonary congestion and edema.
- If recurrent, IV amiodarone or procainamide.
- Consider temporary antitachycardia pacing if recurrent and poorly tolerated.

Preoperative
- For cardiac surgery, convert AFL to NSR if adequate anticoagulation has been achieved, or ensure that ventricular response is well controlled.
- If surgery is elective and AFL is chronic, antiarrhythmic drugs or catheter ablation may be considered. However, anticoagulation should be continued at least 3 weeks after conversion of longer-term (>48 h) AFL prior to elective surgery.
- For more urgent surgery in which anticoagulation cannot be used, consider rate control without cardioversion.
- For short-duration (<48h) AFL, DCC can be performed (may consider heparin prior to DCC with surgical consultation as to risk).

Continued on following page

TABLE 5.9

ATRIAL FLUTTER THERAPY (Continued)

Postoperative	• AFL occurs in 10-20% of all patients after cardiac surgery it typically occurs with AF. Incidence peaks at days 2-3. It is more common in older patients. It rarely occurs after other types of surgery. The AFL may resolve spontaneously; however, the rhythm can increase the length of hospital stay, exacerbate heart failure, slow the recovery process, and cause symptoms.
	• Control rate with β-adrenergic blocker if no CHF or bronchospastic disease and good LVEF (>40%). Diltiazem is often successful as a second-line drug, but use with caution in patients with poor LVEF. Digoxin for rate control is less effective but may be consider particularly in patients with poor LV function.
	• IV amiodarone may be useful for persistent and poorly tolerated AFL; amiodarone, or other antiarrhythmic drugs may be helpful for recurrent episodes.
	• DCC or atrial pace termination (if atrial pacing leads are present) is often successful, especially when employed early after the AFL onset.
	• Discontinue inotropic drugs, if possible.

AFL, Atrial flutter; *AF,* atrial fibrillation; *AV,* atrioventricular; *CHF,* congestive heart failure; *DCC,* direct current cardioversion; *IV,* intravenous; *LVEF,* left ventricular ejection fraction; *LV,* left ventricle; *MI,* myocardial infarction; *MVO2,* myocardial oxygen consumption; *NOAC,* non-vitamin K oral anticoagulants; *TEE,* transesophageal echocardiography.

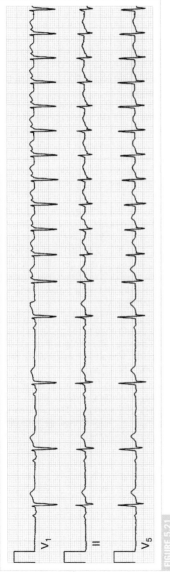

FIGURE 5.21

Atrioventricular nodal reentry tachycardia. This lead V_1, II, and V_5 rhythm strip shows a narrow QRS tachycardia that is AVNRT with antegrade conduction down the slow pathway and retrograde activation up the fast pathway of the AV node (AVN). The tracing begins with four beats of sinus rhythm. A premature atrial complex (seen deforming the T wave of the fourth complex) is conducted to the ventricle with a long PR interval (reflecting conduction down the slow AVN pathway). This is followed by a regular narrow QRS complex tachycardia. After the first beat of the SVT, retrograde P waves are best seen in V_1 as small R'-like deflections at the end of the QRS complexes. This demonstrates the very short RP interval (<90 ms) consistent with AVNRT and helps to distinguish AVNRT from other short RP tachycardias with a longer RP interval (>100 ms), such as AV reentrant tachycardia with an accessory pathway that conducts in the retrograde direction.

pathway conducts antegrade. The fast pathway typically has a longer refractory period than the slow pathway. During sinus rhythm, conduction through the AV node–His-Purkinje system occurs via the fast pathway; however, a premature atrial depolarization (the most common initiating event) that arrives at the fast pathway during its longer refractory period will encounter conduction block but may conduct, with a prolonged PR interval, over the slow pathway. If antegrade conduction is slow enough through the slow pathway that retrograde conduction up the fast pathway can occur, then AVNRT may develop.

In this typical, or common, form of AVNRT, anterograde conduction occurs via the slow AV node pathway and retrograde conduction up the fast pathway, resulting in a (usually) narrow QRS complex tachycardia with no P waves evident (see Fig. 5.21), except possibly at the very end of the QRS complex, which it deforms somewhat relative to the morphology during sinus rhythm. The rate of AVNRT is usually 150 to 200 bpm, although rates can be as high as 250 bpm. Initiation often occurs with a premature atrial (rarely a ventricular) depolarization that is followed by a long PR interval (blocked or delayed conduction in the fast pathway with conduction down the slow pathway) and P waves that are buried in or within 70 ms of the QRS complex. A pseudo-R′ in V_1 and pseudo-S wave in the inferior leads are characteristic features of the ECGs during AVNRT and represent the retrograde atrial activation. The pseudo-S wave in the inferior leads reflects the inverted P waves of retrograde atrial depolarization. Because the precordial leads have an anteroposterior and not a superoinferior axis, the retrograde P waves will not be inverted in V_1.

Another form, atypical, or uncommon, AVNRT, (Fig. 5.22) seen in 5% to 10% of patients with AVNRT is due to antegrade conduction via the fast pathway (producing a normal PR interval) and retrograde conduction via the slow pathway (causing a long RP interval) with negatively directed, inverted, P waves in the inferior leads (II, III, aVF).

A third of AVNRT uses two slow pathways ("slow-slow" AVNRT) and presents as a long RP tachycardia, resembling atypical AVNRT.

Occasionally, AVNRT can display QRS alternans. The precise mechanism is unknown but may relate to tachycardia rate; it does not indicate alternating conduction pathways to the ventricle.

Associated Conditions

AVNRT onset can begin at any age, and it commonly occurs in patients without structural heart disease. Approximately 70% of cases have been reported in women.

Clinical Symptoms and Presentation

AVNRT presentation varies from isolated episodes to incessant recurrences. It can be initiated in some instances by a high catecholamine state. AVNRT is rarely life-threatening but can be highly symptomatic. Symptoms range from palpitations, neck pounding, lightheadedness, weakness, anxiety,

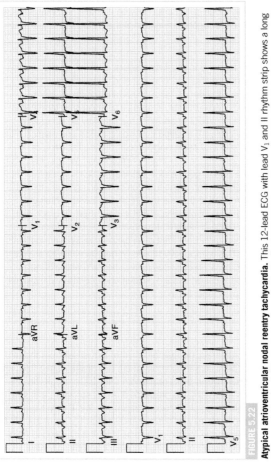

FIGURE 5.22

Atypical atrioventricular nodal reentry tachycardia. This 12-lead ECG with lead V₁ and II rhythm strip shows a long RP narrow complex tachycardia that represents atypical AVNRT (diagnosis made at EP study). Activation proceeds antegrade down the fast pathway of the AV node and then retrograde up the slow pathway, resulting in the long RP interval. The differential diagnosis for a long RP tachycardia includes AT and AV reentry tachycardia mediated by a concealed slowly conducting, decremental retrograde accessory pathway.

shortness of breath, and/or chest pain to angina, pulmonary congestion, near syncope, and frank syncope, depending in part on the presence and severity of underlying heart disease. Syncope can occur from the SVT rate itself as well as from reduction in stroke volume due to atrial contraction against closed AV valves and reflex hypotension due to atrial stretch and intraatrial pressure elevation resulting from the same mechanism. Dizziness and presyncope or syncope can occasionally be due to a period of asystole that sometimes can occur upon termination of the SVT.

Approach to Management (Algorithm 5.11)

Acute episodes can respond to vagal maneuvers, such as carotid sinus massage or the Valsalva maneuver; IV adenosine or IV verapamil (if the rhythm is unresponsive to adenosine) successfully terminates more than 90% of episodes. More than 90% of vagal or adenosine-terminable tachycardias are due to AVNRT or an AVRT mediated by an accessory pathway (discussed later). RF ablation cures both typical and atypical AVNRT in more than 95% of cases and is recommended as first-line therapy for patients with frequent or highly symptomatic recurrences. The approach to ablation is to target the slow pathway, which is located in the posterior-inferior septal portion of the junction between right atrium and right ventricle. Interruption of the reentry circuit disallows maintenance of the arrhythmia. The risk of ablation is that it may cause AV block, but that risk is less than 0.7% (in AVNRT, less in AVRT). Ablation should be considered for the long-term treatment of all patients who have recurrent episodes of AVNRT. This is especially true for young women who are likely to become pregnant, because episodes tend to become worse during pregnancy and medical treatments are difficult and potentially dangerous to the fetus at that time (Table 5.10).

JUNCTIONAL TACHYCARDIA

Description

JT (Fig. 5.23) is an automatic or triggered rhythm that arises from the AV node. It is generally persistent (nonparoxysmal). It is distinguished from an accelerated junctional rhythm by its rate (more than 100 bpm). It may be distinguishable from AVNRT by the presence of AV dissociation, unless it is associated with retrograde atrial depolarization with the P waves buried within the QRS complex. It may be difficult to distinguish JT from low AT. JT typically does not respond to carotid sinus massage. It may respond (slow or terminate) with adenosine, but it will gradually or abruptly reinitiate. Pacing can overdrive suppress this rhythm but will not terminate it.

Associated Conditions

This rhythm tends to occur after cardiac surgery, during acute MI (sometimes after fibrinolytic therapy), after cardioversion of AF, with myocarditis, during exercise (even in otherwise healthy individuals), with sinus node dysfunction,

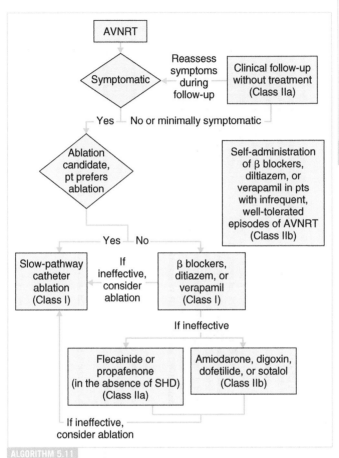

ALGORITHM 5.11

Ongoing management of AVNRT. *AVNRT,* Atrioventricular nodal reentrant tachycardia; *pt,* patient; *SHD,* structural heart disease. (*Reproduced with permission from Page RL et al. 2015 ACC/AHA/HRS Guideline for the Management of Adult Patients With Supraventricular Tachycardia. JACC 2016;67(13):e27-e115.*)

and, rarely today, with digitalis toxicity. The rhythm may be exacerbated by hypokalemia. Its natural history depends on the clinical setting. JT is relatively uncommon in adults and is more common in children.

Clinical Symptoms and Presentation

A loss of AV synchrony, when JT coexists with an independent atrial rhythm, or a loss of optimal AV relationships even when AV synchrony is

TABLE 5.10
ATRIOVENTRICULAR NODAL REENTRANT TACHYCARDIA THERAPY

Acute treatment, stable

- Vagal maneuvers (by physician): Valsalva (with patient in supine position) or carotid sinus massage (if no carotid bruits or history or evidence of cerebrovascular disease). If hypotensive (BP <90–100 mmHg) and rate is >220bpm, carotid massage is unlikely to be effective but Valsalva may work in supine or Trendelenburg positions. If stable, the patient can perform vagal maneuvers at home in the following order: Valsalva maneuver, diving reflex (immerse head in cold water for 1–2 s), gag reflex, cold water on face, and carotid sinus massage, provided that there is no known carotid disease or bruits.

- Adenosine 6-mg rapid IV bolus with a saline flush. If ineffective within 30–60 s, give a 12- to 18-mg bolus. If still ineffective, reassess the rhythm diagnosis. If the tachycardia simply slows in response to adenosine, it may be sinus tachycardia. Adenosine is successful in terminating AVNRT in >90% of patients if given properly. Side effects occur in >40% but usually last <1 min and include flushing, chest pain, and dyspnea (due to bronchospasm). Bronchospasm is the most serious side effect and can require immediate treatment. Drug half-life is 10 s. Adenosine effects are potentiated by dipyridamole and inhibited by (and will not work in the presence of) theophylline. Adenosine can precipitate atrial fibrillation, but this is usually self-limited and tends to occur at large doses. Adenosine should not be given to patients with heart transplant because asystole may ensue.

- Verapamil 5 to 15 mg IV over 5 min. Effect is seen within seconds to minutes. Success rate exceeds 90%. **Do not use in wide complex tachycardia (QRS >0.12 s) because the diagnosis of AVNRT may be incorrect. Verapamil is reserved for patients who have recurrent episodes of AVNRT after termination with adenosine.**

- Other drugs that may be effective but are rarely needed include diltiazem 0.25–0.35 mg/kg IV (compared with verapamil, less effective but also likely to cause hypotension), metoprolol 1–8 mg IV titrated over 15–30 min, or esmolol (50–250 µg/kg/min), especially if the AVNRT is exercise or anxiety induced.

- Nonresponders to above measures: DCC synchronized to the QRS complex (anesthetize, then 50J first shock).

Acute therapy, unstable (chest pain, severe dyspnea, hypotension, syncope, impaired consciousness)

- BP >90 mmHg, awake: Vagal maneuvers, if unsuccessful, adenosine 6 mg (additional 12 mg in 5 min if necessary). If unsuccessful, follow with synchronized DCC with anesthesia.

- BP <90 mmHg but rate >220 bpm and/or highly symptomatic, CHF or severe underlying cardiac disease: DCC.

CHF

- If acute pulmonary edema: Cardiovert.

- If not in pulmonary edema: Vagal maneuvers, as above; adenosine, as above.

Recurrences shortly after conversion to sinus rhythm

* Drug therapy to stabilize: IV diltiazem infusion or IV verapamil (preferable); metoprolol or esmolol if a short-acting β-adrenergic blocker is deemed preferable.

* Further therapy based on frequency of episodes, severity of symptoms, and tachycardia rate.

Chronic prevention (infrequent, well-tolerated, short-lived episodes)

* No specific therapy for a single or first episode.

* Instruct patient to avoid activities and stimulants (including caffeine) that are thought to initiate episodes.

* Instruct patient on vagal maneuvers: See Acute therapy, stable, comments above.

* Consider PRN medications such as β-adrenergic blockers, diltiazem, or verapamil, to be taken when episode occurs.

* EP study with RF ablation—considered as first-line therapy.

Chronic prevention, all others (frequent episodes, poorly tolerated or rapid rates [>220/min])

* **First line:** Catheter ablation of the slow pathway. Slow AV node pathway modification has a success rate >95%, has a low (<1%) risk of the need for a permanent pacemaker, and can be performed on an outpatient (23-h admission) basis. The cost to benefit ratio favors ablation if the patient is young and would otherwise require long-term drug therapy.

* **Second line: Drug therapy**

  ○ No CHF: Preferred drug class: β-adrenergic blocker (atenolol, acebutolol, metoprolol), especially if episodes are exertion or stress related. Alternatives (perhaps less effective but better tolerated): verapamil (long-acting preparation) or diltiazem.

  ○ CHF or decreased LVEF: β-adrenergic blockers, if tolerated, also for survival benefit in heart failure; digoxin (less effective).

  ○ If patient chooses trial of drug therapy but fails more than drugs, proceed to ablation.

Nonresponder

* First line: Catheter ablation.

* **Second line:** Drug therapy: AV nodal blockers first (β-adrenergic blockers, calcium channel blockers, digoxin)

  ○ No structural heart disease: Monotherapy with class IC drug (propafenone, flecainide). Class IC drugs may be initiated in the outpatient setting; they are rarely used and rarely needed. Less desirable alternative: class IA (quinidine, procainamide, disopyramide) given with one of drugs listed above (see Chronic prevention, all others). Disopyramide is not recommended for older males due to the high incidence of urinary retention and exacerbation of CHF. Class IA antiarrhythmic drugs are rarely used any more for AVNRT.

  ○ SHD: Monotherapy with class III drug (sotalol or amiodarone). Sotalol therapy should be initiated in the hospital, and should be avoided in patients with renal insufficiency. Amiodarone may be started as an outpatient. Class IC drugs should not be given to patients with structural heart disease or CAD.

Continued on following page

TABLE 5.10

ATRIOVENTRICULAR NODAL REENTRANT TACHYCARDIA THERAPY (Continued)

MI	• See Acute therapy above.
	• β-adrenergic blocker for 2 months if no prior history of AVNRT. If no previous history, onset after MI is likely due to high catecholamine levels and may not recur.
	• Not a rhythm of acute MI, although the rhythm can cause ischemia or non–Q wave MI (non-QMI).
	• Recurrence late after MI: Radiofrequency or cryo catheter ablation is the preferred option.
Preoperative	• Acute episode: see Acute therapy above.
	• History of AVNRT, now in sinus rhythm: see Chronic therapy. It is best to have this treated preoperative. If present and untreated preoperative, it may become worse in the perioperative period.
Postoperative	• No prior history of AVNRT, acute episode in postoperative period: see Acute therapy.
	• Do not initiate chronic therapy unless recurrence. If recurrence early postoperative, consider β-adrenergic blocker.
	• Surgery of all types is likely to exacerbate the arrhythmia due to high circulating catecholamines.
	• Previous history of AVNRT, acute episode postoperative: see Acute therapy and Chronic prevention.
Pregnancy	• Pregnancy tends to exacerbate the problem.
	• Avoid drug therapy if at all possible. If required, adenosine can be given. Digoxin or low-dose β-adrenergic blockers are probably safe.
	○ Consider RF or cryo catheter ablation after delivery if AVNRT is a major problem during pregnancy.

AV, Atrioventricular; *AVNRT,* atrioventricular nodal reentrant tachycardia; *BP,* blood pressure; *CAD,* coronary artery disease; *CHF,* congestive heart failure; *DCC,* direct current cardioversion; *EP,* electrophysiology; *IV,* intravenous; *LVEF,* left ventricular ejection fraction; *MI,* myocardial infarction; *PRN,* pro rata nata; *RF,* radiofrequency; *SHD,* structural heart disease.

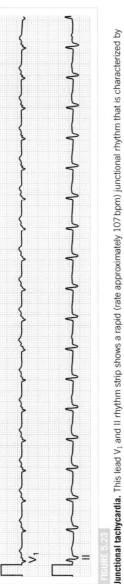

FIGURE 5.23

Junctional tachycardia. This lead V_1 and II rhythm strip shows a rapid (rate approximately 107 bpm) junctional rhythm that is characterized by retrograde P waves or the absence of P waves. These findings are consistent with a JT.

present, due to simultaneous AV activation or retrograde ventriculoatrial activation can cause hypotension, palpitations, fatigue, shortness of breath, low cardiac output, and symptoms of heart failure.

Approach to Management

Return to sinus rhythm may substantially improve hemodynamic function. A β-adrenergic blocker or a calcium channel blocker is the initial drug of choice. Alternatively, class I or class III antiarrhythmic drugs may be attempted. For persistent, recurrent symptomatic JT, ablation of the focal origin can be curative but is associated with a risk of AV block (Table 5.11).

TABLE 5.11

JUNCTIONAL TACHYCARDIA THERAPY

Paroxysmal	• No therapy unless poorly tolerated.
	• Remove offending drugs, such as digoxin.
	• Correct hypokalemia
	• Consider β-adrenergic blocker if frequent episodes.
Sustained	• **First line:** β-adrenergic blocker.
	• **Second line:** Calcium channel blocker. It may be suppressed, if necessary, by digoxin so long as the patient does not have digitalis toxicity.
	• If symptomatic and the above measures are ineffective, it may require suppression with antiarrhythmic drugs. If the patient has no structural heart disease, consider propafenone or flecainide; otherwise, sotalol is the drug of choice. Class IA antiarrhythmic drugs (e.g., procainamide) may also be beneficial. A final alternative is amiodarone.
	• In children (and some adults) with permanent junctional reentrant tachycardia (PJRT), the tachycardia is due to reentry involving a posterior-septal accessory pathway; radiofrequency ablation is curative.
	• The automatic form of JT does not respond to vagal stimulation or atropine.
	• Ablation of the focal origin is curative, although there is a risk of causing AV block.
MI	• If asymptomatic, no therapy. It is a common transient sequelae of inferior infarction. If acute and related to revascularization, it may represent a rhythm of reperfusion injury.
	• If symptomatic, first line is β-adrenergic blocker; second line is calcium channel blocker.
Preoperative	• Rule out digitalis toxicity.
	• If symptomatic, first line is β-adrenergic blocker; second line is calcium channel blocker.
	• This is not a contraindication to surgery.
Postoperative	• If highly symptomatic, first line is β-adrenergic blocker; second line is calcium channel blocker.
	• Can occur after CABG and valvular surgery.
	• Rule out digitalis toxicity.

AV, Atrioventricular; *CABG,* coronary artery bypass graft; *JT,* junctional tachycardia; *MI,* myocardial infarction; *PJRT,* permanent junctional reentrant tachycardia.

"Preexcitation syndrome" is a broad term delineating various conditions that can lead to several forms of SVT. Ventricular preexcitation is due to a connection of muscle fibers between the atria and the ventricles that lies outside the AV node (accessory pathway, Kent bundle). The connection allows conduction often in the antegrade and commonly in the retrograde direction. The accessory pathway can exist anywhere on the right or left side of the heart and/or in the septum. Conduction to the ventricles can occur entirely over the accessory pathway (maximal preexcitation), entirely over the AV node (no preexcitation), or via both pathways (fusion complexes, which can show minimal or more degrees of preexcitation). When conduction of an impulse proceeds antegradely down an accessory pathway and arrives at the ventricular tissue before it arrives via the AV node, there is an aberrant QRS complex because conduction to the ventricles is not proceeding entirely via the normal AV node–His-Purkinje pathway. Because there is little (or no) delay of impulse conduction at the AV node, the PR interval is shorter than normal, and there is a delta wave initiating the QRS complex, reflecting accessory pathway conduction directly from the atria into ventricular tissue. This pattern of a short PR interval and a delta wave is characteristic of WPW syndrome (Figs. 5.24 to 5.26). The vector of the delta wave on the ECG can predict the location of the accessory pathway. Approximately 10% to 15% of accessory pathways are associated with a second accessory pathway; individuals who have more than one pathway generally have a septal accessory pathway.

Ventricular preexcitation may be intermittent (Fig. 5.27) during monitoring and on the ECG, depending on the conduction properties of the accessory pathway and those of the AV node. Both of these can change with rate and with catecholamine levels. Most accessory pathways conduct in both the antegrade and retrograde directions. Accessory pathways that conduct only in the retrograde direction are "concealed" on the ECG. When this occurs, true ventricular preexcitation is not present.

Several tachycardias can arise due to the preexcitation syndrome related to a Kent bundle. The most common is orthodromic AVRT (Fig. 5.28). In orthodromic AVRT, electrical activation proceeds down the AV node–His-Purkinje system to the ventricles and then back retrogradely through the accessory pathway. Because ventricular depolarization occurs along the normal pathways, the tachycardia has a narrow, normal-appearing QRS complex unless BBB exists; ventricular preexcitation is not present, and therefore there will be no delta wave. Compared with AVNRT, this type of AVRT is distinctly different because the P wave may be visualized in the ST segment, rather than within or just after the QRS complex, and there is a short RP interval, but one that is longer than in typical AVNRT.

A less common tachycardia, occurring in only approximately 5% of cases of SVT due to ventricular preexcitation, is antidromic AVRT (Fig. 5.29).

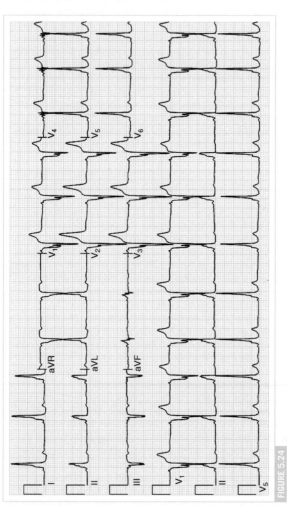

FIGURE 5.24

Wolff-Parkinson-White syndrome. This 12-lead ECG with rhythm strips shows preexcitation with an accessory pathway connecting the right atrium to the right ventricle. This gives rise to a pattern like LBBB because the ventricles are activated over the right-sided accessory pathway. The tracing shows the typical characteristics of WPW syndrome, including a short PR interval, a wide QRS complex, and a delta wave.

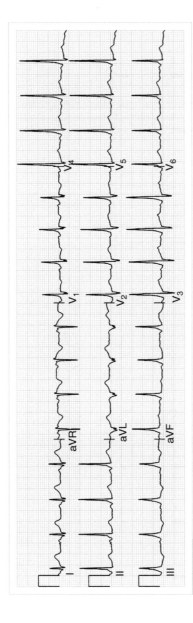

FIGURE 5.25

Wolff-Parkinson-White syndrome with a left lateral accessory pathway. This 12-lead ECG shows preexcitation with an accessory pathway connecting the left atrium to the left ventricle. This gives rise to a pattern like RBBB because the ventricles are activated over the left-sided accessory pathway. The tracing shows the typical characteristics of WPW syndrome, including a short PR interval, a wide QRS complex, and a delta wave. The negative delta wave in leads I and aVL suggest a left lateral accessory pathway that inserts to the lateral free wall of the left ventricle.

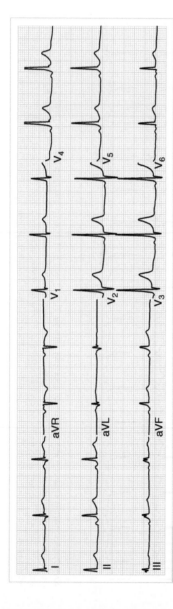

FIGURE 5.26

Wolff-Parkinson-White syndrome with left-sided accessory pathway (fused preexcitation). This 12-lead ECG shows sinus rhythm with preexcitation, but here the findings are more subtle. Although there is a short PR interval and delta wave, which indicate that the patient has WPW syndrome, the degree of preexcitation is less than in the preceding tracing with an intermediate QRS duration of 110ms. Antegrade conduction down the AV node and down the bypass tract fuse in a way that produces a more narrow QRS complex. The positive delta waves in V_1–V_3 suggest that this also is a left-sided accessory pathway. The negative delta waves in I and aVL also are consistent with a left lateral accessory pathway.

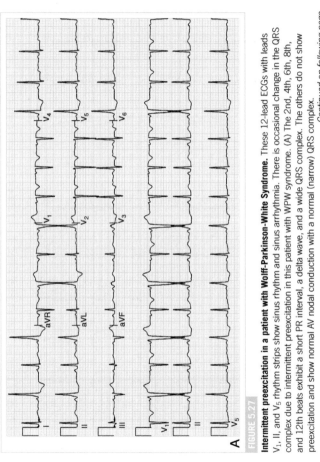

FIGURE 5.27

Intermittent preexcitation in a patient with Wolff-Parkinson-White Syndrome. These 12-lead ECGs with leads V₁, II, and V₅ rhythm strips show sinus rhythm and sinus arrhythmia. There is occasional change in the QRS complex due to intermittent preexcitation in this patient with WPW syndrome. (A) The 2nd, 4th, 6th, 8th, and 12th beats exhibit a short PR interval, a delta wave, and a wide QRS complex. The others do not show preexcitation and show normal AV nodal conduction with a normal (narrow) QRS complex.

Continued on following page

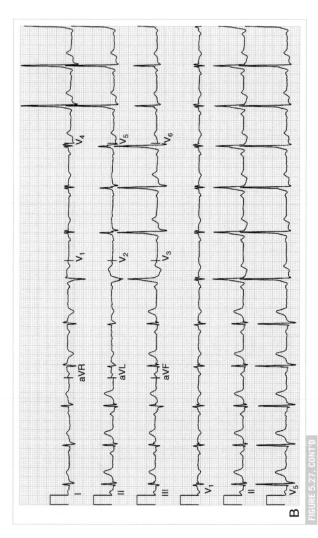

(B) The first five beats are not preexcited, but with sinus slowing, the rest of the tracing shows preexcitation.

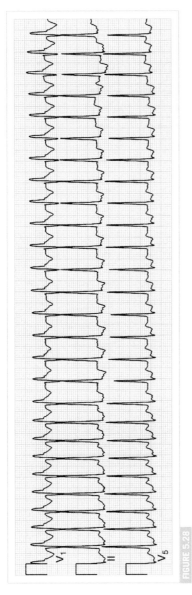

FIGURE 5.28

Atrioventricular reentrant tachycardia. This lead V_1, II, and V_5 rhythm strip shows a short RP narrow QRS complex tachycardia with an RP exceeding 100 ms, consistent with AV reentry tachycardia. The QRS complexes show a typical RBBB morphology. The retrograde limb of the reentry circuit is the accessory pathway. In this case the patient's baseline ECG shows sinus rhythm with no evidence of the delta wave of WPW syndrome conduction, suggesting a "concealed" bypass tract that can conduct only in a retrograde direction.

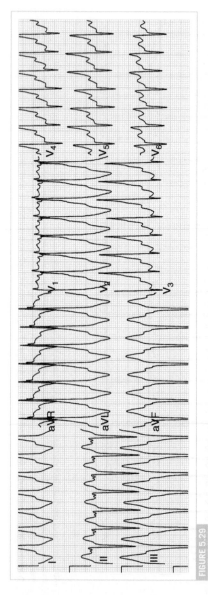

FIGURE 5.29

Ventricular tachycardia mimic: antidromic reentry. This 12-lead ECG tracing shows antidromic SVT in the setting of a bypass tract that was identified at the time of EP study. The QRS complex is wide due to antegrade conduction down a bypass tract. The retrograde activation pathway cannot be determined on this ECG but by an EP study was up the AV node. Antidromic SVT can look identical to VT and can be difficult to distinguish from VT, even by using Brugada criteria for VT.

Antidromic AVRT occurs when antegrade conduction proceeds down the accessory pathway and retrograde conduction proceeds up the AV node or another accessory pathway. It is associated with maximal preexcitation. It is a wide QRS tachycardia that contains a delta wave at its onset; antidromic AVRT can mimic VT.

Accessory pathways can also allow passive activation of a variety of SVTs, such as AFL and sinus tachycardia. By an unknown mechanism, accessory pathways appear to be associated with the existence of AF. Conduction down the accessory pathway is rapid due to the short refractory periods of many of the accessory pathways that are associated with patients who have WPW syndrome together with AF. The accessory pathway in AF tends to conduct antegrade but occasionally can conduct retrograde as well. AF conducting to the ventricles over an accessory pathway is the most feared tachycardia of the preexcitation syndromes because the ventricular rate can be extraordinarily fast (see Fig. 5.13) and can even lead to ventricular fibrillation (VF) (Fig. 5.30). Specific precautions need to be taken when treating these patients with drugs. Acutely, they should not receive digoxin or verapamil and probably also not a β-adrenergic blocker because these drugs delay conduction within

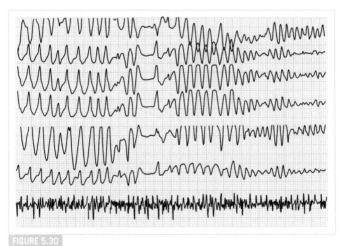

FIGURE 5.30

Atrial fibrillation with preexcitation degenerating to ventricular fibrillation. These six ECG strips and bottom intraatrial electrograms were recorded during an EP study of a patient with WPW syndrome. The tracing shows AF with preexcitation, with a very rapid ventricular response that degenerates to VF. Herein lies the danger of AF in patients with WPW syndrome who exhibit short refractoriness in their accessory pathways. The patient was successfully defibrillated and the pathway was successfully ablated.

the AV node, allowing a greater degree of accessory pathway conduction. Chronically, these patients should not receive digoxin or verapamil. Ablation of the accessory pathway will generally eliminate the AF.

There are accessory pathways that connect the atria to a fascicle (right bundle, atriofascicular fiber, Mahaim fiber) and others that connect a fascicle (peripheral portion of the right bundle) to the ventricular myocardium (fasciculoventricular fibers). There are specific unique properties to the Mahaim fiber. The Mahaim fiber has properties that show progressively slowed conduction with more rapid rates and with early extra stimuli. Indeed the Mahaim fiber acts as a second AV node that connects into the wrong place. Mahaim fibers do not conduct in the retrograde direction. Patients with Mahaim fibers do not necessarily have symptoms. Tachycardias due to Mahaim fibers can be related to conduction down the Mahaim fiber and up the His-Purkinje system and AV node to form a macroreentry circuit. In addition, patients with Mahaim fibers can have dual AV nodal physiology and AVNRT with passive activation down the Mahaim fiber.

Another important form of ventricular preexcitation generally demonstrates only retrograde activation through the accessory pathway; this pathway is a posterior septal slow conducting retrograde pathway. For people with this problem, there can be a unique form of tachycardia known as permanent junctional reciprocating tachycardia (PJRT) (Fig. 5.31). This tachycardia is incessant and often begins in childhood. Over time, patients with this problem often develop tachycardia-induced cardiomyopathy. Individuals with this problem require ablation of the accessory pathway because there is no other treatment. If it is not diagnosed and corrected in time, patients can develop CHF with risk of life-threatening ventricular arrhythmias or symptoms requiring cardiac transplant.

There are other reported forms of ventricular preexcitation that involve rapid conduction via the AV node, leading to a short PR interval but a normal QRS complex. This electrocardiographic finding is not per se the Lown-Ganong-Levine (LGL) syndrome, which, as originally described, involves an SVT and a short PR interval. Indeed a short PR interval need not indicate an accessory pathway at all but could be due to enhanced AV node conduction. With enhanced AV node conduction, the AH interval (i.e., the time it takes to traverse the AV node) is rapid, and the refractory period of the AV node is short so that rapid conduction proceeds very quickly. For people with this condition who develop AF, ventricular response rate can be extremely rapid; because the condition involves the AV node and not an extra AV nodal accessory pathway, there is no delta wave and thus no evidence of ventricular preexcitation. Patients with LGL syndrome may have other accessory pathways involved in reentry tachycardias; however, these are not well characterized. Treatment with either a calcium channel blocker or β-adrenergic blocker may not be effective, and often additional treatment using antiarrhythmic drugs, such as class IC or class III antiarrhythmic drugs is required.

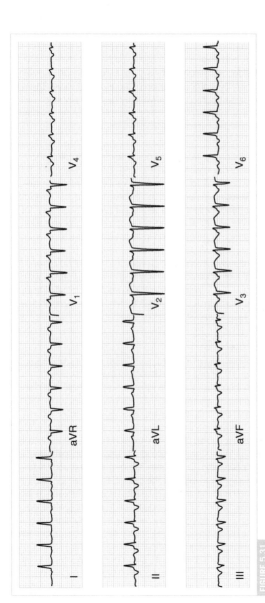

FIGURE 5.31

Permanent junctional reciprocating tachycardia. This 12-lead ECG shows a regular narrow complex SVT with a long RP interval, the differential for which includes atrial tachycardia, atypical AV node reentrant tachycardia, and PJRT. The negative P waves in the inferior leads indicate the atria are being activated in a low-to-high direction. This patient was shown to have PJRT at the time of an EP study. PJRT is a misnomer; it is not a junctional reciprocating tachycardia, but rather it is an orthodromic SVT that involves a septal bypass tract that, unlike other bypass tracts, has decremental conduction with prolonged ventricle to atrium (V-A) conduction.

Associated Conditions

There is no specific association between accessory pathways and any other clinical syndromes or findings. However, ventricular preexcitation is associated with AF, and ablation of accessory pathways can eliminate the AF. Some right-sided accessory pathways are associated with Epstein anomaly, in which there is ventricularization of the tricuspid valve. There is some evidence that hypertrophic cardiomyopathy has an association with left-sided accessory pathways.

Clinical Symptoms and Presentation

Patients with ventricular preexcitation may be completely asymptomatic. This often poses a conundrum with respect to long-term management. Some of these patients may be at risk for AF with rapid ventricular response rate, especially under certain circumstances, such as pregnancy or cardiovascular surgery. On the other hand, patients with ventricular preexcitation may not have arrhythmias. There are those who advocate accessory pathway ablation and elimination of ventricular preexcitation in all patients, including those who are asymptomatic; however, the risk of doing invasive procedures must be recognized. Alternatively, patients at high-risk jobs may not be allowed to continue to work until their accessory pathway is eliminated. Patients with symptomatic ventricular preexcitation generally present as a result of their SVTs (AVRT, AF). Symptoms include palpitations, lightheadedness, dizziness, syncope, weakness, fatigue, and shortness of breath.

Approach to Management (Algorithm 5.12)

The cornerstone to managing ventricular preexcitation is to first understand the mechanism of the arrhythmia and to document that ventricular preexcitation is present because the delta wave may not be easily seen on an ECG or may be confused with a nonspecific interventricular conduction delay. For a patient who presents with a wide QRS complex tachycardia, it may not be possible to know whether it is due to a preexcitation syndrome. In patients presenting with a narrow QRS complex tachycardia, the tachycardia may or may not be due to a retrogradely conducting accessory pathway (concealed accessory pathway). In this case, the best first approach is to perform an EP study after stabilization of the patient. During an EP study, if an accessory pathway is found, it should be eliminated by ablation. If for whatever reason ablation is not recommended, due to patient preference or difficulty in ablating a specific accessory pathway, antiarrhythmic drug therapy can help. The useful drugs include sotalol, flecainide, propafenone, amiodarone, procainamide, and/or quinidine. However, medical management is not the preferred approach. β-adrenergic blockers may be useful in patients who have only orthodromic AVRT. Specific populations, such as pregnant patients and postoperative cardiovascular surgical patients, are at higher risks of problems. If AF occurs in these patient groups, the rapid ventricular rate can be difficult to control (Table 5.12, Algorithm 5.13).

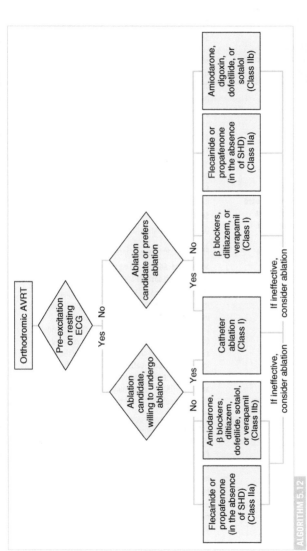

ALGORITHM 5.12

Ongoing management of orthodromic AVRT. *AVRT,* Atrioventricular reentrant tachycardia; *SHD,* structural heart disease (including ischemic heart disease). *(Reproduced with permission from Page RL et al. 2015 ACC/AHA/HRS Guideline for the Management of Adult Patients With Supraventricular Tachycardia. JACC 2016;67(13):e27-e115.)*

PREEXCITATION THERAPY

AF with ventricular preexcitation and rapid ventricular rates: Acute therapy unstable (hypotension, angina, heart failure symptoms)	• **First line:** Synchronized DCC (50–200 J with anesthesia). • **Second line:** IV procainamide or IV amiodarone to block conduction in the accessory pathway, if the patient can tolerate the medication due to low blood pressure and if there is enough time before complete hemodynamic collapse. • Do not give digoxin, adenosine, or verapamil. Avoid β-adrenergic blockers. All these block AV nodal conduction, allowing more impulse conduction down the accessory pathway. • This approach is useful not only for a patient who presents to the emergency department but also for a postoperative patient with rapid rates due to preexcitation.
AF with ventricular preexcitation and controlled ventricular rates without hemodynamic instability: Acute therapy	• **First line:** IV procainamide or IV amiodarone. Procainamide is preferred but may be difficult to find. • **Second line:** Anesthesia and synchronized cardioversion. • Do not give AV nodal blockers.
Orthodromic AVRT: Acute therapy	• **First line:** Carotid sinus massage or Valsalva maneuvers. • **Second line:** Adenosine 6 mg IV and, if ineffective, 12 mg IV. Note that high doses of adenosine may initiate AF. • **Third line:** Verapamil 5–15 mg IV. In many instances it is not clear whether or not the patient will have ventricular preexcitation in sinus rhythm when presenting with orthodromic AVRT. If there is evidence for ventricular preexcitation from ECGs recorded in sinus rhythm, this may not necessarily be the most ideal therapy, but treating this particular rhythm with verapamil does not tend to lead to rapid rates in AF, and if the QRS is narrow during orthodromic SVT, the AV node should be part of the circuit and responsive to verapamil. • **Fourth line:** Intravenous β-adrenergic blockade with esmolol or metoprolol. • **Fifth line:** Synchronized electrical cardioversion; this is first-line therapy if the tachycardia is associated with hemodynamic collapse.
Antidromic AVRT: Acute therapy	• **First line:** IV procainamide or IV amiodarone with procainamide being preferable. May perform carotid massage first if blood pressure is greater than 100 mmHg or Valsalva maneuver.
Long-term therapy: WPW syndrome due to an accessory pathway	• **Second line:** Synchronized electrical cardioversion; this is first line if the patient has hemodynamic collapse. • Avoid digoxin, β-adrenergic blocker, and calcium channel blocker.

TABLE 5.12

PREEXCITATION THERAPY (Continued)

	• **Symptomatic patients:** Catheter ablation is successful in >90% of patients. In patients who present with AF, catheter ablation of the accessory pathway tends to eliminate AF, particularly in those patients without structural heart disease. Ablation is first-line therapy for patients with symptomatic preexcitation syndromes.
	• **Asymptomatic patients:** Consider catheter ablation in young patients, especially if highly active or in a high-risk profession.
	• For those who do not prefer to have ablation or for those patients who have difficult or impossible to correct accessory pathways, drug therapy is second-line treatment. For patients with normal hearts, flecainide, propafenone, sotalol, amiodarone, and procainamide (in that order) could be used should there be no evidence for structural heart disease. In some instances drug therapy is used in lieu of ablation of the pathway in "high risk," such as those accessory pathways that are mid septal and near the His-Purkinje system.
	• For patients who have structurally abnormal hearts, class IC antiarrhythmic drugs are not recommended. For patients with intact ventricular function, sotalol is first-line therapy and if ineffective, amiodarone is second-line treatment.
	• For patients with poor ventricular function in whom ablation is not recommended or is impossible due to other confounding, medical conditions, amiodarone is first-line treatment.
Mahaim fiber tachycardias	• Acute management is similar to that for AVNRT.
	• **First line:** Carotid sinus massage or another vagal maneuver.
	• **Second line:** Adenosine.
	• **Third line:** Procainamide IV or amiodarone IV.
	• Avoid AV nodal blockers.
	• Long-term therapy includes ablation. If ablation is not reasonable due to other concomitant medical problems, is not the patient preference, or is ineffective, first-line treatment includes sotalol, flecainide, or propafenone. β-adrenergic blockers alone may work as well.
LGL syndrome (with SVTs)	EP study followed by ablation of the responsible tachycardia. If the arrhythmia is AF, AFL, or AT with rapid conduction through the AV node, rate control using a β-adrenergic blocker or a calcium channel blocker may be effective.
PJRT	Ablation is first line. Pharmacologic alternatives include AV nodal blockers (β-adrenergic blockers, diltiazem, verapamil, or digoxin), flecainide, propafenone, sotalol, or amiodarone. Flecainide and propafenone should be avoided if there is structural heart disease, such as cardiomyopathy or CAD.

AF, Atrial fibrillation; *AV,* atrioventricular; *AFL,* atrial flutter; *AVRT,* atrioventricular reentrant tachycardia; *DCC,* direct current cardioversion; *ECG,* electrocardiogram; *EP,* electrophysiology; *IV,* intravenous; *LGL,* Lown-Ganong-Levine; *PJRT,* permanent junctional reciprocating tachycardia; *SVT,* supraventricular tachycardia; *WPW,* Wolff-Parkinson-White.

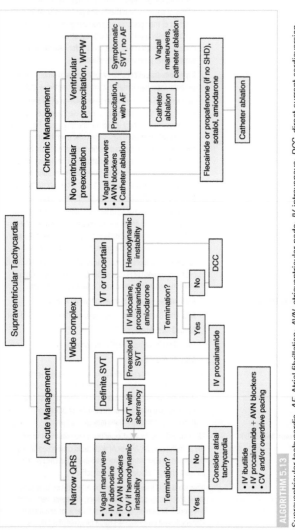

ALGORITHM 5.13

Supraventricular tachycardia. *AF,* Atrial fibrillation; *AVN,* atrioventricular node; *IV,* intravenous; *DCC,* direct current cardioversion; *SHD,* structural heart disease (no overt evidence of myocardial, valvular, congenital or coronary heart disease); *SVT,* supraventricular tachycardia; *VT,* ventricular tachycardia; *WPW,* Wolff-Parkinson-White.

NONSUSTAINED VENTRICULAR TACHYCARDIA

Description

Ventricular tachycardia (VT) is defined as three or more consecutive ventricular beats occurring at a rate of 100 beats or more per minute. Nonsustained ventricular tachycardia (NSVT) (Fig. 6.1) is defined as VT lasting less than 30 seconds and that does not require intervention for termination. The QRS complex morphology may be either monomorphic (e.g., uniform in a given ECG lead) or polymorphic (e.g., variable in a given lead). Polymorphic VT with a normal QT interval is most often ischemic in etiology, and that associated with a prolonged QT is referred to as torsades de pointes (TdP) and is usually nonischemic in etiology. The rate of VT ranges from 100 to 280 bpm. VT complexes are usually wide because of the slower rate of conduction through ventricular tissue compared with that occurring through Purkinje fibers. QRS duration will depend on the origin and mechanism of the VT.

Associated Conditions

NSVT often, but not always, occurs in the presence of structural heart disease. The risk of death in patients with NSVT is disease dependent and is associated with the degree of left ventricular (LV) dysfunction. For example, if coronary artery disease (CAD) is present and if the left ventricular ejection fraction (LVEF) is reduced (<40%), there is a substantial risk of cardiac, especially arrhythmic, death. Up to 95% of patients with dilated cardiomyopathy have NSVT, but this is of unclear prognostic significance; because of its nonsustained nature, it generally does not produce symptoms. The mechanism of NSVT varies if underlying heart disease is present and depends on the disease process, but even for CAD, the mechanism of NSVT may differ from that of sustained VT. Triggered activity or reentry mechanisms may be operative. NSVT also occurs in patients without structural heart disease. Exercise-induced, nonsustained repetitive monomorphic tachycardia is generally catecholamine-dependent. The precise incidence of catecholamine-dependent NSVT is unknown. NSVT occurring in the absence of structural heart disease may arise from the LV or right ventricular (RV) outflow tracts and is characterized by high-amplitude R waves in the inferior leads (II, III, aVF), reflecting base to apex depolarization. Idiopathic LV fascicular tachycardia may also manifest as runs of NSVT; these usually have a superior mean frontal plane QRS axis and right bundle branch block (RBBB) morphology. The QRS complexes of fascicular tachycardias

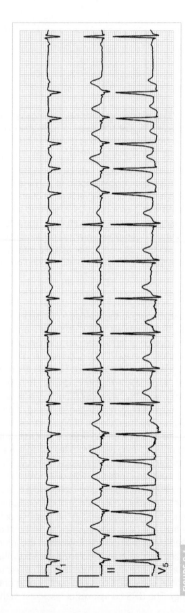

FIGURE 6.1

Nonsustained Ventricular Tachycardia. This lead V$_1$, II, and V$_5$ rhythm strip shows repetitive runs of nonsustained wide QRS complex tachycardias (5-6 beats long, rate ~125-135 bpm) that represent nonsustained ventricular tachycardia. The second run is followed by a compensatory pause. There is AV dissociation evident in the first run on lead V$_1$.

are not as wide as VTs originating in ventricular tissue because ventricular depolarization proceeds, at least in part, through the Purkinje system.

Clinical Presentation and Symptoms

Most episodes of NSVT are asymptomatic; however, NSVT is not only a harbinger of sudden death in select patient populations but also may be highly symptomatic, causing palpitations, dyspnea, chest discomfort, lightheadedness or dizziness, and frank syncope. Postextrasystolic beats may be perceived as forceful "thumps" in the chest.

Approach to Management (Algorithm 6.1)

Unless NSVT produces symptoms or is related to CAD with LV dysfunction or other structural heart disease, the risk of death is low, and there is no need for treatment. However, new-onset NSVT may be an indication of developing structural heart disease. Investigation for specific risk factors and disease entities should be undertaken. Evaluation should initially include an ECG with specific attention to entities such as epsilon waves, QT interval, and Brugada patterns, as well as echocardiography, to assess ventricular structure and function. Other appropriate tests include Holter monitoring, event monitoring, treadmill testing, and possibly signal-averaged electrocardiography. If these tests document abnormalities consistent with significant structural heart disease, cardiac catheterization or imaging studies, such as magnetic resonance imaging (MRI), may be appropriate.

Empiric treatment of NSVT may be worse than the arrhythmia itself and should be reserved for patients who are highly symptomatic, who have high risk for sudden death, or who have a high enough NSVT burden that it contributes to a tachycardia-induced cardiomyopathy. Palpitations in NSVT are not generally a sufficient indication to plan aggressive suppressive therapy, and reassurance may be all that is needed. For symptomatic idiopathic NSVT, various therapies, including β-adrenergic blockers, class I antiarrhythmic drugs, sotalol, or amiodarone may be helpful in reducing symptoms. Radiofrequency (RF) ablation is an alternative approach if symptoms are refractory to drug therapy or if the frequency of NSVT and ectopy contribute to a tachycardia-induced cardiomyopathy (typically requiring high premature ventricular contraction [PVC] burden, such as greater than 25% of ventricular complexes or greater than 10,000 PVCs/24-hour period).

Polymorphic NSVT is not necessarily a harbinger of sustained VT. Torsades de pointes ventricular tachycardia (TdP VT) tends to occur in repetitive, nonsustained paroxysms, although sustained VT and ventricular fibrillation (VF) can occur. Structural heart disease is commonly absent. Catecholaminergic polymorphic ventricular tachycardia (CPVT) is a cause of exercise-induced NSVT and has been associated with mutations in genes controlling intracellular calcium. These patients may respond to β-adrenergic blockers, and in high-risk patients with syncope or family

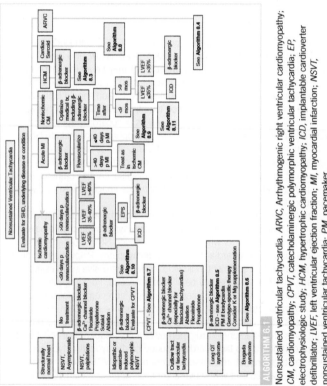

ALGORITHM 6.1

Nonsustained ventricular tachycardia. *ARVC,* Arrhythmogenic right ventricular cardiomyopathy; *CM,* cardiomyopathy; *CPVT,* catecholaminergic polymorphic ventricular tachycardia; *EP,* electrophysiologic study; *HCM,* hypertrophic cardiomyopathy; *ICD,* implantable cardioverter defibrillator; *LVEF,* left ventricular ejection fraction; *MI,* myocardial infarction; *NSVT,* nonsustained ventricular tachycardia; *PM,* pacemaker.

history of sudden death, implantable cardioverter defibrillator (ICD) implantation may be warranted. Bidirectional VT is currently more commonly associated with this type of VT than with digitalis toxicity, which is now infrequent. LV and right ventricular outflow tract (RVOT) NSVT, as well as idiopathic LV fascicular tachycardia, may be amenable to medical therapy (β-adrenergic blockers, calcium channel blockers [especially verapamil], class I or class III antiarrhythmic drugs) or cure by catheter ablation techniques (Table 6.1).

Description

VT is defined as sustained (Fig. 6.2) if it persists for more than 30 seconds or requires early or immediate termination (cardioversion or antitachycardia pacing) for hemodynamic instability. VT can be monomorphic (single QRS morphology in a given ECG lead) or polymorphic (multiple QRS morphologies in a given ECG lead). Monomorphic VT can be regular or irregular in rate and can display a "warm-up" phenomenon in which the tachycardia cycle length gets shorter after its onset. Multiple monomorphic morphologies can be present in a single patient at different times. Polymorphic VT is usually irregular in rate. Polymorphic VT with normal QT interval (Fig. 6.3) most often occurs in the setting of myocardial ischemia or infarction. Polymorphic VT associated with long QT interval is termed *TdP VT.* VT rates range from 100 to 280 bpm, thereby differentiating it from accelerated ventricular rhythm. Sustained VT is a serious and potentially life-threatening problem, particularly when it coexists with structural heart disease. Hemodynamic stability depends on rate, underlying heart disease, ventricular function, ventricular activation patterns, atrioventricular (AV) relationships, and concomitant drug therapy. AV dissociation occurs in up to 60% to 70% of patients but is clearly evident on the ECG in less than 30% of patients because the rapid VT rate and the wide QRS morphology "buries" the P waves. Mimics of VT include sinus tachycardia and other supraventricular tachycardias (SVTs) with preexisting or rate-related bundle branch block (BBB) (Fig. 6.4A and B), hyperkalemia (Fig. 6.5), antidromic AV reentrant tachycardia with antegrade activation through an accessory pathway (see Fig. 5.29), and artifact (Fig. 6.6).

Associated Conditions

There are multiple potential mechanisms of VT. Understanding the underlying mechanism(s) is important when planning therapy, both acutely and for the long term. Monomorphic VT can be due to microreentry or macroreentry in the ventricular myocardium, usually around a scar. It can also be due to bundle branch reentry (especially in patients with dilated cardiomyopathy, in whom more than 5% of VTs are due to this mechanism). It can be due to triggered activity resulting from delayed afterdepolarizations (DADs), such as has been postulated in RVOT

TABLE 6.1

MANAGEMENT OF NONSUSTAINED MONOMORPHIC AND POLYMORPHIC VENTRICULAR TACHYCARDIA

Setting	Therapy	Comments
Normal LV function	• No symptoms, no heart disease: no therapy	• Multiple clinical scenarios exist depending on the age of patient, heart disease, and symptoms.
	• Young patient with bidirectional (or polymorphic) VT that may be life-threatening (CPVT): β-adrenergic blocker	• Idiopathic VT may occur in repetitive monomorphic variety and be symptomatic.
	• Symptoms of palpitations, no heart disease: β-adrenergic blocker (e.g., acebutolol, 200-800 per day)	• Not life-threatening.
		• Is exacerbated by exercise, mental stress, and catecholamines.
	• Idiopathic LV fascicular tachycardia (RBBB left axis QRS morphology): verapamil	• Idiopathic polymorphic VT in the young can be potentially life-threatening.
	• If LBBB (inferior axis morphology), β-adrenergic blocker is first line. Other drugs: sotalol (started in hospital), propafenone, flecainide, amiodarone.	• Treat with β-adrenergic blocker.
		• Consider genotyping for CPVT.
	• RF ablation is curative for this type of VT in more than 95% if it can be initiated and mapped in the EP laboratory.	• Consider RV cardiomyopathy (dysplasia) with LBBB/noninferior axis morphology.
	• CAD, no symptoms: β-adrenergic blocker, no additional antiarrhythmic therapy	• Consider ischemia.
	• CAD with symptoms, β-adrenergic blocker, sotalol, amiodarone (started in the hospital)	• The 12-lead morphology is helpful.
	• Polymorphic NSVT	• If LBBB with inferior axis, it is likely from the RV or LV/aortic cusp outflow tract in normal hearts and is ablatable.
	• In the setting of the long QT with syncope, treatment is required.	• If QRS is negative in I and aVL, it may be arising from the septum.
	• Genotyping is available.	• If it is positive in these leads, it may be arising from the free wall and may be adenosine sensitive.
	• β-Adrenergic blockers are the first choice for long QT type I.	• VTs may respond to β-adrenergic blockers, verapamil, and most antiarrhythmic drugs.
	• With syncope or family history of sudden death, LQT2, or LQT3: ICD.	

	• If it is a RBBB left axis QRS pattern, it may be a reentrant idiopathic VT from the LV apical septum.
	▪ Thought to be due to fascicular reentry.
	▪ Can be cured with RF ablation.
	▪ Is sensitive to verapamil (only use if known to be this type of VT).
	• Even patients with normal hearts may be at slightly higher risk for CA compared with the general population, but further evaluation and therapy is not beneficial.
	• Polymorphic tachycardia may be due to ischemia or infarction and may be transient.
	• Increased risk of sudden and total death.
	• Increased risk is not related to length of episodes.
	• EP testing may risk stratify.

Ischemic cardiomyopathy	• For LVEF ≤30%, more than 1 month after MI, 3 months after revascularization, ICD implantation.
	• For LVEF ≤35%, NYHA FC II–III, ICD implantation is recommended.
	• For LVEF ≤40%, EP study is recommended, and if sustained VT is induced, ICD should be implanted.
	• For NYHA FC III–IV heart failure, LVEF ≤35%, and QRS duration >120 ms, cardiac resynchronization therapy is recommended.

Nonischemic cardiomyopathy	• β-adrenergic blockers, ACE inhibitors, and other optimal therapies for heart failure
	• For LVEF ≤35%, NYHA FC II–III, ICD is recommended.
	• For NYHA FC III–IV heart failure, LVEF ≤35%, and QRS duration >120 ms, cardiac resynchronization therapy is recommended.

Continued on following page

TABLE 6.1

MANAGEMENT OF NONSUSTAINED MONOMORPHIC AND POLYMORPHIC VENTRICULAR TACHYCARDIA (Continued)

Setting	Therapy	Comments
HCM	<ul><li>β-adrenergic blocker, especially if symptomatic</li><li>Memory loop event recorders may be beneficial in correlating symptoms with arrhythmias.</li><li>No indication for amiodarone or other antiarrhythmic drugs if asymptomatic</li><li>Start amiodarone, if symptomatic, in the hospital.</li><li>ICD if<ul><li>Septum > 30 mm</li><li>Syncope</li><li>NSVT</li><li>Family history of sudden death</li><li>High-risk genotype</li><li>If prior CA</li><li>Sustained VT/VF</li></ul></li></ul>	<ul><li>Potentially indicative of a malignant, life-threatening ventricular arrhythmia.</li><li>EP testing of no proven benefit in this setting.</li></ul>
MI	<ul><li>No specific therapy</li><li>Assess LV function.</li><li>β-Adrenergic blocker as part of the post-MI regimen</li><li>If continued NSVT and impaired LV function (LVEF < 0.40) after 4-6 weeks, consider ICD and suppressive antiarrhythmic therapy to slow VT rate and prevent shocks.</li></ul>	<ul><li>Little prognostic meaning early after MI. Predictive value increases with increasing time from MI.</li><li>If polymorphic, consider ischemia (or electrolyte disturbance if the QT interval is prolonged).</li><li>May represent a coronary reperfusion injury rhythm.</li></ul>

Pre-op
- If noncardiac surgery planned, assess symptoms, longevity of the problem, drugs
  - If recent onset: assess LV function
  - If LVEF ≤0.40, and if CAD, consider EP test
  - If no CHF LVEF ≤0.30, ICD. If CHF and LVEF ≤0.35, ICD

Post-op
- No therapy
  - Has little prognostic meaning early after surgery
  - Resolves spontaneously in the great majority
  - Evaluate for underlying heart disease if risk factors are present.
  - Plan follow-up Holter monitor. If episodes continue, consider EP test. If induced VT, consider ICD if LVEF ≤0.40 or other criteria met (ischemic, nonischemic cardiomyopathy; discussed previously).
    - If asymptomatic, treat based on monitor results or based on EP test results.

ACE, Angiotensin-converting enzyme; *CA,* cardiac arrest; *CABG,* coronary artery bypass graft; *CAD,* coronary artery disease; *CPVT,* catecholaminergic polymorphic ventricular tachycardia; *EP,* electrophysiologic; *FC,* functional class; *HCM,* hypertrophic cardiomyopathy; *ICD,* implantable cardioverter defibrillator; *LBBB,* left bundle branch block; *LV,* left ventricular; *LVEF,* left ventricular ejection fraction; *MI,* myocardial infarction; *NSVT,* nonsustained ventricular tachycardia; *NYHA,* New York Heart Association; *RBBB,* right bundle branch block; *RF,* radiofrequency; *RV,* right ventricular; *VT,* ventricular tachycardia.

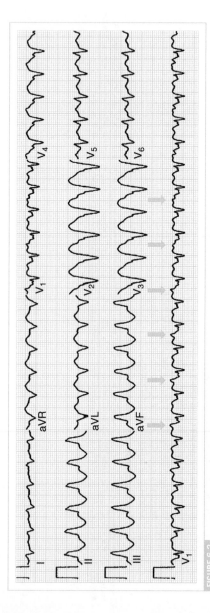

FIGURE 6.2

Sustained Monomorphic Ventricular Tachycardia. This 12-lead ECG with V₁ rhythm strip shows a wide QRS complex tachycardia (rate of ~140 bpm) that has features of ventricular tachycardia including wide (0.16 sec) QRS complexes and atrioventricular (AV) dissociation (arrows show sinus P waves at a rate of ~72 bpm).

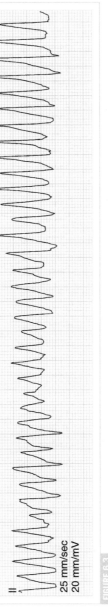

FIGURE 6.3

Polymorphic Ventricular Tachycardia. This lead II rhythm strip shows polymorphic VT. This VT occurred in a patient with myocardial ischemia who did not have QT prolongation.

25 mm/sec
20 mm/mV

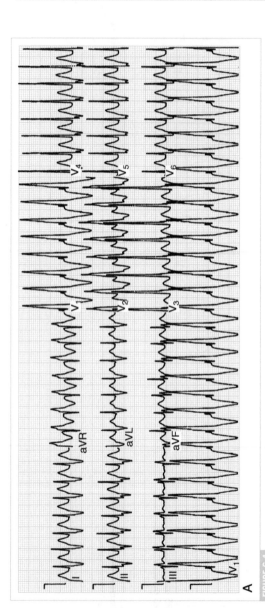

FIGURE 6.4

A) Ventricular Tachycardia Mimic: Sinus Tachycardia with Bundle Branch Block. This 12-lead ECG with rhythm strips shows a rapid wide QRS complex tachycardia that looks like ventricular tachycardia. However, on closer inspection, there is typical right bundle branch block morphology, and there may be retrograde P waves in the terminal part of the QRS. In this case the rhythm is a supraventricular tachycardia and the wide QRS complex is due to an underlying right bundle branch block. **B) Ventricular Tachycardia Mimic: Sinus Tachycardia with Left Bundle Branch Block** This 12-lead ECG with rhythm strips shows a wide QRS complex tachycardia that looks like ventricular tachycardia. However, there is typical left bundle branch block morphology, and there are P waves before each QRS complex. The rhythm is sinus tachycardia and the wide QRS complex is due to left bundle branch block.

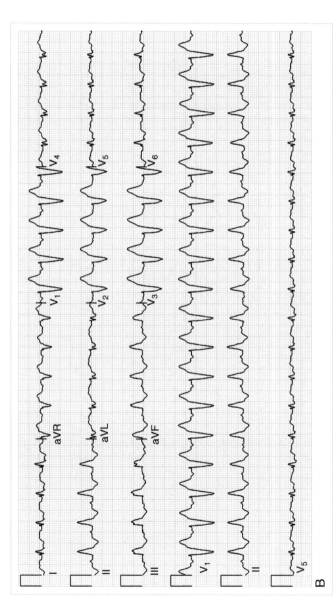

FIGURE 6.4, CONT'D

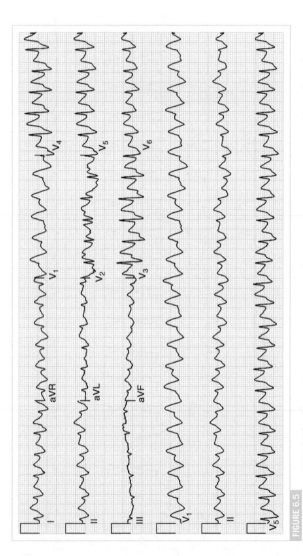

Ventricular Tachycardia Mimic: Hyperkalemia. This 12-lead ECG tracing with leads V_1, II, and V_5 rhythm strips shows a wide complex tachycardia in a patient with renal failure whose serum level potassium was >7 mmol/L. Note the very wide QRS complex and the suggestion of a sine wave pattern. With treatment of the hyperkalemia, the QRS duration decreased back to normal.

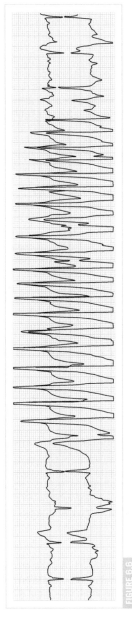

Ventricular Tachycardia Mimic: Normal Sinus Rhythm with Artifact. This 2-lead rhythm strip shows an apparent rapid polymorphic wide complex rhythm that looks very much like ventricular tachycardia (VT). However, there is obvious noise abutting the second and third QRS complexes and last 3 QRS complexes. The QRS complexes march through the noise, most evident at the end of the rhythm strip. The noise on the baseline at the end may appear to be ventricular complexes or ventricular fibrillation, but occur immediately through and after normal QRS complexes, which would be during ventricular refractoriness. These findings are all consistent with sinus rhythm with artifact. Artifact can be misdiagnosed as VT. Distinguishing features include a lack of compensatory pause after the tachycardia and the finding that, on closer examination, the QRS complexes of the intrinsic rhythm appear to "walk through" the tachycardia (as is the case here). This may be associated with rapid movement, such as toothbrushing.

idiopathic VT, or early afterdepolarizations (EADs), such as in TdP. Although rarely seen nowadays, VT caused by digitalis toxicity, including bidirectional tachycardia (see Fig. 9.4), can also result from triggered activity.

The most common causes of sustained monomorphic VT are structural abnormalities resulting from CAD with myocardial infarction (MI), dilated cardiomyopathy, valvular heart disease, proarrhythmia caused by antiarrhythmic drug use, and arrhythmogenic right ventricular cardiomyopathy (ARVC). VT can be the cause for or the effect of ischemia and/or congestive heart failure (CHF) even if it does not cause hypotension.

Sustained monomorphic VT that occurs in the absence of structural heart disease is termed "idiopathic" VT. There are two common forms of idiopathic VT: (1) outflow tract VTs, most commonly arising from the RVOT (typically left bundle branch block [LBBB], inferior axis morphology) but also from the left ventricular outflow tract (LVOT)/aortic cusp (LBBB or RBBB morphology, inferior axis) or mitral annulus, and (2) LV fascicular tachycardia, most commonly RBBB-superior axis morphology, arising from the LV inferoapical wall due to reentry within the fascicles. However, these specific morphologies do not indicate that the tachycardia is necessarily idiopathic in origin or that it is even VT. Nonetheless, monomorphic VT should always be the suspected cause for a wide QRS complex (more than 0.12 seconds) tachycardia, particularly if the patient has structural heart disease, prior MI, or the 12-lead ECG pattern differs significantly from the baseline ECG. If the QRS complex morphology in wide complex tachycardia does not resemble classical RBBB or LBBB, it is likely VT.

Polymorphic VT is almost always life-threatening and requires emergent treatment. Long QT interval polymorphic VT (TdP) (Fig. 6.7) can be due to an acquired long QT syndrome precipitated by certain drugs (e.g., class IA or III antiarrhythmic drugs) or other conditions that prolong the QT interval, such as hypokalemia and hypomagnesemia. A catecholamine-dependent form of TdP also exists. TdP is usually initiated by a long–short ("pause-dependent") sequence that causes further prolongation of the QT interval and enhancement of the TU or U wave and increasing bizarre QRSTU complexes. The U wave in TdP is thought to reflect the magnitude of the EAD, which is the cellular basis of the arrhythmia. TdP may be due to a genetic abnormality, most commonly mutations in potassium or sodium channel–associated genes. The congenital disorder is most commonly autosomal dominant (Romano-Ward syndrome), but rare recessive forms have been described and associated with deafness (Jervell and Lange-Nielsen syndrome). Polymorphic VT with a normal QT interval is most often ischemic in etiology.

Clinical Presentation and Symptoms

VT can be well or poorly tolerated, presenting as a stable monomorphic or poorly tolerated VT presenting as hemodynamic collapse and degeneration to VF or cardiac arrest (CA). Hemodynamic stability is not a criterion for determining tachycardia origin (e.g., SVT vs. VT) because a hemodynamic

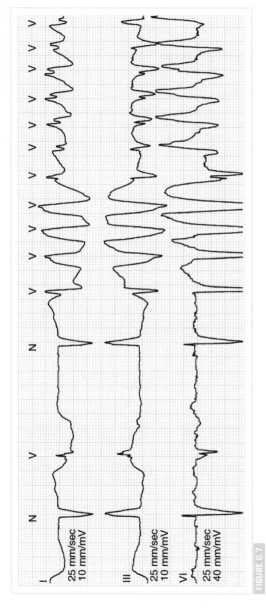

FIGURE 6.7

Torsades de Pointes. This lead I, III, and V_1 rhythm strip shows sinus bradycardia with left bundle branch block and marked QT prolongation with premature ventricular contractions (R-on-T) that initiates a very rapid polymorphic ventricular tachycardia with the characteristic twisting of the QRS complex around the isoelectric baseline. Torsades des pointes literally means "twisting of the points."

state depends not only on the rate but also on the nature of the underlying cardiac disease, ventricular function, and concomitant drugs. However, in general, the faster the VT and the worse the LV function, the more poorly VT is tolerated. Very rapid VT is known as ventricular flutter; it is diagnosed if the VT rate is greater than 280 bpm or if there is no obvious isoelectric baseline of the ECG.

Approach to Management

First, it is critical to determine hemodynamic stability. If the VT is causing hemodynamic instability, urgent direct current (DC) shock is required. Assessing whether the mechanism of a wide QRS complex tachycardia is due to a ventricular or SVT is essential. Sinus tachycardia with aberrancy will not respond to a DC shock. SVT requires a different treatment pathway than VT, and ultimately the distinction between the two will be important.

Because 70% to 90% of wide QRS complex tachycardias are VT and not SVT, even with hemodynamic tolerance, the tachycardia should be treated as VT. However, if the patient is tolerating the tachycardia and SVT is strongly suspected, it is acceptable to attempt vagal maneuvers or give adenosine 6 mg intravenous (IV) followed by 12 mg IV before administering lidocaine or DC cardioversion. Adenosine may also induce ventriculoatrial conduction block, which indicates that VT is the mechanism of the tachycardia. Adenosine can terminate some RVOT idiopathic VTs. Thus tachycardia termination by adenosine is not 100% specific for the diagnosis of SVT. Although verapamil may occasionally terminate idiopathic VT, it is contraindicated in any wide QRS complex tachycardia that is of uncertain etiology or is known to be VT.

Acute Management (Algorithm 6.2)

Always consider emergent electric (DC) shock to stop VT. Even if the VT is tolerated, an external cardioverter defibrillator should always be close at hand and ready to be used by knowledgeable personnel because hemodynamic collapse can occur without warning or change in VT rate. The advanced cardiac life support (ACLS) protocol must be known and followed. If the sustained VT terminates spontaneously and/or recurs, an IV antiarrhythmic drug may be effective (e.g., amiodarone) in suppressing it. Cardioversion (synchronized to the QRS complex) can be performed for slower VTs if there is a distinct isoelectric interval, even if the tachycardia is well tolerated but has not responded to IV antiarrhythmic drugs. If the patient is awake, IV anesthesia should be administered promptly before cardioversion. In patients with severe hypotension (e.g., pulseless VT), a nonsynchronized DC shock should be performed, similar to defibrillation for VF. For VT without hemodynamic impairment, the initial energy to cardiovert is 50 to 100 J, delivered from a biphasic cardioverter. For those who do not tolerate the VT, an unsynchronized DC shock should be delivered at 200 J. If that is ineffective, increase to 300 J, and if that is ineffective, then deliver 360 J. If a second shock at 360 J is ineffective,

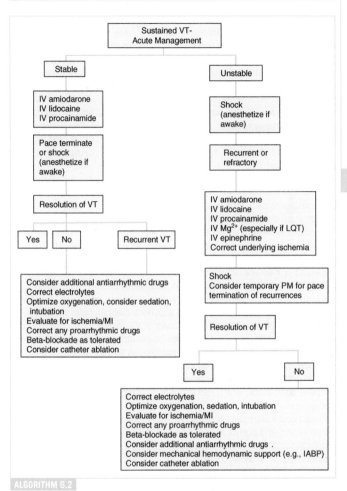

ALGORITHM 6.2

Sustained ventricular tachycardia—acute management. *IABP,* Intra-aortic balloon pump; *IV,* intravenous; *LQT,* long QT interval; *MI,* myocardial infarction; *PM,* pacemaker; *VT,* ventricular tachycardia.

additional therapy with IV drug infusions must be considered. A widely patent IV must be in place and the patient monitored carefully and continuously.

IV antiarrhythmic drugs that can potentially convert or prevent recurrences of VT include amiodarone, lidocaine, and procainamide. Used acutely, these drugs can also prevent VT from recurring after the rhythm is converted with a DC shock. Although they may not convert the rhythm, these drugs may nonetheless still effectively suppress arrhythmias after sinus rhythm has been achieved by other means. IV amiodarone, 150 mg over 10 minutes, is the recommended antiarrhythmic drug of first choice. Lidocaine 1.5 mg/kg, repeated at a 0.5- to 1-mg/kg dose may be effective to facilitate VT termination. Procainamide 10 to 15 mg/kg given at 25 mg/min may facilitate conversion or slow the VT rate so that it can be pace terminated; however, the class I antiarrhythmic drugs can increase the energy required to cardiovert and defibrillate. Procainamide can be negatively inotropic and can precipitate hypotension. It (and its renally excreted metabolite, N-acetyl-procainamide) can cause QT interval prolongation and TdP.

If the VT rate is less than 200 bpm but recurs persistently, consider placement of a temporary transvenous pacemaker to rapidly pace the ventricles to pace terminate VT. If an ICD is already in place, antitachycardia pacing may be programmed.

If a shock is ineffective, additional drug therapy for VT includes epinephrine 1 mg IV, which may be repeated once, or vasopressin. Use epinephrine very rarely and with extreme caution if an acute infarction is suspected or if severe ischemia is present based on symptoms or ECG findings. Further drug use depends on the clinical situation (discussed later), the type of VT, the underlying cardiac diagnosis, and the LV function.

There are several important clinical situations that can have special implications regarding long-term treatment of VT. Rarely, VT is due to digitalis intoxication. This VT, which can be bidirectional, may not respond to DC shock. Digoxin antibodies are indicated, as well as correction of electrolyte disturbances, such as low potassium and magnesium. This must be done cautiously and gradually to avoid potassium-induced complete heart block, which can occur at high potassium levels in digitalis toxicity.

VT can occur after cardiac surgery. This is often transient, but if it is monomorphic and occurs after the first 24 to 48 hours or if it is associated with important LV functional impairment (LVEF ≤ 0.40), there is a high likelihood that VT may recur.

Chronic Management

In the setting of MI, transient VT episodes are not rare. Polymorphic VT with a normal QT interval may be due to ischemia. VT can also represent reperfusion injury. These VTs, although transient, especially if they occur within the first 48 hours of the MI, may indicate future arrhythmic risk if they are associated with impaired LV function (LVEF ≤ 0.40). Evaluation can include electrophysiologic (EP) testing to assess long-term implications, especially if the patient is not a candidate for revascularization. However, late (>48 hours) sustained VT generally indicates significant residual risk for sudden cardiac death, and ICD implantation is indicated for secondary prevention of sudden cardiac death.

All patients with structural heart disease and new onset of VT should undergo careful reevaluation of their underlying disease. If there is evidence of progression of CAD or valvular disease, cardiac catheterization may be needed. If the patient has a dilated cardiomyopathy, evaluation of LV function is indicated. In all cases, episodes of sustained monomorphic VT require long-term treatment when not associated with an acute event, such as drug toxicity, MI, myocardial trauma, and cardiac surgery. EP testing may be indicated in these patients. Long-term therapy usually includes ICD implantation and ablation, and/or adjunctive antiarrhythmic drug (Table 6.2).

Survivors of hemodynamically compromising sustained VT/VF or aborted sudden cardiac death (in the absence of reversible causes or acute MI) are at high risk for recurrence. Before long-term therapy for VT is planned, assessment of the underlying structural heart disease must occur. If there is structural heart disease with LVEF ≥ 0.35. The patient is at high risk for CA and death within 1 year (rate: 15% to 30%). These patients require aggressive long-term therapy. Randomized studies, including the Antiarrhythmics versus Implantable Defibrillator (AVID) trial, have demonstrated superiority of ICDs over medical therapies (using antiarrhythmic drugs) in these patients. Antiarrhythmic drugs, such as amiodarone and sotalol, may be used as adjunctive therapy to prevent multiple recurrent shocks. Recurrences of VT may also be treated with catheter ablation to decrease the number of ICD shocks.

Patients with normal LV function, no structural heart disease, and slower monomorphic VTs have a good prognosis. These patients may respond to an antiarrhythmic drug or ablation.

Patients with the congenital long QT syndrome (LQTS) type 1 often respond to β-adrenergic blockade. Some may respond to class IB antiarrhythmic drugs (LQT3, in particular). For those who are bradycardic (<60 bpm at rest with a long QT), a permanent DDD pacemaker is often effective. For patients with CA, recurrent syncope, or recurrent polymorphic VT, an ICD is recommended.

VENTRICULAR FIBRILLATION

Description

VF (Fig. 6.8) is the most common rhythm associated with sudden cardiac death and the most common cause of death due to cardiovascular issues.

VF is an irregular and rapid polymorphic ventricular tachyarrhythmia that is associated with no effective cardiac contractions and thus no cardiac output. Death will occur unless a perfusing rhythm is restored within seconds to minutes; 0.1% to 0.2% of the population has CA due to rapid ventricular VT or VF each year. It is potentially, but not always, correctable by defibrillation, and it is not clear how often the rhythm is actually treatable. It may be initiated by a long–short sequence of ventricular ectopic beats or by a monomorphic or polymorphic VT.

TABLE 6.2

MANAGEMENT OF SUSTAINED VENTRICULAR TACHYCARDIA

Setting	Therapy	Comments
Acute therapy		• Assess cause and hemodynamic tolerance.
• Monomorphic VT well tolerated (patient awake and alert, no angina, no CHF, stable BP)	• First line: Amiodarone 150 mg over 10 minutes followed by 1 mg/min for 6 h followed by 0.5 mg/min	• Guidance of therapy is dependent on the clinical status of the patient.
	• May combine amiodarone IV with oral drug and with IV lidocaine if needed	• VT can always degenerate to VF even if it is at first stable.
	• Lidocaine 1.5-2 mg/kg (but only effective in <15%)	• IV amiodarone is emerging as first-line therapy for sustained monomorphic VT due to lack of efficacy of other drugs.
	• Second line: Procainamide 10-15 mg/kg at 25 mg/min (or less), assessing the BP carefully	• Procainamide has a negative inotropic effect.
	• Procainamide can slow VT and may be effective in an additional 20% to 30%	• Temporary transvenous pacing requires time and experienced personnel to accomplish.
	• Amiodarone is probably more effective than procainamide, safer, and better tolerated	
	• Third line: Cardioversion after adequate anesthesia	
	• Do not cardiovert while awake	
	• Fourth line: Antitachycardia pacing via a temporary transvenous pacing lead	
Acute therapy, MI	• Same as above but degree of urgency in treatment is greater	• Monomorphic VT
	• The length of time in VT, even if apparently tolerated, should be minimized	• May not increase long-term mortality.
	• Lidocaine is associated with no improvement in mortality	• Can be ischemia induced but this is rare (<3% of all MIs).
		• Tends to indicate "an electrical reentry circuit" of damaged myocardium.

Acute therapy, polymorphic VT

- Normal QT interval
  - Assess cause and hemodynamic tolerance.
  - Rule out ischemia, infarction, electrolyte abnormality (low K^+ or Mg^{2+}), or adverse drug effect.
- Patient stable
  - Assess age, underlying disease process and LV function, potential causative factors (e.g., exercise).
  - Therapy depends on the clinical status, which can always degenerate to VF even if it appears to be stable.
  - IV amiodarone may be effective, but there are no data on well-tolerated polymorphic VT.

- If stable and the patient is awake (very rare):
  - If ineffective, DC shock (200 J > 300–360 J) after anesthetized
- IV β-adrenergic blockade as tolerated
  - Monomorphic VT can be highly symptomatic but is almost never "malignant" and life-threatening.
  - LBBB/inferior axis VT is usually from the outflow tract.
    - If the QRS is negative in I and aVL, suspect a septal or LV origin.
    - If it is positive in these leads, suspect a free wall origin.

Chronic prevention

- No structural heart disease
- Idiopathic VT, usually in young patient
- Often exercise or stress induced
- Rule out RV cardiomyopathy (dysplasia) with MRI

- First line: β-adrenergic blocker titrated to the highest tolerated dose
- If recurrent episodes (with moderate or severe symptoms) occur: RF catheter ablation
- The success for LBBB inferior axis and for RBBB superior axis VT ablation is 90% to 95%
- RF ablation is first line if patient has syncope, hemodynamic intolerance, or patient preference
  - The mechanism may be due to triggered automaticity. Highly amenable to RF ablation.
  - RBBB/superior axis VTs are likely due to reentry in the Purkinje system.
    - Are verapamil sensitive.
    - Can be successfully ablated.
  - For LBBB, noninferior axis morphology VTs, r/o ARVC.

Continued on following page

TABLE 6.2

MANAGEMENT OF SUSTAINED VENTRICULAR TACHYCARDIA (Continued)

Setting	Therapy	Comments
Prior MI, ischemia can be provoked	• If monomorphic, suspect a substrate that is due to scar, not ischemia	• May also be associated with VF.
	• If polymorphic, suspect ischemia or infarction	• Rarely, monomorphic VT is due to ischemia alone, but always suspect substrate even if episodes occur relatively soon after infarction.
	• Consider a functional stress test or coronary angiogram and revascularization if ischemic	• If an antiarrhythmic drug is being used, consider the possibility of a proarrhythmic effect.
	• ICD implantation if hemodynamically significant sustained VT/VF	• Most patients (>95%) with chronic VT due to CAD will be inducible in the EP laboratory, but this does not change treatment strategy.
	• Ablation can be successful in >50% but with a high rate of long-term recurrence	
	• Used as adjunctive therapy to ICD implantation	
	• May be used to reduce recurrent ICD shocks	
	• Adjunctive antiarrhythmic drugs include amiodarone or sotalol	

ARVC, Arrhythmogenic right ventricular cardiomyopathy; *BP*, blood pressure; *EP*, electrophysiologic; *ICD*, implantable cardioverter defibrillator; *IV*, intravenous; *LBBB*, left bundle branch block; *LV*, left ventricular; *MI*, myocardial infarction; *MRI*, magnetic resonance imaging; *RBBB*, right bundle branch block; *RF*, radiofrequency; *RV*, right ventricular; *VF*, ventricular fibrillation; *VT*, ventricular tachycardia.

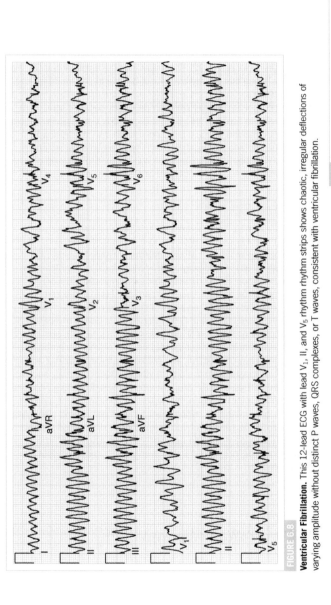

FIGURE 6.8

Ventricular Fibrillation. This 12-lead ECG with lead V₁, II, and V₅ rhythm rhythm strips shows chaotic, irregular deflections of varying amplitude without distinct P waves, QRS complexes, or T waves, consistent with ventricular fibrillation.

A patient who has VF will collapse and lose consciousness within seconds. Patients who have out-of-hospital CA due to VF are rarely resuscitated because it takes only minutes before resuscitation attempts become futile. The best chance for successful resuscitation is when VF, rather than asystole, is present. The longer the time a patient is in VF, the greater the chance that the rhythm will not be able to be terminated and the patient will die.

In addition, monitoring may provide challenges because some "fine" VF (as opposed to "coarse" VF) (Fig. 6.9) can look like asystole. In some instances, such as the LQTS, a rapid polymorphic VT mimicking VF will self-terminate and be associated with syncope; in most instances, patients with VF die. In other instances noise with lead hook-up or other recording artifacts, such as movement of electrodes, can mimic VF (Fig. 6.10).

Associated Conditions

Most individuals who have VF have some underlying cardiovascular cause. Common associated cardiovascular conditions include (1) CAD (ischemia, with or without an MI or underlying myocardial scar); (2) valvular heart disease (especially aortic stenosis); (3) nonischemic dilated cardiomyopathy; (4) hypertrophic cardiomyopathy (HCM); (5) ARVC congenital heart disease; (6) cardiovascular and coronary artery abnormalities; and (7) a variety of channelopathies, such as Brugada syndrome, LQTS, and CPVT. Rarely, VF is due to myocarditis, commotio cordis, or the short QT interval syndrome. VF may also be the terminal rhythm in other conditions, such as pulmonary embolism, stroke, acute airway obstruction, and pulmonary hypertension of any etiology. VF may result from the proarrhythmic effects of drugs, such as antiarrhythmic drugs, specific drug overdoses, illicit drugs (e.g., cocaine or methamphetamine), hypoxia, hypovolemia, acidosis, toxins, cardiac tamponade, pneumothorax, hypoglycemia, hypothermia, and electrolyte abnormalities. If the patient is hypothermic or has drowned in cold water, prolonged resuscitation may be needed, as the "diving reflex" in cool water may improve long-term survival even with no cardiac output for many minutes.

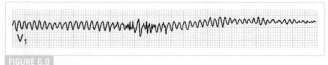

FIGURE 6.9

Ventricular Fibrillation. This rhythm strip shows ventricular fibrillation that degenerates further into fine ventricular fibrillation.

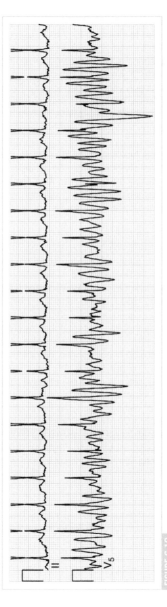

FIGURE 6.10

Ventricular Fibrillation Mimic: Artifact. The lead II and V₅ rhythm strip shows an apparent wide complex polymorphic tachycardia in lead V₅ that has characteristics of ventricular fibrillation and torsades de pointes. However, closer inspection of the tracing reveals that there are some rapid QRS-like deflections that walk through the rhythm completely in sync with the underlying sinus rhythm seen on lead II. This represents artifact that is superimposed on sinus rhythm.

Assess the patient, manage the arrhythmia, and stabilize the patient. Attempt to make a diagnosis as to the cause for the VF (e.g., by prior history, witness testimony, known prior disease). Assess the need for a long-term treatment plan, but consider that aggressive resuscitation attempts may not be successful if prolonged VF has occurred.

Begin chest compressions and ventilate periodically. Record a rhythm strip as soon as feasible, making sure that electrical noise is not present. Determine whether VF or asystole is present. If it is not possible to determine, assume that it is VF, and deliver a defibrillating shock.

In an unwitnessed CA, apply "quick look" paddles before shock delivery, recognizing that the time to first shock is critical. *Do not delay* or cease chest compressions while awaiting the defibrillator. An automatic external defibrillator (AED) can be attached quickly during cardiopulmonary resuscitation (CPR) and can provide an accurate view of whether or not VF is present.

During CPR, frequent respirations are not as necessary as once thought; however, chest compression is required. It should be begun immediately before an AED is attached or external defibrillation performed unless the latter can be performed immediately. The ACLS recommends the following for witnessed or unwitnessed CA due to VF: DC shock 200 to 300 J, 300 J, 360 J, 360 J, adequate CPR, central-line intubation, IV magnesium, amiodarone (300-mg IV push may be helpful, especially through central line, but do not delay shock for this reason).

If defibrillation is ineffective, give IV epinephrine, IV magnesium sulfate, and possibly IV vasopressin and continue CPR. After return to a stable rhythm, obtain a 12-lead ECG, place in an acute (intensive care unit) bed. Assess potential causes for arrest. If there is evidence for ischemia or infarction, emergent cardiac catheterization may be necessary. There is no evidence that prophylactic antiarrhythmic drugs are beneficial. It is best to proceed with IV amiodarone if VF is resistant to shock or if it recurs. Insufficient data support the use of antiarrhythmic drugs, including amiodarone, to prevent the long-term recurrence of VF and to improve long-term prognosis.

After defibrillation, additional management includes optimizing cardiopulmonary function, attempting to identify the precipitant, instituting measures to prevent recurrence, and starting therapy that may prolong long-term neurologic function, including hypothermia. Short-term memory loss is common after resuscitation and is common in survivors.

Poor prognostic indicators include absent corneal reflex in 24 hours, absent pupillary response at 24 hours, absent withdrawal response to pain at 24 hours, a lack of motor response at 24 hours, a lack of motor response at 72 hours, and an electroencephalogram (EEG) at 24 to 48 hours showing absence of brain activity.

It is important to recognize that after resuscitation from VF, patients can be comatose for a long period. Hemodynamic instability because of multiorgan system failure is common. Electrolyte shifts (e.g., hypokalemia, hypomagnesemia, and hypocalcemia) may occur but do not necessarily determine the etiology of the VF. Hypokalemia is common and may be due to a catecholamine effect that drives potassium into cells; in such patients there may be a rapid return of potassium levels to normal without the need for large supplementation (and therefore hypokalemia can be assumed not to be the cause for the VF).

If the cause for VF can be determined and corrected (rarely), no additional therapy may be required; however, should a patient survive VF with no correctable condition present and there is a reasonable chance of long-term survival, an ICD should be implanted.

SPECIFIC VENTRICULAR ARRHYTHMIA SYNDROMES

Specific ventricular tachyarrhythmia syndromes in patients with structural heart disease include ventricular arrhythmias in the setting of ischemic and nonischemic dilated cardiomyopathies, HCM, and ARVC. Ventricular arrhythmia syndromes in patients without structural heart disease include normal heart or idiopathic VTs; these encompass outflow tract VTs (from the right or LVOT, aortic cusp, mitral annulus, or aortic-mitral annulus isthmus) and LV fascicular VTs (idiopathic left VT or idiopathic left ventricular tachycardia [ILVT]). Polymorphic VT associated with LQTS (TdP), CPVT, and Brugada syndrome also typically occur in patients with structurally normal hearts.

VENTRICULAR TACHYARRHYTHMIAS IN THE SETTING OF STRUCTURAL HEART DISEASE

Ventricular Arrhythmias Associated with Ischemic Cardiomyopathy

Mechanisms of ischemic ventricular arrhythmias include reentry (particularly around myocardial scar border zones), triggered activity, or enhanced automaticity (e.g., during reperfusion or ischemia). Early (<48 hours after MI) sustained ventricular arrhythmias are associated with increased in-hospital mortality and likely reflect electrical instability due to the acute infarct. Acute therapy includes cardioversion or defibrillation for sustained VT or VF, antiarrhythmic drugs, correction of metabolic imbalances, and treatment for recurrent or ongoing ischemia, including revascularization.

Long-term management includes risk stratification in an attempt to assess arrhythmia recurrence. For survivors of hemodynamically significant sustained VT or VF occurring more than 48 hours after acute MI, ICD implantation is indicated for secondary prevention of sudden cardiac death. Risk factors for sudden death include frequent PVCs, NSVT, VT/VF more than 48 hours after MI, low LVEF, or inducible sustained ventricular arrhythmias at EP study. After MI, episodes of NSVT are common; however, empiric suppression of PVCs or NSVT using antiarrhythmic drugs has been shown to be associated with an increased mortality, with the possible exception of amiodarone. Primary prevention studies of ICDs have demonstrated that in selected patients with NSVT with LVEF less than or equal to 40% after MI, ICDs can confer a survival benefit. Cardiac resynchronization therapy (CRT) is indicated in selected patients with low LVEF and wide QRS duration.

For primary prevention of sudden cardiac death in patients after MI with ischemic cardiomyopathy, ICD implantation is indicated in patients with LVEF less than or equal to 35% and New York Heart Association (NYHA) functional class (FC) II and III heart failure symptoms; ischemic cardiomyopathy with LVEF less than or equal to 30%; ischemic cardiomyopathy, LVEF less than or equal to 35%; NYHA FC III and IV and QRS duration greater than or equal to 120 ms receiving CRT; and NSVT and LVEF of 36% to 40% who have inducible sustained VT or reproducibly inducible VF at EP study. β-adrenergic blockers and angiotensin-converting enzyme (ACE) inhibitors also have been associated with improved survival rates and should be routinely used in the absence of contraindications.

Ventricular Arrhythmias Associated with Nonischemic Cardiomyopathy

VT or VF has been reported to be the cause of death in 8% to 50% of patients with nonischemic cardiomyopathy. Mechanisms of ventricular arrhythmias associated with nonischemic cardiomyopathy include reentry, triggered activity, and enhanced automaticity.

Bundle branch reentrant VT (BBRVT) is a form of macroreentry occurring within the bundle branches that has been described in patients with nonischemic cardiomyopathy who have evidence of His-Purkinje conduction system disease (e.g., an intraventricular conduction defect). More than 5% of VTs in these patients are due to this mechanism. The typical form is a very rapid monomorphic VT with LBBB and a superior axis morphology, although rare RBBB morphologies have been described. In LBBB morphology BBRVT, the anterograde limb is the right bundle branch, and the retrograde limb is the left bundle branch. This form can be treated effectively by ablation of one of the bundle branches (most commonly the right bundle).

For survivors of hemodynamically significant sustained VT or VF, ICD implantation is indicated for secondary prevention of sudden cardiac death. Various noninvasive and invasive tests have been proposed to risk stratify patients who have not yet had a sustained ventricular arrhythmia event. These include (1) Holter monitoring; (2) signal-averaged ECG; (3) QT dispersion (the difference in milliseconds between the longest and shortest QT intervals on a 12-lead ECG, which reflects the degree of homogeneity of ventricular repolarization); (4) T-wave alternans; and (5) EP study (even though this evaluation is less predictive of arrhythmic events than it is in patients with ischemic cardiomyopathy). CRT is indicated in selected patients with low LVEF and wide QRS duration (more than 120 ms).

For primary prevention of sudden cardiac death in nonischemic cardiomyopathy, ICD implantation is indicated in patients with LVEF less than or equal to 35% and NYHA FC II and III heart failure symptoms and in those with LVEF $\leq$35%, NYHA FC II to IV and QRS duration $\geq$120 ms who are candidates for CRT. Because β-adrenergic blockers and ACE inhibitors have been shown to improve survival in heart failure, these drugs are also indicated. In patients with ICDs and frequent appropriate shocks for NSVT and sustained VT, antiarrhythmic drugs and VT ablation can be used as adjunctive therapy to reduce the frequency of shocks.

Hypertrophic Cardiomyopathy

HCM (Fig. 6.11) is caused by mutations in genes encoding protein components of the cardiac sarcomere with autosomal dominant transmission. Genetically and phenotypically heterogeneous, more than 20 associated genes have been reported. These mutations are characterized by a highly variable expression and clinical course. Depending on the mutation, phenotypic penetrance varies from 30% to 80%.

Sudden death can occur in asymptomatic young individuals, including athletes, even as the initial presentation. Symptoms may result from diastolic dysfunction and LV outflow obstruction in the obstructive form of HCM; however, HCM can also be compatible with normal longevity. Risk factors for sudden cardiac death include prior VT/VF/CA, recurrent syncope, strong family history of sudden cardiac death, a decrease or attenuation of the increase of blood pressure (BP) on exercise, severe LV hypertrophy (e.g., 3-cm septum thickness), NSVT, end-stage cardiomyopathy, or high-risk genotype. Ventricular arrhythmias are often polymorphic. ICD implantation is indicated if CA or sustained VT/ spontaneous VF have occurred and can be considered if at least one high-risk factor is present (see Algorithm 8.3).

Arrhythmogenic Right Ventricular Cardiomyopathy

ARVC, sometimes referred to as arrhythmogenic RV dysplasia, is a cardiomyopathy that predominantly involves the right ventricle with fibrous, fatty infiltration, thinning, or hypokinetic areas of the RV; the left ventricle can also be involved in this process. Clinically, ARVC can present with symptomatic ventricular arrhythmias or sudden death and is a cause of sudden death in athletes. During sinus rhythm, the ECG may show anterior T-wave abnormalities such as T-wave inversion, mainly involving leads V_1 to V_3, reflecting the RV; occasionally an epsilon wave (Fig. 6.12) can be seen at the end of the QRS complex at the beginning of the ST segment, most obvious in lead V_1 or V_2. The signal-averaged

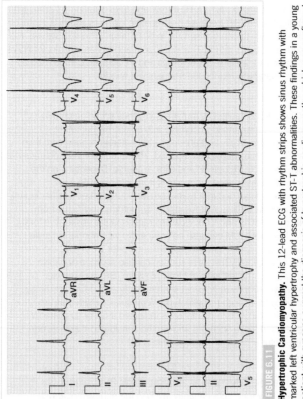

FIGURE 6.11

Hypertrophic Cardiomyopathy. This 12-lead ECG with rhythm strips shows sinus rhythm with marked left ventricular hypertrophy and associated ST-T abnormalities. These findings in a young patient with syncope suggest the diagnosis of hypertrophic cardiomyopathy, which was confirmed by echocardiography.

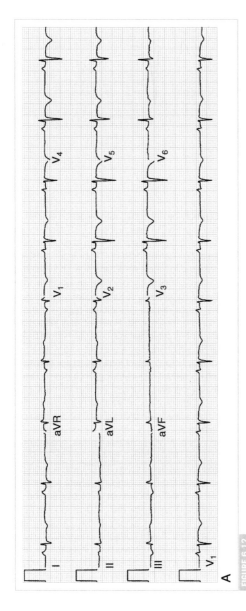

Continued on following page

FIGURE 6.12

Arrhythmogenic Right Ventricular Cardiomyopathy—Epsilon Wave. This 12-lead ECG tracing with lead V₁ rhythm strip (A) shows sinus rhythm with T-wave inversion over the right precordial leads. In addition, there is an epsilon wave (small deflection at the end of the QRS complex), evident in lead V₁ (B), which is characteristic of arrhythmogenic right ventricular cardiomyopathy.

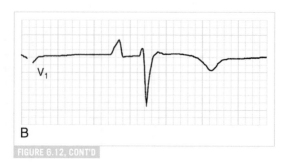

B

FIGURE 6.12, CONT'D

electrocardiogram (SAECG) may be abnormal, with evidence of late potentials. In general, the VTs or PVCs have multiple LBBB morphologies (Fig. 6.13) and are often precipitated by exercise. Both polymorphic and monomorphic VT can occur. Cardiac MRI or CT are more sensitive than echocardiographic imaging to detect ARVC and may show the high signal intensity fatty infiltration, thinning, hypokinesis, aneurysmal areas or dyskinetic bulges of the RV, RV dilation, or RVOT ectasia. The changes typically involve the inferior, apical, and/or infundibular regions of the RV, but the left ventricle can also be involved. However, fatty infiltration of the RV alone is not sufficient for the diagnosis because normal hearts may have intramyocardial fat, which increases with age and weight. Gadolinium enhancement may help to detect intramyocardial fibrosis. On endomyocardial biopsy, characteristic histopathology includes replacement-type fibrosis and myocyte degenerative changes. Fat replacement, clusters of myocyte death, myocardial atrophy, and inflammatory infiltrates may be seen. Changes in the intercalated disk proteins may be detected on immunohistochemical staining.

Criteria for clinical diagnosis of ARVC include two major, one major plus two minor, or four minor criteria. Major criteria include severe RV dilation or reduction in right ventricular ejection fraction (RVEF) with normal or only mildly reduced LV function, localized RV aneurysms, severe segmental RV dilation, fibrofatty replacement of myocardium on biopsy, epsilon waves or localized QRS prolongation of more than 110 ms in V_1 to V_3, or familial disease confirmed at necropsy or surgery. Minor criteria include mild RV dilation or reduction in RVEF with normal or only mildly reduced LV function, mild segmental RV dilatation, regional RV hypokinesis, late potentials on SAECG, sustained or nonsustained LBBB type VT, frequent PVCs (>1000 per 24 hours), inverted T waves in V_2 to V_3 in patients over age 12 in the absence of RBBB, family history of premature sudden death (under age 35 years) due to suspected ARVC, or family history with a clinical diagnosis.

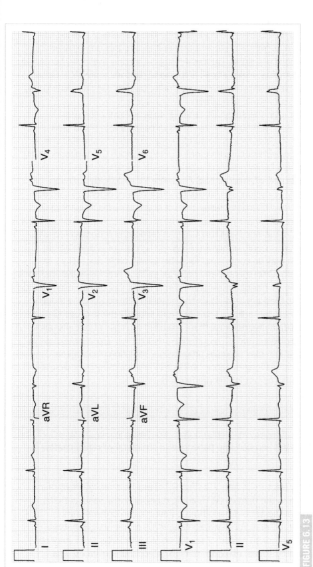

FIGURE 6.13

Arrhythmogenic right ventricular dysplasia/cardiomyopathy with premature ventricular complexes (PVCs). This 12-lead ECG and rhythm strips show precordial T wave inversion and PVCs with multiple left bundle branch block morphologies that have a superior (not inferior) axis. The non-inferior directed axis contrasts with the inferior axis of outflow tract PVCs that have high positive QRS complexes in the inferior leads II, III and AVF (See Figure 6.14).

There is strong familial transmission with autosomal dominant, variable penetrance inheritance patterns and mutations in desmosomal genes in approximately half of patients. Desmosomes are specialized intercellular junctions that anchor intermediate filaments of the cytoskeleton to the cytoplasmic membrane in adjoining cells. These are most prevalent in tissues, such as myocardium and skin epithelium, that are exposed to frictional and shear stress. Genetic testing is clinically available. Screening of family members, especially all first-degree relatives, may allow earlier diagnosis; manifestations usually occur after puberty. Genetic testing may provide reassurance of noncarriers.

Pharmacologic therapy, ICDs, and RF ablation have been used as treatments of ventricular arrhythmias in patients with ARVC (see Algorithm 8.7). Risk factors for sudden death or appropriate ICD shocks in ARVC from retrospective analyses include previous CA, syncope, young age, malignant family history of sudden death, participation in competitive sports, sustained VT, frequent NSVT, severe RV systolic dysfunction, LV involvement, LV dysfunction, late gadolinium enhancement on cardiac MRI, and QRS dispersion greater than or equal to 40ms or marked QRS prolongation. ICD implantation is recommended for patients meeting strict diagnostic criteria who have had CA, spontaneous or inducible rapid VT, depressed LV function, or familial ARVC at high risk of sudden death. ICD implantation may be considered for patients with other risk factors for sudden death. Drug therapy and catheter ablation are adjunctive therapies for increased VT frequency. Antiarrhythmic drugs that can be used include β-adrenergic blockers or class III drugs (sotalol, amiodarone), although data do not support a survival benefit from antiarrhythmic drugs. Catheter ablation is adjunctive because there are often multiple VT circuits, and progressive disease and VT recurrence are common. Because excessive myocardial strain may promote progression, limitation of competitive athletics, such as long-distance biking, running, swimming, or weight training, is also commonly recommended.

VENTRICULAR ARRHYTHMIAS IN STRUCTURALLY NORMAL HEARTS

Syndromes of repetitive, monomorphic, nonsustained, or sustained VT and paroxysmal VTs can occur in patients with structurally normal hearts.

Outflow Tract Ventricular Tachycardias

The outflow tract PVCs and VTs (Fig. 6.14) are focal tachyarrhythmias that arise from the right or LVOT, aortic cusp, or mitral valve annulus, commonly at the aortomitral isthmus. Patients can present with frequent symptomatic or asymptomatic PVCs or frequent, repetitive, or paroxysmal nonsustained or sustained VT. The PVCs or VT may be precipitated by stress, exercise, or high catecholamine states. The arrhythmia may suppress with exercise and return during recovery periods. Vagal maneuvers or adenosine may terminate the tachycardias.

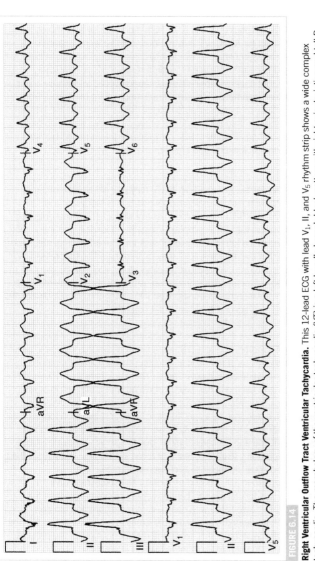

FIGURE 6.14

Right Ventricular Outflow Tract Ventricular Tachycardia. This 12-lead ECG with lead V_1, II, and V_5 rhythm strip shows a wide complex tachycardia. The morphology of the ventricular tachycardia (VT) is a left bundle branch block pattern with right axis deviation and tall R waves in II, III, and aVF localizing the site of VT initiation to the right ventricular outflow tract.

The PVCs or VTs are monomorphic and characterized by left BBB morphology with an inferior axis (e.g., tall positive R waves in aVF, II, and III). RBBB morphologies may also occur and suggest a left-sided origin. LBBB morphology PVCs or VT with a noninferior axis should lead to an evaluation for ARVC. VT may not be inducible with programmed ventricular extrastimulation at electrophysiology study but may occur during rapid pacing or infusion of isoproterenol. PVCs or NSVT may be so frequent that a tachycardia-induced cardiomyopathy may ensue (e.g., with persistent bigeminy). The arrhythmia mechanism may result from triggered activity or increased automaticity. RF catheter ablation has been curative in greater than 90%. LVOT or aortic cusp sites have also been targets for ablation. Treatment also may include β-adrenergic blockers, calcium channel blockers, and type I or III antiarrhythmic drugs.

Idiopathic Left Ventricular or Fascicular Tachycardia

ILVT or fascicular tachycardia (Fig. 6.15) may present as a paroxysmal VT in patients with a structurally normal heart. This tachycardia is characterized by RBBB morphology, usually with a left superior axis (e.g., left-axis deviation with QRS complexes negative in leads II and aVF). ILVT usually arises in the left inferoposterior septum. The arrhythmia mechanism is reentry within the fascicles. ILVT may be terminated or suppressed by verapamil or diltiazem. At electrophysiology study, ILVT can be induced by programmed ventricular extrastimulation, rapid pacing, isoproterenol, or exercise. RF ablation has been successful in curing this VT, usually at sites where the VT is preceded by a fascicular potential.

Long QT Syndrome

The long QT syndromes (Fig. 6.16) are a family of syndromes due to genetic mutations on various chromosomes affecting several cardiac channels responsible for ventricular repolarization. There are more than 10 clinical syndromes, and each one has been associated with mutations in specific genes or loci; however, the specific mutation can vary tremendously even though it may involve a specific gene. The most common forms of LQTS are LQT1, LQT2, and LQT3. These syndromes are associated with episodic syncope and CA caused by VF due to TdP VT. There are unique electrocardiographic features of each of these syndromes. In addition, there are specific clinical characteristics of each syndrome.

First described in 1957 based on familial autosomal recessive inheritance was the Jervell and Lange-Nielsen syndrome in which the prolonged QT is associated with deafness. A more common familial disorder without deafness and with autosomal dominant inheritance is the Romano-Ward syndrome; this syndrome represents most of the patients with the LQTS. In such patients there may be a relationship between the length of the QT interval at rest and exercise and outcomes, but this is not always the case. There can be different phenotypic expressions and unique electrocardiographic characteristics of each long QT syndrome, but some

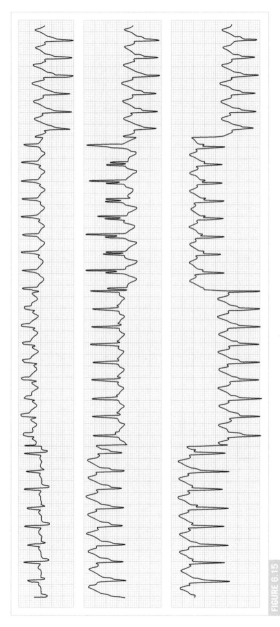

FIGURE 6.15

Idiopathic Left Ventricular or Fascicular Tachycardia. This 12-lead ECG shows a very rapid wide complex tachycardia with a right bundle branch block morphology and left superior axis (negative QRS complexes in leads II and aVF) that is due to reentry within the left ventricle fascicles.

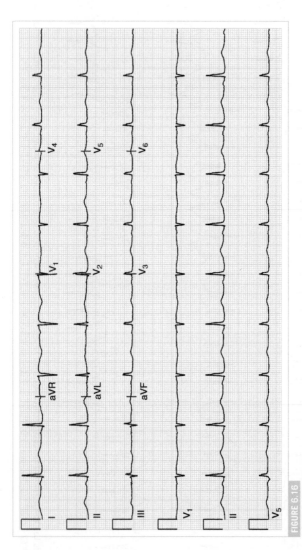

Long QT Syndrome. This 12-lead ECG with lead V$_1$, II, and V$_5$ rhythm strip shows normal sinus rhythm. There is marked QT prolongation.

individuals are genotypically negative for LQTS known gene mutations though phenotypically positive for LQTS and vice versa. The phenotype and genotype may be predictive of outcomes.

In LQT1 (decreased I_{Ks} current), the QT fails to shorten with exercise, and episodes of sudden death tend to occur with activities, such as swimming. In LQT2 (decreased I_{Kr} current), loud noises and emotional distress are associated with sudden death, and the VT episodes tend to follow pause-dependent QT prolongation. In LQT3 (slowly inactivating Na current), episodes tend to occur at night and at slower rates. For this less common group, exercise shortens the QT, and class IB antiarrhythmic drugs are being studied. β-adrenergic blockers may be helpful for the patient with LQT1 and LTQ2. Although there is a direct relationship between the QT interval and death, it can be difficult to predict which patient is at greatest risk before an episode ultimately occurs. The highest risk groups are those with LQT1 and 2 syndromes when the QT interval is greater than 500 ms and males with LQT3. Risk factors for cardiac events include (1) the length of the corrected QT interval (QTc); (2) LQT1 and LQT2 with long QTc; (3) males with LQT3; (4) adolescence; (5) males before puberty; (6) females during adulthood; (7) pregnancy and postpartum period; (8) family history; (9) syncope; (10) resuscitated CA; and (11) genotype.

TdP VT (see Fig. 6.7) is a form of polymorphic VT associated with prolonged QT intervals, reflecting prolonged cardiac repolarization. TdP is potentially life-threatening and can be sustained or degenerate to VF. It is most commonly seen as a complication of QT-prolonging medications or in association with acquired or congenital long QT syndromes. The mechanism is attributed to triggered activity due to EADs. The heart rate ranges from 150 to 250 bpm, with twisting of the QRS complexes around the baseline. QT prolongation and QTU abnormalities are characteristic but may be present only in QRST complexes preceding TdP. Giant U waves (U waves taller than the T waves in a given ECG lead) may be present. These U waves may reflect the amplitudes of the cellular EADs. TdP typically is rate dependent. Sinus bradycardia (SB), bradycardia resulting from AV block, or abrupt prolongation of the RR interval (e.g., with a pause after a premature complex or nonconducted atrial premature depolarization) can trigger its onset. TdP typically initiates with a long–short coupled interval, which may occur because of a PVC on the previous, long QT-associated T wave; a pause followed by a subsequent sinus or supraventricular beat and another PVC with a short coupling interval then may initiate TdP.

Evaluation of the LQTS includes an ECG, ambulatory monitoring to detect variability of the QT interval, including diurnal variation, PVCs and nonsustained TdP VT, and exercise testing. There is no role for EP testing. Genetic testing is available. A careful history for QT-prolonging drugs (prescription and over the counter), diet, and circumstances surrounding symptoms is important. Acquired LQTSs, many of which are associated with drugs that can prolong repolarization, are more commonly encountered than are congenital syndromes, but most are likely associated with similar ion channel abnormalities. Acquired LQTS may represent uncovering of a previously undetermined congenital long QT variant.

Acute treatment for TdP includes discontinuation and avoidance of offending drugs and correction of electrolyte imbalances. Patients with normal serum Mg^{2+} may nonetheless have total body depletion; IV Mg^{2+} is thus extremely useful to treat TdP. Acceleration of the heart rate shortens the QT interval and may be accomplished using pharmacologic drugs (e.g., isoproterenol in selected patients, especially those without ischemic heart disease) or pacing. Lidocaine, mexiletine, or phenytoin can be tried as well.

Long-term management includes ICD implantation for life-threatening arrhythmias (see Algorithm 8.5). β-adrenergic blockers can be used for patients with less severe presentations and possibly for asymptomatic family members (e.g., with LQT1). Genotype-specific therapies are being studied. Supplemental potassium and magnesium can be considered, and electrolyte abnormalities should be corrected promptly, especially in case of acute illnesses, such as may occur with diarrhea, vomiting, or other metabolic conditions. Evaluation of first-degree relatives is advised. QT-prolonging drugs should be avoided. Patients may be directed to http://www.crediblemeds.org for listings of drugs to be avoided. Avoidance of genotype-specific triggers, such as strenuous swimming in LQT1 or loud noises in LQT2, may be helpful.

Brugada Syndrome

The Brugada syndrome (Fig. 6.17) is a cause of sudden death, often at night, and a common cause of nocturnal sudden cardiac death in young healthy males in Southeast Asia (sudden unexpected nocturnal death syndrome). It may cause some cases of sudden infant death syndrome. Primary VF and rarely sustained VT may occur in up to one-third of patients. The ECG shows RBBB-like morphology with J-point elevation in leads V_1 to V_3 and persistent descending ST elevation in the right precordial leads. These characteristic changes may not be present at all times and may be worsened or unmasked by sodium channel blockers (e.g., flecainide, procainamide, ajmaline). AV conduction abnormalities and atrial arrhythmias are common. This ECG pattern can also occur during acute ischemia, fever, and with certain drugs, such as tricyclic antidepressants; however, the clinical syndrome of syncope, VT, and sudden death is rare in these cases. Thus the ECG pattern is not equivalent to the syndrome. The ST elevation over the right precordial ECG leads can lead to the mistaken diagnosis of anterior wall MI and hyperkalemia.

The clinical diagnosis of Brugada syndrome can be confirmed with a type 1 ECG (J wave ≥2 mm; negative T waves; coved, gradually descending ST in more than one right precordial lead V_1 to V_3, with or without a sodium channel blocker) and either an SCN5A mutation and/or at least one of the following: documented VF, self-terminating polymorphic VT, a family history of sudden death before age 45, coved-type ECGs in family members, EP inducibility, or syncope or nocturnal agonal respiration.

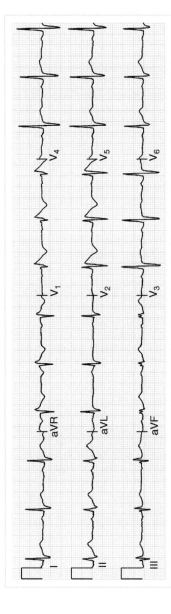

FIGURE 6.17

Brugada Syndrome. This 12-lead ECG shows the distinctive right bundle branch block-like QRS complex and ST elevation that is consistent with Brugada syndrome. Here there is an R' and ST elevation in lead V_1 as well as in lead V_2. Patients are considered to have the unique clinical presentation of Brugada syndrome when this ECG pattern is associated with ventricular tachycardia or ventricular fibrillation, which can result in syncope or sudden cardiac death. This ECG pattern has been associated with SCN5A gene mutations that affect the sodium channel and is associated with life-threatening ventricular arrhythmias and sudden death in otherwise healthy individuals.

The diagnosis of Brugada syndrome can be strongly considered with a type 2 ECG (J wave ≥2 mm, positive or biphasic T wave, "saddle-back" ST elevation greater than or equal to 1 mm in more than one right precordial lead V_1 to V_3 at baseline and converted to a type 1 ECG after challenge with a sodium channel blocker [e.g., flecainide, ajmaline, procainamide]), or a type 3 ECG (J wave ≥2 mm, positive T, saddle-back ST elevated less than 1 mm in more than one lead at baseline with conversion to type 1 ECG after challenge with a sodium channel blocker) (Figs. 6.18 and 6.19).

Loss-of-function mutations in the SCN5A gene, which codes for the α-subunit of the sodium channel (the same gene that causes LQT3 but with loss of function rather than gain of function) have been identified in Brugada syndrome with autosomal dominant inheritance, although genetic heterogeneity and variable penetrance have been identified. Mutations in SCN5A have been identified in 20% to 25% of cases. There is at least one other locus described. Inheritance is in an autosomal dominant pattern though with penetrance of approximately 30%. Thirty percent of patients with this mutation have diagnostic ECGs, and challenge with sodium channel blocker can increase the diagnostic ECG rate to 80%.

High-risk factors include a history of aborted sudden cardiac death, syncope, prior ventricular arrhythmias, spontaneous ST elevation, and inducible VT/VF. The role of EP testing is controversial. Lower risk indicators are asymptomatic patients with a diagnostic ECG only after provocative challenge. There has been no effective drug therapy identified. Amiodarone and β-adrenergic blockers are inadequate. Isoproterenol has been used for electrical storms. ICD implantation is appropriate for those surviving aborted sudden cardiac death or sustained VT/VF or for those who have syncope (see Algorithm 8.9). ICD implantation in asymptomatic patients is controversial but may be considered in patients with a strong family history of sudden death or syncope or inducible VT/VF (in asymptomatic patients EP studies have been reported to be predictive of events, but this is controversial). Quinidine may prevent symptoms because of its inhibition of I_{to} and quinidine or isoproterenol have been helpful in VT/VF electrical storm. Catheter ablation of the RVOT epicardium has been reported as a potential therapy for recurrent ICD shocks or electrical storm.

Drugs or circumstances that should be avoided in Brugada syndrome include high fevers, excessive alcohol intake and large meals, vagotonic drugs, α-adrenergic antagonists, tricyclic antidepressants, first-generation antihistamines, cocaine toxicity, class IC antiarrhythmic drugs (flecainide, propafenone), and class IA antiarrhythmic drugs (procainamide, disopyramide). Patients may be directed to http://www.brugadadrugs.org for listings of drugs to avoid.

Catecholaminergic Polymorphic Ventricular Tachycardia

Polymorphic VT not associated with long QT may be associated with ischemia or electrolyte abnormality, but the syndrome of CPVT (Fig. 6.20) is a cause of exercise-induced polymorphic VT. CPVT may present with

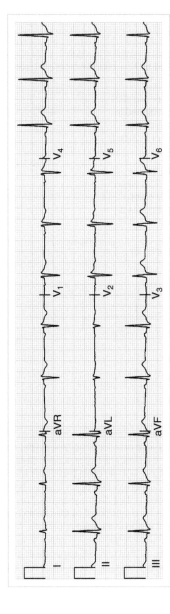

FIGURE 6.18

Type II Brugada pattern ECG. This 12-lead ECG shows a type II Brugada pattern in leads V_1 and V_2. While a type I ECG pattern (Figure 6.17) supports a diagnosis of Brugada syndrome, Brugada syndrome can be considered for type 2 or 3 ECG patterns (Figure 6.19) if the ECG pattern converts to a type 1 pattern after challenge with a sodium channel blocker.

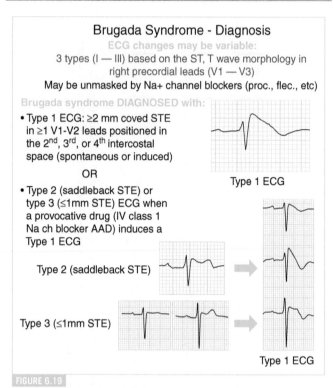

Brugada Syndrome - Diagnosis

ECG changes may be variable:

3 types (I — III) based on the ST, T wave morphology in right precordial leads (V1 — V3)

May be unmasked by Na+ channel blockers (proc., flec., etc)

Brugada syndrome DIAGNOSED with:

- Type 1 ECG: ≥2 mm coved STE in ≥1 V1-V2 leads positioned in the 2nd, 3rd, or 4th intercostal space (spontaneous or induced)

OR

- Type 2 (saddleback STE) or type 3 (≤1mm STE) ECG when a provocative drug (IV class 1 Na ch blocker AAD) induces a Type 1 ECG

Type 1 ECG

Type 2 (saddleback STE)

Type 3 (≤1mm STE)

Type 1 ECG

FIGURE 6.19

Brugada ECG patterns. A type 1 ECG pattern supports diagnosis of Brugada syndrome. Brugada syndrome can be considered for type 2 or 3 ECG patterns if ECG pattern converts to a type 1 pattern after challenge with a sodium channel blocker.

syncope, polymorphic VT during exercise or acute emotion, absence of structural heart disease, and a family history of sudden death. The age of onset is usually in childhood, but late onset (fourth decade) has been reported. CPVT can cause sudden cardiac death and has been postulated to cause some cases of sudden infant death syndrome. Supraventricular arrhythmias are common. A family history of sudden death in relatives less than 40 years old is present in about one-third of patients. An exercise stress test may provoke the arrhythmia, which is characterized by a rapid, bidirectional, or polymorphic VT that may self-terminate or degenerate to VF. The mechanism is postulated to be due to DADs and triggered activity. Mutations in genes controlling intracellular calcium (e.g., ryanodine receptor 2 [RYR2] or calsequestrin 2 [CASQ2]) have been identified.

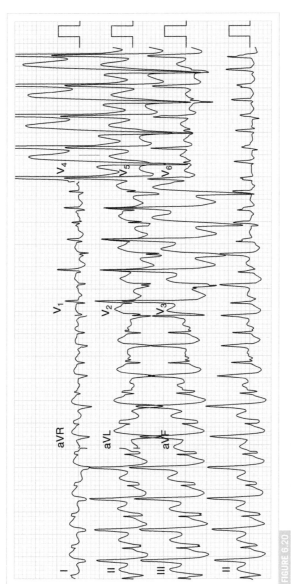

FIGURE 6.20

Catecholaminergic Polymorphic Ventricular Tachycardia. This 12-lead ECG and lead II rhythm strip show bidirectional ventricular tachycardia in a patient with catecholaminergic polymorphic VT (CPVT). *(Courtesy Dr. Peter Aziz).*

Other loci have been postulated. A form of ARVC (ARVC2) associated with apical morphologic changes and CPVT has been associated with RYR2 mutation. Genetic testing is available. β-adrenergic blockers are effective in approximately 60% to 70% of patients, and repeat stress testing can help to assess efficacy. Calcium channel blockers, sodium channel blockers, and amiodarone are less or not effective. ICDs are indicated for CA survivors, sustained VT/VF, or recurrent syncope or sustained VT while on β-adrenergic blockers (see Algorithm 8.10). There may be a role for flecainide in reducing ventricular arrhythmias and may be considered in patients who continue to have incomplete control of their arrhythmias on β-adrenergic blockers.

Drug- and Metabolic-Induced Torsades de Pointes

TdP, a potentially life-threatening polymorphic VT associated with prolonged QT intervals, can occur as a result of medications (see Fig. 6.7) and/or congenital long QT syndromes. TdP has a rate of 150 to 250 bpm, with twisting of the QRS complexes around the baseline. Drug-induced TdP may represent a *forme fruste* of a congenital LQTS, but it is not clear that a genetic abnormality is necessary to cause QT prolongation and TdP in the great majority of patients who develop this arrhythmia because of drugs or electrolyte abnormalities.

TdP may be related to low potassium and/or magnesium levels; however, a normal Mg^{2+} level does not preclude low total body Mg^{2+}, as serum Mg^{2+} represents only 1% to 2% of total body stores. Drug-induced TdP is more common in women, especially older women, and it is more likely to occur during critical illnesses or with malnutrition or high-protein diets. Other causes for prolonged QT interval that may predispose to TdP include structural heart disease, cerebrovascular accident (head trauma, stroke), impaired metabolism or clearance of QT interval-prolonging drugs, pH imbalance, hypothyroidism, altered nutritional states, bradycardia (<50 bpm) or pauses, and hypothermia. In many cases TdP is multifactorial.

QT prolongation and QTU abnormalities (e.g., giant U waves, which exceed the height of the T wave in a given ECG lead) are characteristic but may be present only in QRST complexes preceding TdP.

Drug-induced TdP is typically rate and pause dependent. The pause may be extrasystolic, with the extraasystole arising either from atrial or ventricle, and can follow a nonconducted atrial premature depolarization. It usually initiates with long-short coupled intervals (see Fig. 6.7).

Some drugs have a marked effect on prolonging the QT interval but do not usually induce TdP; this is commonly seen in patients receiving amiodarone. Conversely, some drugs that do not prolong the QT interval substantially can cause TdP. The actual risk of TdP appears to be drug dependent (and for some drugs, dose dependent). It appears that most drug-induced TDP is related to blockade of the HERG potassium channel (i.e., I_{Kr}), but it is not clear that this is related to a specific congenital abnormality. The absolute risk of TdP may be low but is still consequential. This has led to some drugs being removed from the market due to the risk of TdP even if only a few patients out of several million developed the arrhythmia; in part, this is related to TdP being potentially life-threatening, and many drugs that are associated with it are used for relatively innocuous non–life-threatening conditions.

When considering QT prolongation and the risk of TdP, it must be recognized that this risk is a drug-dependent and condition-dependent issue. For example, several antiarrhythmic drugs can prolong the QT interval (e.g., amiodarone, sotalol) but still have potential benefit and therefore should be considered for use but with caution. Therefore, when considering use of a specific drug for a specific problem, it becomes important to recognize the risk of TdP and select the drug that is associated with the lowest risk in that drug class, unless the drug is found to be ineffective, in which case more risky drugs need to be used. In many if not most instances, it cannot be determined with certainty which drug will cause TdP in which specific patient. A normal ECG does not necessarily ensure that TdP will not occur at some later time under differing conditions. A drug that has been used successfully for many years can still cause TdP as a person ages, has changes in autonomic tone, develops extrasystoles with postextrasystolic pauses, or develops abnormalities in electrolyte balance or renal insufficiency.

The Food and Drug Administration considers QT interval prolongation a major issue, and it is a major reason drugs do not get approved.

It is important to recognize the variety of medications and conditions that can lead to QT interval prolongation and the potential for TdP. Drugs and conditions associated with TdP include the following:

- Antiarrhythmic drugs
  - Quinidine
  - Procainamide (including its metabolite N-acetylprocainamide)
  - Disopyramide
  - Sotalol
  - Amiodarone
  - Ibutilide
  - Dofetilide
- Tricyclic antidepressants
- Phenothiazines
- Antibiotics
  - Erythromycin
  - Pentamidine
  - Trimethoprim-sulfamethoxazole
  - Ampicillin

- Ketoconazole
- Itraconazole
- Spiramycin
- Clarithromycin
- Fluconazole
- Moxifloxacin
- Other QT-prolonging drugs
  - Diuretics (lowering potassium)
- Organophosphates
- Electrolyte abnormalities
  - Hypokalemia
  - Hypomagnesemia
  - Hypocalcemia (uncommon)
- Bradyarrhythmias
- Hypothyroidism
- Liquid protein and other diets, anorexia, bulimia
- Central nervous system abnormalities, particularly affecting sympathetic outflow
  - Subarachnoid hemorrhage
  - Brainstem, cervical cord lesions
- Cocaine

Useful sources of information on QT-prolonging drugs may be found at www.torsades.org and www.qtdrugs.org (Table 6.3).

PRIMARY AND SECONDARY PREVENTION OF SUDDEN CARDIAC DEATH

Sudden, unexpected death is a common cause of death. It is often cardiac and arrhythmic in nature. Because of its abrupt and unexpected occurrence, a ventricular tachyarrhythmia, such as VF, is often the etiology. However, sudden death presumed to be due to a cardiac cause is not necessarily due to VF, and even if VF is the terminal rhythm, this does not necessarily mean that the VF caused the death or that its termination would have prevented the death. Despite these caveats, the role in the prevention of sudden death for medications (β-adrenergic blockers, ACE inhibitors, aldosterone antagonists, statins), AEDs, wearable cardioverter defibrillators, and ICDs have become better defined based on controlled clinical trials. A potential way to reduce risk is to identify which patients can benefit from specific long-term therapeutic strategies. Assessing which patients are at highest risk for sudden cardiac death (but not death from other causes) can modify outcomes and improve long-term prognosis.

Secondary prevention of sudden cardiac death involves reduction of risk and prevention of death after an episode of CA (usually out-of-hospital CA) due to sustained VT with hemodynamic collapse or VF (see Algorithm 8.2). Well over 70% of such individuals have ischemic heart disease with or without LV dysfunction. Most commonly, there is a history

Continued on following page

TABLE 6.3

MANAGEMENT OF SPECIFIC VENTRICULAR ARRHYTHMIA SYNDROMES

Setting	Therapy	Comments
Prior MI, discrete LV aneurysm or scar	First line: ICD implantation	Due to a reentry substrate.
	Second line: Amiodarone or sotalol	Reentry circuit is usually around the rim of the aneurysm (border zone).
	Third line: Mapping and RF ablation in the EP lab	Can be ablated by aneurysmectomy with (better) or without map-guided resection in the operative room with cryoablation and/or endocardial resection.
	Fourth line: Consider map guided resection in the OR	Success rate for tachycardia cure is high, albeit with a 10%–15% mortality.
	Mortality is 10–15%	
	Indicates an advantage only to patients with frequently recurrent, resistant VT	
Structural heart disease	ICD implantation is the first line approach for prevention of sudden cardiac death	Patient with sustained monomorphic VT without provoked ischemia will likely have several recurrences.
Ischemia cannot be provoked	EP testing is highly sensitive and specific in patients with CAD, but not with valvular cardiomyopathy or dilated cardiomyopathy	Rate of VT inducibility at EP study is less in nonischemic cardiomyopathy than in ischemic cardiomyopathy.
No aneurysm	ICD implantation is considered first line therapy for hemodynamically significant sustained VT with reduced LV function without need for EP study	In idiopathic dilated cardiomyopathy, a cause of VT may be bundle branch reentry VT, which may be ablated at one of the involved bundle branches.
	If LV function is reduced, ICD implantation is best approach	
Nonischemic or idiopathic dilated cardiomyopathy	If LV function is normal, consider EP study with mapping and ablation	
	If LV function is reduced due to frequent PVCs or VT and there is a suspicion that the cardiomyopathy is tachycardia-induced, EP study with mapping and ablation may not only cure the VT but may improve LV function	
	Adjunctive antiarrhythmic therapy to reduce recurrences include β-adrenergic blockers, sotalol, or amiodarone	

TABLE 6.3

MANAGEMENT OF SPECIFIC VENTRICULAR ARRHYTHMIA SYNDROMES (Continued)

Setting	Therapy	Comments
HCM	• Often polymorphic • Potentially life-threatening • Urgent early cardioversion even if apparently well tolerated • ICD implantation for sustained VT or other major high risk factors	• Genetically and phenotypically heterogeneous. • Autosomal dominant transmission. • Caused by mutations in genes encoding protein components of the cardiac sarcomere. • Highly variable clinical course. • Sudden death frequent in asymptomatic young patients <35 years. • May occur in young athletes. • May be the initial presentation. • Symptoms may also result from diastolic dysfunction and outflow obstruction in obstructive form. • Compatible with normal longevity. • Risk factors for sudden cardiac death (indications for ICD implantation) • Prior VT/VF/CA • Recurrent syncope • Strong family history of sudden cardiac death • Failure to raise BP on exercise • Very thick ventricle (e.g., 3-cm septum) • NSVT • High-risk genotype

ARVC (dysplasia)

- ICD for spontaneous or inducible rapid sustained VT, CA, depressed LV function, or familial ARVC at high risk of sudden death
- Antiarrhythmic drugs and catheter ablation are adjunctive for increased VT frequency
- Sotalol (initiate in hospital) 80 mg to start but preferably 120–240 mg bid
- Amiodarone or β-adrenergic blockers may be effective
- Catheter ablation is adjunctive, but multiple VT circuits, recurrences, and progressive disease are common

- Predominant RV cardiomyopathy with fibrous, fatty infiltration, thinning, or hypokinetic areas of the RV.
- May involve the LV.
- A cause of ventricular arrhythmias in patients with apparently normal LV.
- A cause of sudden death in athletes.
- VTs generally have multiple LBBB morphologies and are often precipitated by exercise.
- MRI more sensitive than echocardiography.
  - The SAECG is often positive.
  - There can be an epsilon wave seen in V_1-V_3.
- Strong familial transmission (>50% of patients) is present with autosomal dominant, variable penetrance patterns, and mutations in desmosomal system genes reported.
  - Genetic testing is clinically available.

Tetralogy of Fallot

- If severe RV and/or pressure overload, surgical repair of anatomic abnormalities is required
- If surgery planned, consider mapping and ablation around the ventricular septal defect
- If no surgery is planned, consider RF ablation of the macroreentry circuit
  - First line: Amiodarone
  - Second line: ICD

- Polymorphic VT and monomorphic VT can both occur.
- Due to reentry around ventricular septal defect or its repair.
- Often related to dilatation of the RV, which may be due to pulmonary hypertension.
- Assess hemodynamics and need for surgical repair.

Continued on following page

TABLE 6.3

MANAGEMENT OF SPECIFIC VENTRICULAR ARRHYTHMIA SYNDROMES (Continued)

Setting	Therapy	Comments

Bidirectional VT	• If due to digoxin toxicity (rare):
	   ○ Observe in an intensive care unit
	   ○ Correct hypokalemia and hypomagnesemia
	   ○ Give digoxin antibodies (especially if sustained or poorly tolerated or if degenerate to VF)
	 • If the patient is on digoxin and the episodes are nonsustained, dig antibodies are not indicated
	 • If catecholamine-sensitive VT occurs in children or young adults, β-adrenergic blockers and ICD are indicated
		• Generally indicates digoxin toxicity.
		 • Administration of digoxin antibodies should be considered.
		 • In children, this may be the forme fruste of congenital LQTS.

CPVT	• β-adrenergic blockers are effective in approximately 60% of cases • Use re-exercise stress test to assess efficacy • ICDs are indicated for recurrent CA	• A cause of exercise-induced polymorphic VT. • Mutations in genes controlling intracellular calcium have been reported. • For example, ryanodine release channel RYR2, calsequestrin CASQ2. • Other loci postulated.

Long QT syndrome	• Involves acute management of TdP
	 • Avoid offending drugs
	 • Correct electrolyte imbalances
	 • Accelerate heart rate to shorten QT interval (e.g., pacing, isoproterenol)
	 • Use IV Mg^{2+}
		• Inherited ion channel disorder (Na^+ and K^+ channels).
		 • Autosomal dominant inheritance most common (Romano-Ward syndrome), clinical features vary with genetic mutation.
		   ○ LQT1 (55%–60% of autosomal dominant LQTS)—KCNQ1 mutations (decreased I_{Ks} α-subunit)—events with exercise, swimming; broad T wave.
		   ○ LQT2 (35%–40%)—KCNH2 (HERG). KCNE2 mutations (decreased I_{Ks} α-subunit)—events with auditory, startle, emotional stimuli; notched/bifid or low T wave.
		   ○ LQT3 (3%–5%)—SCN5A mutations (increased I_{Na} α-subunit)—events during sleep, bradycardia; long flat ST segment.

- Consider lidocaine, mexiletine, phenytoin

- No role for EP study

- Use ICD for recurrent life-threatening arrhythmias or VF

- Use β-adrenergic blockers for patients with less severe presentations and possibly asymptomatic family members (e.g., LQT1)
  - Genotype-specific therapy is being studied
  - Consider supplemental K^+ and Mg^{2+}
  - Evaluate (history, ECG) first-degree relatives for presence of LQTS

- Rare autosomal recessive with congenital deafness (Jervell and Lange-Nielsen syndrome).

- Clinical features can vary with genetic mutation.
  - Variable expression of severity.

- Syncope and sudden death increased frequency in adolescence.

- Risk factors for cardiac events:
  - QTc duration
  - LQT1 and LQT2 with long QTc
  - Males LQT3, adolescence
  - Males before puberty
  - Females during adulthood, pregnancy, and postpartum period
  - Family history
  - Syncope
  - Resuscitated CA
  - Genotype

- Acquired long QT syndrome (e.g., drug-induced TdP) may represent the uncovering of a previously undetermined congenital long QT variant.

ARVC, Arrhythmogenic right ventricular cardiomyopathy; *bid,* twice a day; *BP,* blood pressure; *CA,* cardiac arrest; *CAD,* coronary artery disease; *CPVT,* catecholaminergic polymorphic ventricular tachycardia; *EP,* electrophysiologic; *HCM,* hypertrophic cardiomyopathy; *ICD,* implantable cardioverter defibrillator; *IV,* intravenous; *LBBB,* left bundle branch block; *LQTS,* long QT interval syndrome; *LV,* left ventricular; *MI,* myocardial infarction; *MRI,* magnetic resonance imaging; *NSVT,* nonsustained ventricular tachycardia; *PVCs,* premature ventricular contractions; *QT_c,* corrected QT interval; *RF,* radiofrequency; *RV,* right ventricular; *SAECG,* signal-averaged electrocardiogram; *TdP,* torsades de pointes; *VF,* ventricular fibrillation; *VT,* ventricular tachycardia.

of a prior MI; acute ischemia is not necessarily the trigger. Nonischemic cardiomyopathy, another common cause of out-of-hospital CA, is generally idiopathic but may be related to viral myocarditis, alcohol, or toxins, such as cocaine. The remainder of out-of-hospital CA includes various genetic and congenital conditions, acute myocarditis, valvular heart disease, HCM, RV cardiomyopathy (dysplasia), infiltrative heart diseases (e.g., amyloidosis, hemochromatosis), and sarcoidosis. Some conditions are poorly understood. For example, idiopathic VF may be related to triggers in the His-Purkinje system that could be ablated and potentially cured.

For patients with ischemic or nonischemic cardiomyopathy and sustained monomorphic VT, catheter ablation may be an effective strategy to reduce the risk of recurrent episodes. Endocardial and epicardial ablation strategies are now available to attempt to eliminate VT originating in either the right or left ventricles; however, patients with ablated VT who continue to have ventricular dysfunction remain at risk for sudden cardiac death. Catheter ablation strategies for VT where structural heart disease is present have not yet been shown to reduce the risk of sudden cardiac death or total mortality. Such patients should be considered for ICD implantation, even if ablation appears to be successful.

Several triggers other than VT/VF may initiate out-of-hospital CA, including electrolyte disorders (e.g., severe hypokalemia) and myocardial ischemia; however, revascularization to prevent myocardial ischemia does not eliminate it entirely and may not fully normalize any associated LV dysfunction. Most patients with out-of-hospital CA do not have acute MI. Several noncardiac causes for out-of-hospital CA also exist, such as aspiration, pulmonary embolus, sepsis, ruptured aortic aneurysm, and intracerebral bleed. If the etiology can be correctly identified and appropriately and effectively treated, long-term preventive strategies may not be necessary.

Patients who have had an out-of-hospital CA due to VF who do not have an obvious reversible cause are likely to have recurrences and are good candidates for an ICD for secondary prevention. This represents the minority of ICD implants, as most such individuals are not resuscitated.

The need for an ICD after an acute MI with resuscitated VF is not completely resolved, and long-term mortality benefits have not been demonstrated. In some instances a wearable cardioverter defibrillator can be used in the short term after MI if LV dysfunction is present. Wearable cardioverter defibrillators are only a short-term solution because they are not always actually worn by the patient and long-term mortality benefit has not been proven. It is best to err in favor of the patient and consider placing an ICD in the patient for whom the cause for the resuscitated VF is not known with certainty and who otherwise has a reasonable chance of a good long-term prognosis.

Primary prevention of sudden cardiac death refers to prophylactic strategies in patients who have not yet had a CA or hemodynamically decompensating sustained ventricular arrhythmias. Primary prevention patients represent a much larger group at risk for sudden cardiac death due to VF. Factors associated with risk for out-of-hospital CA have been identified. Patients at high risk of sudden arrhythmic death but otherwise not at high risk of overall death are excellent candidates for an ICD to allow reasonable and functional long-term survival (see Algorithm 8.1).

Clinical risk factors include male gender, older age, diabetes, systolic CHF (especially NYHA FC II to IV on optimal medical treatment), hypertension, syncope in patients with heart disease, AF, renal insufficiency, increased heart rate, smoking, and an abnormal 6-minute walk test. However, all clinical predictors suffer from lack of sensitivity, specificity, and predictive accuracy.

Both noninvasive and invasive tests have been used to assess risk for sudden cardiac death. Most noninvasive tests are also nonspecific and lack sensitivity, specificity, and adequate predictive accuracy. Nevertheless, they can help to clarify long-term prognosis. Such tests include an abnormal ECG (specifically, the presence of LBBB or Q-wave MI), PVCs on Holter monitor, a positive signal averaged ECG, abnormal baroreceptor sensitivity, decreased heart rate variability, increased QT dispersion, abnormal spectral turbulence, abnormal T-wave alternans, or an abnormal high-sensitivity CRP. Many of these tests reveal markers and not predictors of event and are often population and disease specific. The highest risk individuals may already be identified as being at high risk based on LVEF and underlying disease. Furthermore, such patients may be at higher risk for total mortality independent of the risk for sudden cardiac death. There has been recent interest in using T-wave alternans to identify arrhythmic risk, but its role is not completely defined. In general, the benefit of noninvasive and even invasive EP testing is not completely defined. Such tests are best used when patients are at borderline or intermediate risk (moderately impaired ventricular function or mild-to-moderate CHF).

Because all individuals are at some risk for sudden cardiac death even without any risk factor, identification of risk is a complex and difficult issue. Although risk factors can identify the individuals at highest risk for sudden cardiac death due to VF, these patients are often also at great risk for dying of nonarrhythmic death, and they represent a small percentage of all patients who are at risk for out-of-hospital CA.

Much of the clinical decision about who should get aggressive therapy and who should receive an ICD remains incompletely defined. Clinical decisions regarding use for an ICD are generally based on two clinical variables (NYHA FC and LVEF [$\leq$0.40] after optimal medical therapy, no matter how nonspecific these predictors might be) and on the results of randomized clinical trials.

EP testing has been used to attempt to quantify risk; however, the results depend on the underlying disease and the predictive accuracy is not that high. The EP test is best used in NYHA FC I patients with CAD when NSVT is present and the LVEF is 30% to 40%. If there is CAD or a nonischemic cardiomyopathy, NYHA FC II and III CHF, and an LVEF less than or equal to 0.35, an ICD should be implanted without specific need for an EP test. Patients with CAD and LVEF less than or equal to 0.30 are candidates for an ICD regardless of the presence or absence of symptoms due to the systolic LV dysfunction. Patients without CAD but with LVEF less than or equal to 0.35 and NYHA FC II-III CHF symptoms may also be considered candidates for an ICD.

Although patients with CHF symptoms, diastolic dysfunction, and preserved LVEF are at risk for out-of-hospital CA, they have not been shown to benefit from an ICD.

Several clinical syndromes are associated with sudden cardiac death (e.g., LQTS, Brugada syndrome, ARVC, HCM). In these syndromes the risk of total mortality aside from sudden cardiac death is low. Therefore it makes perfect sense to consider an ICD implant when the risk for sudden death is high enough. This becomes a complex issue because even if the risk appears low (e.g., 1% to 2% per year), the risk of other causes of death is so extremely low that the relative risk of death from an out-of-hospital CA is quite high; these patients can benefit substantially from an ICD. The specific clinical syndromes associated with sudden cardiac death are often in a population of structural heart disease.

SPECIAL CIRCUMSTANCES

An "individualized" approach is required for circumstances in which patients have survived VT and/or VF or are at potential risk for future VT/VF but in whom long-term risk may be uncertain or available data are lacking, confusing, and contradictory. Specific circumstances include: (1) postoperative, perioperative, and intraoperative VT or VF; (2) well-tolerated sustained VT; (3) drug interventions that can exacerbate VT or VF; (4) VT/VF early after acute cardiac interventions, such as percutaneous coronary intervention or surgical coronary revascularization (see Algorithm 8.4); (5) acute cardiac and cardiopulmonary conditions that may resolve or stabilize over a period of time, including myocarditis, acute MI (see Algorithm 8.3), pulmonary embolus, bacterial endocarditis, acute valvular lesions, "holiday heart syndrome," and newly diagnosed cardiomyopathy (see Algorithm 8.5) of uncertain etiology; and (6) infiltrative conditions (e.g., sarcoidosis, amyloidosis).

For each circumstance, acute stabilization, treating the underlying condition, and management of risk for future VT/VF are the primary goals. Acute precipitating conditions may exacerbate an arrhythmia of any sort, but CA and similar potentially life-threatening and seriously hemodynamically impairing arrhythmias need to be suppressed acutely regardless of etiology.

With regard to intraoperative and perioperative arrhythmias, the problem becomes complex. Cardiac interventions can lead to shifts in electrolyte and fluid balance and can lead to fluctuations in autonomic tone, creation of an ischemic substrate, and the use of drugs that may have potential proarrhythmic effects. Cardiac surgery can exacerbate a variety of arrhythmias, including VT (see Table 6.1), VF, and more commonly atrial arrhythmias, including atrial flutter and atrial fibrillation (see Tables 5.7 and 5.8).

A wearable cardioverter defibrillator, a defibrillator that is worn externally, can detect and treat VT and VF. It is reasonable to consider a wearable cardioverter defibrillator for individuals at risk for sudden cardiac death due to VT or VF and for whom an implantable defibrillator may ultimately be required. The patient should also have their underlying medical and arrhythmia conditions stabilized.

Chapter 7

Cardiac Pacing and Pacemaker Rhythms

Cardiac pacing systems are described by a three- or four-letter code. The first letter indicates the chamber in which pacing stimuli are delivered (atrium, A; ventricle, V; or both, D). The second letter indicates the chamber in which sensing of the intracardiac electrical signal is occurring (atrium, A; ventricle, V; or both, D). The third letter indicates the response of the device to a sensed signal (inhibition of pacing stimulus output, I; triggering [causing to occur] of stimulus output, T; or both, D). The fourth letter, R, indicates that the device is rate adaptive—that is, it uses one or more sensors to achieve increases and decreases in pacing rate to mimic normal physiologic responses to changes in metabolic need. Commonly used sensors are body motion sensors (e.g., accelerometers) and minute ventilation sensors; one or more sensors can be programmed to be used simultaneously ("blended" sensors).

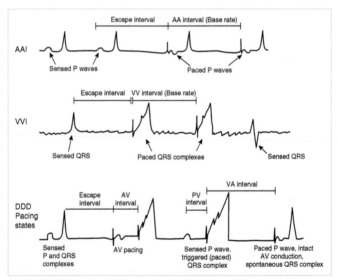

From Olshansky B, Chung M, Pogwizd S, Goldschlager N. Arrhythmia Essentials. Sudbury, MA: Jones & Bartlett Learning; 2012:241.

The usual pacing system implanted in patients who do not have chronic atrial fibrillation (AF) is DDD(R), in which both sensing and pacing occur in both atria and ventricles; AAI(R) systems (Fig. 7.1), which sense and pace only in the atrium, are still in use for patients with sinus node dysfunction and atrioventricular (AV) conduction, and there are systems that can switch between AAI(R) and DDD(R), or AAI(R) and VVI. VVI(R) systems (Fig. 7.2), which sense and pace only in the ventricles, are generally reserved for patients with chronic atrial fibrillation or very old, infirm patients, although they may be used in some young patients with the rare need for backup pacing. Examples of standard dual-chamber pacemakers are shown in Figs. 7.1, 7.3, and 7.4.

The *base rate* (lower rate limit, standby rate) of a pacing system is that programmed rate at which pacing will occur if there is no spontaneous cardiac depolarization. In devices programmed to rate responsiveness, the base rate is the lowest programmed rate at rest. The *upper rate limit*, which is either atrial (native P wave) based or sensor based, is the programmed maximum pacing rate that can occur. The maximum *tracking* rate is that rate at which ventricular pacing will be triggered by native P waves in a 1:1 relationship (atrial based); the maximum sensor-based rate is the highest programmed rate dictated by sensor input to the pulse generator. Whereas these rates are often programmed to be the same, the sensor-based rate can be programmed to exceed the tracking rate in response to exercise, thereby avoiding rapid ventricular paced rates triggered by supraventricular tachycardias.

The *magnet* rate (designated AOO, VOO, or DOO, as sensing, and therefore response to a sensed signal, do not occur; thus, the letter "O"— an asynchronous mode) is that nonprogrammable rate that occurs when a magnet is placed over the pulse generator. It varies with the manufacturer; several manufacturers set a constant magnet rate well above the expected spontaneous rate (e.g., 100 beats per minute) in order to allow myocardial depolarization (pacing) to be confirmed (Fig. 7.5A); other manufacturers set a rapid magnet rate for a specific number of cycles, followed by a slower rate (see Fig. 7.5B). Because magnet placement eliminates sensing, pacing output occurs despite the existence of a spontaneous cardiac rhythm; repetitive atrial or ventricular beating is only very rarely a clinical consequence.

The programmed AV or PV intervals, independently programmable, define the interval between an atrial and ventricular stimulus or a sensed P wave (atrial electrogram) and the triggered ventricular stimulus, respectively. In DOO mode, the AV interval is generally shortened in order to usurp intact AV conduction and allow confirmation of ventricular pacing; some manufacturers design a lengthening of this interval after a specified number of cycles in order to assess native AV conduction (see Fig. 7.5B).

After a sensed or paced event, an independently programmable refractory period ensues in each channel (atrial, ARP; and ventricular,

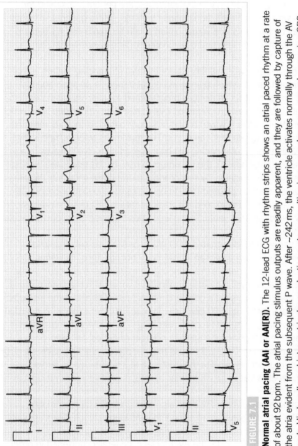

FIGURE 7.1

Normal atrial pacing (AAI or AAI[R]). The 12-lead ECG with rhythm strips shows an atrial paced rhythm at a rate of about 92 bpm. The atrial pacing stimulus outputs are readily apparent, and they are followed by capture of the atria evident from the subsequent P wave. After ~242 ms, the ventricle activates normally through the AV node-His bundle and intraventricular conduction system, resulting in a normal narrow, normal-appearing QRS complex. This rhythm could represent a single-chamber atrial pacemaker or a dual-chamber pacemaker in which the intrinsic QRS activates the ventricle without the need for ventricular pacing.

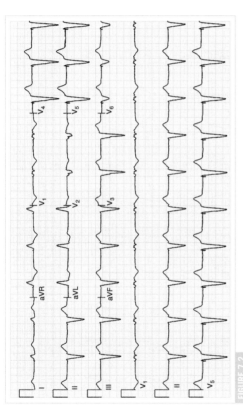

FIGURE 7.2

Normal ventricular pacing (VVI or VVI[R]). This 12-lead ECG tracing with rhythm strips shows a ventricular paced rhythm at a rate of 60 bpm. There is no preceding atrial activity and no preceding atrial stimulus outputs, indicating that this represents a single-channel pacemaker in a VVI or VVI(R) mode. The left bundle branch block pattern of the QRS with superior axis is consistent with pacing from the right ventricle apex. Note the 1:1 ventriculoatrial conduction best seen in leads II, III, and aVF, and the absence of visible pacing stimuli in some leads (e.g., II, III, aVL, aVF, and V3). This is a common finding and explained by digital sampling techniques; significant confusion can be caused by the absence of visible pacing stimuli.

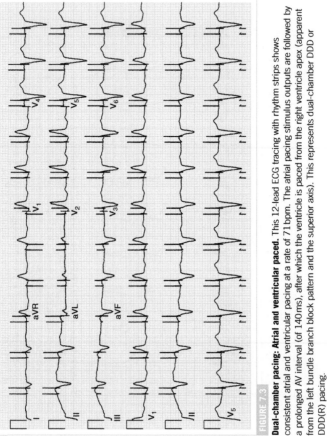

Dual-chamber pacing: Atrial and ventricular paced. This 12-lead ECG tracing with rhythm strips shows consistent atrial and ventricular pacing at a rate of 71 bpm. The atrial pacing stimulus outputs are followed by a prolonged AV interval (of 140 ms), after which the ventricle is paced from the right ventricle apex (apparent from the left bundle branch block pattern and the superior axis). This represents dual-chamber DDD or DDD(R) pacing.

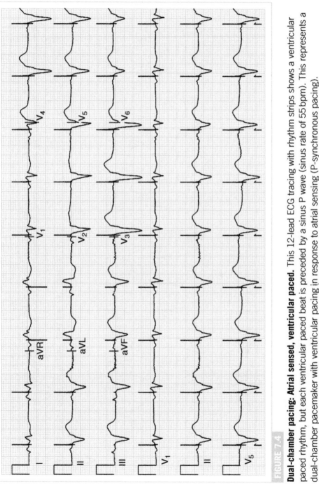

FIGURE 7.4

Dual-chamber pacing: Atrial sensed, ventricular paced. This 12-lead ECG tracing with rhythm strips shows a ventricular paced rhythm, but each ventricular paced beat is preceded by a sinus P wave (sinus rate of 55 bpm). This represents a dual-chamber pacemaker with ventricular pacing in response to atrial sensing (P-synchronous pacing).

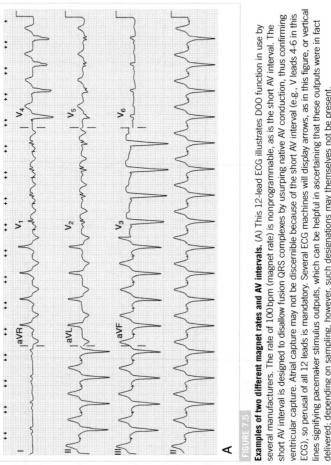

FIGURE 7.5

Examples of two different magnet rates and AV intervals. (A) This 12-lead ECG illustrates DOO function in use by several manufacturers. The rate of 100 bpm (magnet rate) is nonprogrammable, as is the short AV interval. The short AV interval is designed to disallow fusion QRS complexes by usurping native AV conduction, thus confirming ventricular capture. Atrial capture may not be discernible because of the short AV interval (e.g., V leads 4-6 in this ECG), so perusal of all 12 leads is mandatory. Several ECG machines will display arrows, as in this figure, or vertical lines signifying pacemaker stimulus outputs, which can be helpful in ascertaining that these outputs were in fact delivered; depending on sampling, however, such designations may themselves not be present.

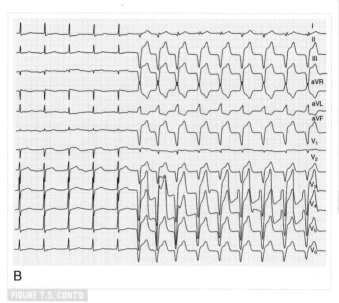

B

FIGURE 7.5, CONT'D

(B) This ECG displays simultaneously recorded 12 leads, run as a rhythm strip. The usefulness of recording all 12-leads as a rhythm strip allows identification of paced complexes in all ECG leads. In this manufacturer's magnet mode, 3 AV outputs are delivered at 100 bpm and short AV interval, followed by outputs delivered at 85 bpm at the programmed AV interval, designed to evaluate native AV conduction. Had a regular 12-lead ECG been performed, the initial 3 beats at 100 bpm and short AV interval would have been missed, and ventricular capture not confirmed.

VRP), during which the device will not respond to electrical signals. In DDD pacing systems, a programmable postventricular atrial refractory period (PVARP) is designed to prevent tracking of early P waves, which can be retrogradely conducted, thus avoiding "pacemaker-mediated tachycardia" and rapid paced ventricular rates.

Failure to capture, noncapture (Fig. 7.6) indicates that a pacing stimulus output does not depolarize myocardial tissue. This can occur because of too low a programmed voltage output, an increase in myocardial stimulation threshold (such as occurs during hyperkalemia or flecainide treatment), pacing lead insulation break or fracture, lead dislodgement, or battery end of life; failure to capture may also be "functional" due to refractoriness of the myocardial tissue. Pacing system interrogation through manufacturer-specific programmers is often necessary to define the nature of the problem.

Undersensing (Fig. 7.7) refers to failure to sense the intracardiac signal and is usually due to a poor signal rather than a pacing system failure; it

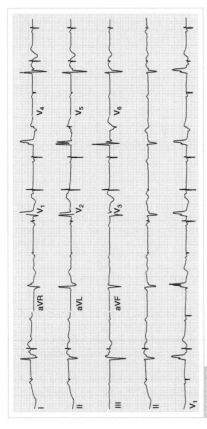

FIGURE 7.6

Failure to capture (ventricle). The 12-lead ECG shows an underlying sinus rhythm with complete heart block and a fascicular escape rhythm (right bundle branch block and left anterior fascicle block patterns at a rate of about 29 bpm). A VVI mode of function is present, evident from ventricular stimulus outputs that do not regularly follow sinus P waves. There is clear failure to capture with absence of paced QRS complexes. The second QRS complex could represent pseudofusion; "pseudofusion" describes the situation in which a pacemaker stimulus is superimposed on the native QRS complex but does not contribute to depolarization. Pseudofusion complexes can be seen with normally functioning pacemakers, and they differ from true fusion complexes, in which the intrinsic and paced depolarizations merge, leading to a QRS complex intermediate in morphology between native and paced ventricular beats. *(From Olshansky B, Chung M, Pogwizd S, Goldschlager N. Arrhythmia Essentials. Sudbury, MA: Jones & Bartlett Learning; 2012:247.)*

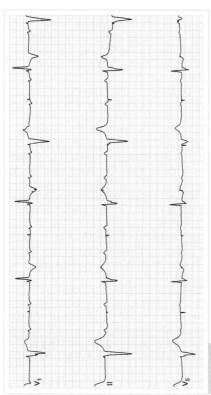

FIGURE 7.7

Undersensing (Failure to sense and failure to capture). This 12-lead ECG shows an underlying sinus rhythm (rate 88 bpm) with complete heart block and a ventricular escape rhythm (rate of 29 bpm). There is a ventricular paced rhythm with intermittent failure to sense (undersensing). Undersensing is evident from the premature ventricular pacing stimulus outputs that are superimposed on the T waves of the first, second, and fifth QRS complexes (best seen in lead II). These pacing stimuli occur prematurely relative to the base VV interval due to their failure to reset after the native QRS complex, due in turn to undersensing. There is also intermittent failure to capture, evident from the multiple pacemaker stimulus outputs that fall outside of tissue refractory periods and thus would be expected to capture but are not followed by QRS complexes. (*From Olshansky B, Chung M, Pogwizd S, Goldschlager N. Arrhythmia Essentials. Sudbury, MA: Jones & Bartlett Learning; 2012:248.*)

can often be corrected by appropriate programming. Undersensing can also result from lead fracture or insulation break or lead dislodgment; interrogation will be necessary to confirm this diagnosis; if present, lead revision will be required.

Oversensing (Fig. 7.8) is the sensing of electrical signals that are not actually generated within the cardiac chamber, or sensing unwanted signals, such as a T wave in the ventricle. The oversensed signal can come from the patient (e.g., myopotentials; Fig. 7.9), the environment (e.g., electronic article surveillance devices, electrocautery, ionizing radiation), and the pacing system itself (e.g., a lead insulation break or fracture that generates electrical signals due to potential differences within the leads). The oversensed signals will cause inhibition of pacing output or, if occurring in the atrial channel in DDD systems, triggering of an earlier-than-expected ventricular pacing stimulus.

Rapid paced ventricular rates generally occur in response to supraventricular tachycardias (Fig. 7.10), in which the sensed atrial signals trigger ventricular pacing; this can cause hemodynamic compromise and may need to be emergently managed by programming or by placing a magnet over the pulse generator to eliminate sensing. Devices in use today have a programmable function that changes the mode of pacemaker function from DDD(R) to DDI(R) or VVI(R) or VDI(R) in response to sensing of rapid atrial rates (automatic mode switch) to prevent this complication, but the function must be programmed "on" and the parameters for the mode switch programmed; device interrogation is necessary to assess all programmed parameters and functions.

Occasionally, a rapid paced ventricular rate can result from pacemaker-mediated tachycardia (PMT) (Fig. 7.11). In this circumstance, a paced ventricular depolarization is conducted retrogradely to the atrium, and the sensed atrial electrical signal triggers another ventricular paced event, which leads again to retrograde ventriculoatrial (VA) conduction and subsequent triggering of a ventricular paced event and so forth. The rapid paced ventricular rate, as well as the VA conduction, can cause unwanted hemodynamic consequences; application of a magnet will prevent sensing and thus terminate the PMT. Subsequent pacemaker programming to eliminate sensing of the retrograde P wave (increase in PVARP) can resolve the problem.

Paced QRS complexes resulting from right ventricular outflow tract or apical pacing sites are generally broad (>120 ms) and have an left bundle branch block (LBBB) pattern as depolarization is originating from the right ventricle. The frontal plane axis will be inferiorly directed if the outflow tract is being paced and superiorly directed if the apex is being paced. Unintended left ventricle (LV) pacing is suggested by paced complexes with a right bundle branch block (RBBB) pattern (Fig. 7.12A and B).

Biventricular pacing systems (Fig. 7.13), in which right and left ventricles are stimulated simultaneously or in proximity, will be narrower and may have a rightward axis due to the LV stimulation; they may also have RBBB

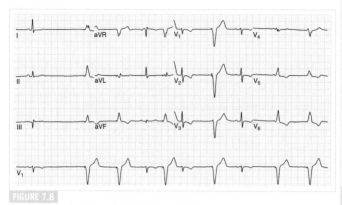

FIGURE 7.8

Oversensing (and undersensing). The 12-lead ECG with lead V_1 rhythm strip shows an intrinsic marked sinus bradycardia with an irregular rhythm composed of native and ventricular paced complexes. The VV interval of the pacemaker, evident from the interval between the first and second ventricular pacing stimulus outputs (preceding the second and third QRS complexes), represents the key timing interval of the pacemaker. The pause between the first and second QRS complexes exceeds the VV interval, indicating oversensing of electrical activity with subsequent inhibition of pacemaker output, resulting in an inappropriate pause in rhythm. In addition, the pacemaker fails to sense the second native QRS complex (the fourth QRS complex of the tracing), resulting in premature firing of the pacemaker relative to the VV interval. However, the undersensing is intermittent since the sixth and eighth QRS complexes are appropriately sensed. *(From Olshansky B, Chung M, Pogwizd S, Goldschlager N. Arrhythmia Essentials. Sudbury, MA: Jones & Bartlett Learning; 2012:249.)*

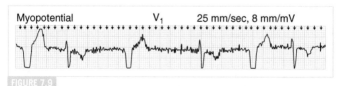

FIGURE 7.9

Myopotential inhibition. V1 rhythm strip illustrating myopotential oversensing, in which irregular and longer-than-programmed ventricular stimuli occur. Note that the escape intervals (measured from the spontaneous QRS complexes to the paced complexes) vary due to the oversensed signals that, after the sensed event, set up a new escape interval measured from the oversensed event. Here myopotentials (muscle potentials from arm movement) are sensed as electrical potentials by the pacemaker leads and result in inhibition of pacemaker output (oversensing). Oversensing is more common with unipolar than with bipolar pacing leads.

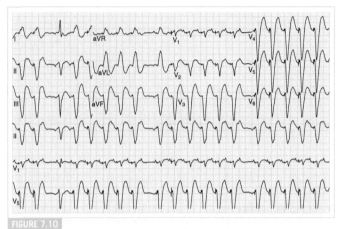

Upper rate pacing with atrial tachycardia. This 12-lead ECG tracing with rhythm strips shows an atrial tachycardia (140 bpm) evident from the negative P waves in leads II, III, and aVF. There is group beating and variable AV conduction with an overall ventricular rate of ~118 bpm. Pacing stimulus outputs are observed before each QRS complex, but no pacing stimulus is present before the P waves, consistent with a dual-chamber pacemaker that is sensing the atrium and pacing the ventricle. There is gradual prolongation of the AV delay so that the ventricular response is at or just below the upper rate limit of the pacemaker (likely 120 bpm). The pacemaker is demonstrating upper rate behavior pacing, in which the ventricular rate cannot exceed the upper programmed rate for the pacemaker even though the atrial rate is more rapid (in this case 140 bpm). To maintain the ventricular rate at or under the upper programmed rate, "electronic" AV Wenckebach occurs, as depicted on this ECG. This represents normal pacemaker behavior. *(From Olshansky B, Chung M, Pogwizd S, Goldschlager N. Arrhythmia Essentials. Sudbury, MA: Jones & Bartlett Learning; 2012:251 [Figure 7-9].)*

morphology. Morphology in biventricular pacing is dependent on lead location and the programmed relative timing of right and left ventricular pacing impulses.

All pacing systems can store in memory episodes of rapid heart rates, provided they are appropriately programmed to do so. High rates in either atrium or ventricle can be interrogated, and stored intracardiac electrograms can be viewed for confirmation of the rhythm and appropriate management undertaken. Pacing devices also store other clinically relevant information, such as heart rate histograms, percentage of atrial and ventricular pacing and sensing, and number of mode switches. Evaluation of such data can have direct effects on patient management.

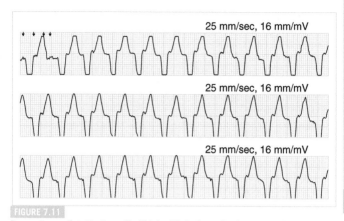

25 mm/sec, 16 mm/mV

25 mm/sec, 16 mm/mV

25 mm/sec, 16 mm/mV

FIGURE 7.11

Pacemaker-mediated tachycardia. This lead II rhythm strip shows a rapid paced ventricular rhythm that represents pacemaker-mediated tachycardia (PMT). The characteristics of PMT are a rapid paced ventricular rhythm (usually near the programmed upper rate limit of the pacemaker) in which retrograde atrial activity (seen here in the down-sloping segment of the T waves of the ventricular paced beats) originating from ventricular paced beats is then sensed by the pacemaker, triggering a subsequent ventricular paced activation, the rhythm then becoming sustained. In the acute situation, placing a magnet over the pulse generator eliminating all sensing will terminate the rhythm. In the long term, the problem can be corrected by increasing the postventricular atrial refractory period of the pacemaker such that any retrograde P waves fall within it and are not tracked. Contemporary pacing systems also have automatic PMT-terminating algorithms to break the rhythm without specific intervention. In this case, retrograde ventriculoatrial conduction occurred because of a long programmed AV interval, during which time the atria recovered their ability to depolarize retrogradely.

Pacemakers nearing end of life from battery depletion can present with marked slowing of the paced rate (Fig. 7.14). Interrogation of the device often alerts the clinician to this problem via text on the programmer's screen; inability to interrogate due to insufficient battery voltage and current is also a clue to end of life. If interrogation can be accomplished, pulse generators nearing end of life ("elective replacement time") will display a warning.

INDICATIONS FOR PACING

Indications for Temporary Transvenous Cardiac Pacing

- In patients with medically refractory symptomatic bradycardia or high risk of bradycardia of any etiology
- In patients in whom a permanent cardiac pacing system is necessary but cannot be implanted expeditiously

- In patients with LBBB in whom a right heart catheter is to be inserted (risk of development of complete AV block due to catheter-induced trauma to the right bundle)
- In patients with new AV block, including progressive first-degree AV block, developing during infections (e.g., aortic valve endocarditis, Lyme disease)
- In patients undergoing electrical cardioversion who have known sinus node dysfunction
- In patients for whom only temporary pacing is needed (drug-induced bradycardia, transient heart block post inferior myocardial infarction [MI], preoperatively in a patient who needs a valve replacement, endocarditis, lead extraction)
- In patients with pause-dependent ventricular tachycardia (VT) for treatment and prevention

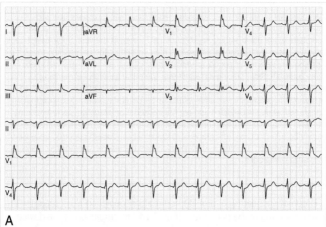

A

FIGURE 7.12

Unintended left ventricular pacing. (A) This 12-lead ECG tracing with rhythm strips shows sinus rhythm (rate of 83 bpm) with a ventricular paced rhythm. There are small pacing stimulus outputs preceding each wide QRS complex (best seen in leads V_3 to V_6) and no pacing stimulus outputs before the P waves. Unlike normal ventricular pacing from the right ventricle, which exhibits a left bundle branch block pattern, these ventricular paced beats show a right bundle branch block pattern. The reason for this is that the ventricular lead is in the left ventricle (instead of the normal location in the right ventricular apex). The ventricular pacing lead in this patient was inadvertently passed through a patent foramen ovale into the left atrium, through the mitral valve, and into the left ventricle. It was subsequently repositioned. *(From Olshansky B, Chung M, Pogwizd S, Goldschlager N. Arrhythmia Essentials. Sudbury, MA: Jones & Bartlett Learning; 2012:254-255.)*

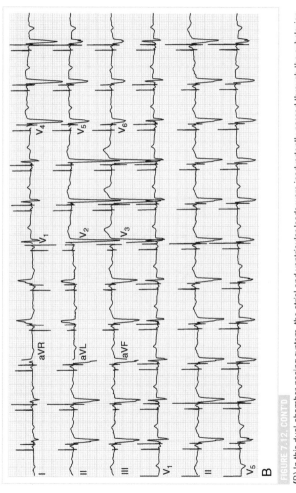

FIGURE 7.12, CONT'D

(B) In this dual-chamber pacing system, the atrial and ventricular leads were inadvertently passed through the subclavian artery. Pacing in the proximal aorta and left ventricle resulted in this paced morphology unexpected from right atrial and right ventricular pacing.

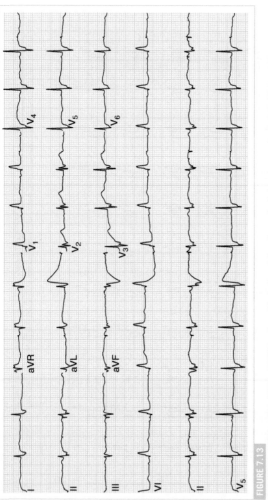

FIGURE 7.13

Biventricular pacing. This 12-lead ECG tracing with rhythm strips shows dual-chamber pacing from both the atrium and the ventricle. However, unlike the prior ECG tracings in which the QRS complex shows a right bundle branch block pattern, this tracing shows a narrower QRS complex with a right superior axis. This represents biventricular pacing from the right ventricular apex and an epicardial left cardiac vein. *(From Olshansky B, Chung M, Pogwizd S, Goldschlager N. Arrhythmia Essentials. Sudbury, MA: Jones & Bartlett Learning; 2012:256.)*

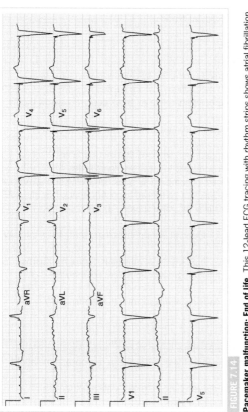

FIGURE 7.14

Pacemaker malfunction: End of life. This 12-lead ECG tracing with rhythm strips shows atrial fibrillation with a ventricular paced rhythm at a rate of 47 bpm. Sensing cannot be evaluated because there are no native QRS complexes to be sensed. The problem is the rate. As pacemakers near their end of life, the pacing rate decreases. In this case, a paced rate of 47 bpm is lower than the programmed rate of 60 bpm and reflects that the battery is near depletion and that replacement of the pacemaker generator is necessary. Interrogation of the pacing system if remaining battery energy allows it will document battery depletion. (*From Olshansky B, Chung M, Pogwizd S, Goldschlager N. Arrhythmia Essentials. Sudbury, MA: Jones & Bartlett Learning; 2012:257.*)

- In high-risk, post-MI patients (uncommon in current MI treatment era) with medically refractory symptomatic bradycardia
- Hemodynamically destabilizing AV block at any level (use caution in patients undergoing percutaneous intervention due to bleeding risk; pacing lead should be placed prior to the percutaneous coronary intervention (PCI)
- New bundle branch block (BBB) with Mobitz type II second-degree AV block
- Alternating BBB or fascicular block

Indications for Permanent Cardiac Pacing

Atrioventricular Block

- Advanced second-degree or complete AV block with symptoms of bradycardia or if due to medications that are needed for some other reason
- Advanced second-degree or complete AV block occurring below the AV node
- Advanced second-degree or complete AV block with an escape pacemaker with rate of <40 bpm
- Asystolic periods of more than 3 seconds that recur and are unpredictable and are unrelated to hypervagotonic states
- Second-degree, advanced, or complete AV block developing during exercise
- After ablation of the AV junction performed to control ventricular rate in AF
- Post-op AV block (usually aortic valve surgery) that is not expected to resolve
- Second-degree AV block found at electrophysiologic study to be infra-AV nodal
- Neuromuscular disease (e.g., myotonic muscular dystrophy, Kearns-Sayre syndrome), because progression to advanced or complete AV block is unpredictable
- First-degree AV block causing symptoms due to suboptimal AV relationships

Sinus Node Dysfunction

- Symptomatic bradycardia or pauses in rhythm, including chronotropic incompetence (inability to increase sinus rate in response to metabolic needs)
- Symptomatic bradycardia resulting from medications otherwise necessary to treat other conditions
- Questionably symptomatic bradycardia, but with a rate of <40 bpm
- Syncope of unclear etiology with evidence for sinus node dysfunction
- Prolonged pauses occurring on termination of atrial arrhythmias, such as atrial fibrillation

Carotid Sinus Syndrome

- Recurrent syncope in a patient with documented carotid sinus hypersensitivity (>3-sec pause in rhythm whether due to sinus bradycardia or AV block)

Neurocardiogenic Syncope

- Symptomatic patient with prolonged pauses or asystole and recurrent, otherwise refractory, syncope occurring spontaneously in whom hypotension alone is not the cause for collapse

Bifascicle Block

- Occurring with Mobitz type II, advanced second-degree, or complete AV block
- Occurring with alternating BBB
- Syncope if other arrhythmic causes (e.g., VT) have been excluded
- Prolonged His-ventricle conduction time (>100 ms) found at EP study in patients with symptoms

Post-Myocardial Infarction

- Persistent second-degree or complete AV block that is infra-AV nodal, with or without symptoms
- Transient advanced or complete AV block in presence of BBB in patients with anterior MI
- Persistent second-degree or complete AV block that is intra-AV nodal but causes symptoms in patients with inferior MI

To Prevent Tachyarrhythmias (Usually with an Implantable Cardioverter Defibrillator)

- Pause-dependent VT (e.g., torsades de pointes)
- Congenital long QT syndrome

Systolic Heart Failure (Biventricular Pacing, "Cardiac Resynchronization" Therapy; Usually Implanted with ICD)

- LBBB with QRS ≥120 ms, left ventricular ejection fraction (LVEF) ≤35%, New York Heart Association (NYHA) class II, III, or ambulatory class IV heart failure symptoms on guideline-directed medical therapy (GDMT)
- Non-LBBB with QRS ≥120 ms, LVEF ≤35%, NYHA class III-ambulatory class IV heart failure symptoms on GDMT
- LBBB, LVEF ≤30%, ischemic systolic heart failure, NYHA class I symptoms on GDMT
- Non-LBBB with QRS ≥150 ms, LVEF ≤35%, NYHA class II heart failure symptoms on GDMT
- LVEF ≤35% on GDMT, with anticipated requirement for significant (>40%) ventricular pacing, or with atrial fibrillation if patient requires ventricular pacing, AVN ablation, or pharmacologic rate control that will allow near 100% ventricular pacing

Conditions for Which Permanent Cardiac Pacing Is Not Indicated

Atrioventricular Block

- Asymptomatic first-degree AV block
- Mobitz type I second-degree AV block that is intra-AV nodal and not symptomatic
- Sleep apnea, high vagal tone (e.g., sleep), or conditions likely to resolve (e.g., drug toxicity)

Sinus Node Dysfunction

- For an asymptomatic patient
- When it is due to nonessential drug therapy that can be discontinued
- When it is due to a condition that can be corrected

Carotid Sinus Hypersensitivity

- Where carotid sinus massage is abnormal (>3 seconds of asystole due either to sinus bradycardia/arrest or AV block) but patient is asymptomatic; the hypersensitivity response must be distinguished from carotid sinus syndrome, in which the patient is symptomatic *and* has an abnormal response to carotid sinus massage

Neurocardiogenic Syncope

- Situational syncope where avoidance of the triggering situation is effective

Fascicle Block

- Asymptomatic patient, without or with first-degree AV block

Post-Myocardial Infarction

- When AV block is transient and unaccompanied by bi- or trifascicular or BBB
- Transient AV block with unifascicular block
- New BBB or fascicular block without AV block
- Asymptomatic first-degree AV block with fascicular or BBB

Chapter 8

Implantable Cardioverter Defibrillators

An implantable cardioverter defibrillator (ICD) is a device that is placed subcutaneously or submuscularly, with leads that are positioned within the heart (or, more recently, subcutaneously). In contrast to a pacemaker that primarily delivers pacing stimuli to treat bradyarrhythmias, the primary purpose of an ICD is to prevent tachyarrhythmic death due to ventricular tachycardia (VT) or ventricular fibrillation (VF). This is done by continuously monitoring the heart rhythm and delivering antitachycardia pacing (ATP) stimuli or shocks to terminate VT with ATP or VT/VF with shocks. Current ICDs incorporate fully functional pacing support, thereby also treating bradyarrhythmias, including asystolic pauses that can result from shock delivery. Because of the need for capacitors that store large amounts of electrical energy necessary to defibrillate, an ICD is larger than a pacemaker.

The implant procedure is similar to that for a pacemaker, except for the size of the device and the need for special leads that incorporate defibrillation coils along the body of the leads. The typical device has one to three transvenous leads placed, including a pace/sense defibrillation lead in the right ventricle (RV). Dual-chamber ICDs also have a pacing/sensing lead in the right atrium. Devices that incorporate cardiac resynchronization therapy (CRT) have a lead placed in a ventricular branch of the coronary sinus to stimulate the left ventricle (LV) or a lead placed on the LV epicardial surface.

The device senses the ventricular rhythm through the right ventricular lead and then can rapidly pace or deliver a shock to defibrillate or cardiovert. The shock configuration includes the defibrillation coils on the transvenous lead(s) and often the ICD pulse generator ("can") itself. Fortunately, modern implantable defibrillators use a biphasic shock, and this is highly effective to stop VT and VF, but for patients who have higher energy requirements for termination of their ventricular arrhythmias or who have older systems with epicardially placed defibrillation patches, additional shocking electrode hardware may include subcutaneous coils or patches and separate coils in the superior vena cava/brachiocephalic vein or azygos vein. The atrial lead (or a sensing electrode in the right atrium) is used to detect atrial electrical activity and pace the atria if necessary. It can help detect and discriminate atrial from ventricular tachyarrhythmias (via automatic detection algorithms or via manual analysis of stored data), thus helping prevent "inappropriate shocks" (i.e., shocks not given to stop otherwise sustained ventricular tachyarrhythmias). The LV lead is used for purposes of cardiac resynchronization to improve ventricular function and symptoms in patients with heart failure who have electrical dyssynchrony due to conduction system abnormalities.

The ICD is multiprogrammable. A series of tachycardia "zones" can be programmed to detect VF and VTs of varying rates. Most devices can be programmed from one to three zones. A slower zone can be programmed "on" for purposes of arrhythmia detection only, but generally zones are programmed to determine the type of therapy that will be delivered. The fastest zone is considered a VF zone. Rate alone is considered the main criterion for arrhythmia "diagnosis," but a certain number of beats or arrhythmia duration need to be satisfied before therapy is actually delivered.

The way the ICD works is as follows: After tachyarrhythmia detection criteria are satisfied, the capacitors are charged, and the device delivers a shock (Figs. 8.1 and 8.2). Most modern devices take a second look (reevaluation of the heart rhythm) after charging up for a shock ("noncommitted") to avoid delivering a shock if the arrhythmia is not sustained. The shock energy is programmable and in some instances can exceed 40 J. The shock waveform is biphasic; biphasic shocks need less energy to terminate ventricular arrhythmias than monophasic shocks and are thus more effective. Most modern devices can deliver four to six consecutive shocks as needed before being required to see a normal rhythm and reattempting to shock. ICDs also have the capability to pace for slow and for fast rhythms.

The subcutaneous ICD (SICD) is not a leadless ICD but has leads placed subcutaneously with the ICD. It is larger than the transvenous ICD and cannot detect atrial activity. Nevertheless, it is highly effective with specific algorithms to discriminate atrial from ventricular arrhythmias. It cannot pace the heart for long periods of time with present technology.

ICDs can be programmed in a manner similar to pacemaker programming to deliver pacing stimuli for bradyarrhythmias, but they can also overdrive pace (ATP) in attempts to terminate VT. Some devices are capable of attempting to pace terminate VT while charging to deliver a defibrillating shock if necessary. Some ICDs can also deliver ATP to treat atrial arrhythmias. The time required to detect a tachycardia and the characteristics of the atrial and ventricular relationships are programmable for each tachycardia zone to help discriminate SVT from VT.

ICDs are not perfect in discriminating SVT from VT simply by rate criteria or in determining whether an arrhythmia is nonsustained. As such, some shocks are "inappropriate"—that is, given for non-life-threatening SVTs, for sinus tachycardia faster than the programmed rate criterion, for self-terminating VTs, or for electrical noise (e.g., for noise from a fractured lead; Figs. 8.3, 8.4, and 8.5). Inappropriate shocks may occur in up to one-third of patients receiving ICDs. To minimize the occurrence of inappropriate shocks, various algorithms have been used to discriminate atrial fibrillation (AF), atrial flutter (AFL), sinus tachycardia, or other SVT from VT. These

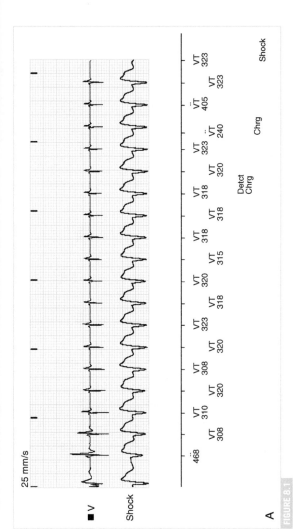

FIGURE 8.1

Implantable cardioverter defibrillator shock for ventricular tachycardia. This rhythm strip shows a run of sustained ventricular tachycardia (VT) (A) that is successfully cardioverted by an implantable cardioverter defibrillator (ICD) with the return of normal rhythm (B).

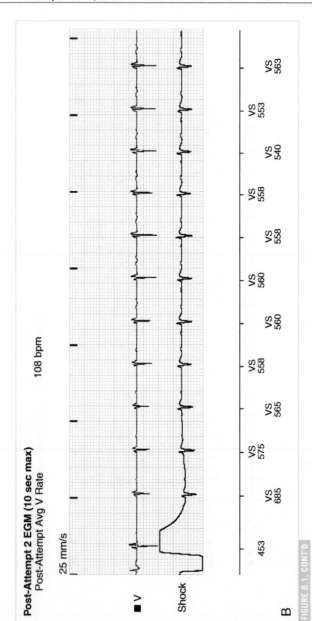

Post-Attempt 2 EGM (10 sec max)
Post-Attempt Avg V Rate

108 bpm

25 mm/s

V
■

Shock

	453
VS 685	
VS 575	
VS 565	
	VS 558
VS 560	
	VS 560
	VS 558
	VS 558
	VS 540
VS 553	
	VS 563

B

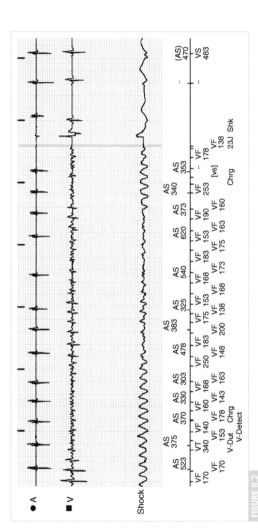

FIGURE 8.2

Implantable cardioverter defibrillator shock for ventricular fibrillation. An episode of ventricular fibrillation (VF) terminated by an implantable cardioverter defibrillator (ICD) shock, recorded from the ICD and downloaded from its memory. The top recording is the intracardiac atrial electrogram ("AS" indicates atrial sensed electrogram), the middle one is the intracardiac ventricular electrogram (closely spaced bipole), and the bottom one is the farfield electrogram from the shocking coil electrodes. "VF" indicates ventricular fibrillation is present. A vertical dashed line indicates delivery of a defibrillating 23-J shock from the ICD, returning the patient to a slower rhythm. *ICD,* Implantable cardioverter defibrillator; *LV,* left ventricle; *VF,* ventricular fibrillation; *VT,* ventricular tachycardia.

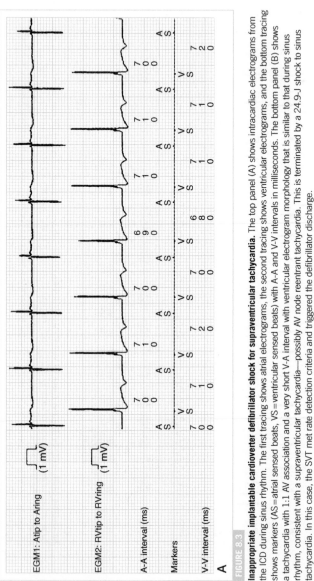

EGM1: Atip to Aring (1 mV)

EGM2: RVtip to RVring (1 mV)

A-A interval (ms)

Markers

V-V interval (ms)

A

FIGURE 8.3

Inappropriate implantable cardioverter defibrillator shock for supraventricular tachycardia. The top panel (A) shows intracardiac electrograms from the ICD during sinus rhythm. The first tracing shows atrial electrograms, the second tracing shows ventricular electrograms, and the bottom tracing shows markers (AS = atrial sensed beats, VS = ventricular sensed beats) with A-A and V-V intervals in milliseconds. The bottom panel (B) shows a tachycardia with 1:1 AV association and a very short V-A interval with ventricular electrogram morphology that is similar to that during sinus rhythm, consistent with a supraventricular tachycardia—possibly AV node reentrant tachycardia. This is terminated by a 24.9-J shock to sinus tachycardia. In this case, the SVT met rate detection criteria and triggered the defibrillator discharge.

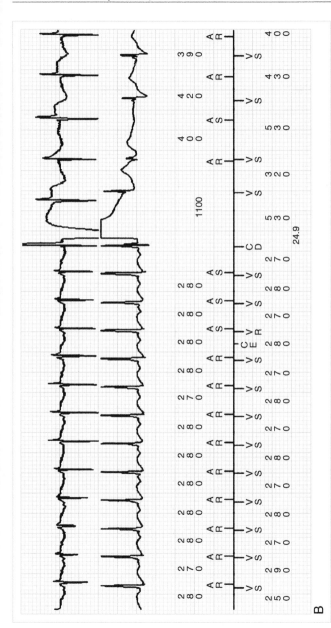

FIGURE 8.3, CONT'D

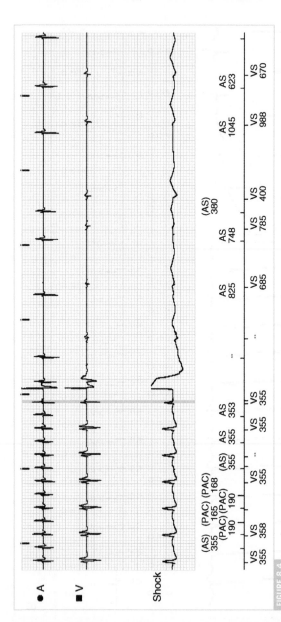

FIGURE 8.4

Shock for atrial flutter. This intracardiac electrogram tracing shows atrial electrograms (*top strip*), ventricular electrograms (*second strip*), farfield shock electrode electrograms (*third strip*), and the marker channel (*bottom strip*). The electrograms show atrial flutter (AFL) with 2:1 AV conduction that is terminated by a shock, indicated by the vertical line, restoring sinus rhythm with atrial ectopy.

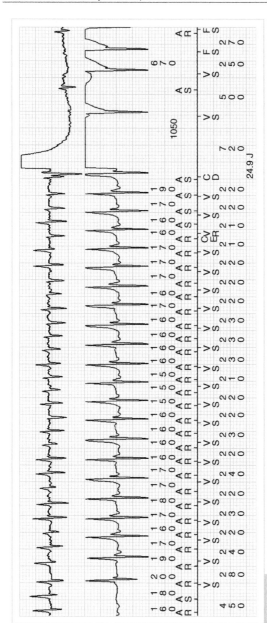

FIGURE 8.5

Shock for dual tachycardia: atrial fibrillation and ventricular tachycardia. This intracardiac electrogram tracing shows atrial electrograms at the top, ventricular electrograms in the middle, and a marker channel at the bottom. There is atrial fibrillation evident on the atrial electrogram with initiation of a regular monomorphic ventricular tachycardia (VT) that triggers a 24.9-J shock that terminates both rhythms.

discriminating algorithms commonly use specific rhythm characteristics, such as atrial and ventricular relationships, irregularity of the rhythm, suddenness of onset, or electrogram morphology. The atrial and ventricular relationships may help discriminate 1:1 A-V relationships (as may be seen in SVT) from V-A dissociation (as may be seen in VT). Irregularity of the intervals between beats is used to distinguish AF from the more regular ventricular tachyarrhythmia. Sudden-onset criteria are used to discriminate gradual-onset sinus tachycardia from a sudden-onset VT characterized by an abrupt increase or jump in rate. Some ICDs have special template-matching algorithms to assess the ventricular electrogram morphology and help discriminate atrial from ventricular rhythms.

Although programming of discrimination algorithms is intended to improve the specificity of shocks, inherent to this strategy is a potential trade-off in sensitivity for true life-threatening ventricular arrhythmias. As the goal of ICD therapy is to treat all life-threatening arrhythmias, and as the consequences of missing out on treating one of these true arrhythmias could be sudden death, the VF rate zone may be programmed without many SVT discriminators, which are reserved for slower VT detection zones. Another strategy is to defer programming of discriminators unless there is a clinical occurrence or history of supraventricular arrhythmias causing inappropriate shocks, or rapid rates that could overlap with a VT zone. Other strategies may also use longer detection intervals. Because devices are multiprogrammable, each device can be tailored to a specific patient's needs and clinical arrhythmias.

Other functions included in ICDs are automatic capacitor reforms and advanced recordings and diagnostics that generally include the capability of transtelephonic monitoring to send information to clinicians caring for the patient. The average battery life of an ICD is 5 to 10 years. The devices can now automatically maintain the capacitors regularly and can monitor lead functional parameters (e.g., impedance) and intracardiac electrogram characteristics (e.g., ventricular and atrial electrogram size). Modern ICDs can allow this information to be downloaded via a programmer or remotely via an external device that communicates with the ICD and transmits information to a central station. Remote monitoring is highly valuable, as it can provide the clinician with continuous information, should there be failure of a device or a component, such as a lead. Furthermore, it can provide information about the frequency of ventricular pacing and sensing.

Device interrogation can be performed with a wand placed over the device or remotely transtelephonically to determine if a tachyarrhythmia occurred, what type of therapy was delivered, and whether the therapy was successful in terminating the arrhythmia. In addition, interrogation can provide the frequency and duration ("burden") of atrial arrhythmias, such as AF. It can also provide the heart rate and rate variation over time. Device interrogation is useful to determine the need for pacing and the frequency of pacing at different programmed rates. The relationship between pacing timing is adjustable. These adjustments include lower (base) rate; rate responsiveness; upper tracking rate at which the ventricles are paced in 1:1 relationship to atrial activity; an upper sensor-based rate, if necessary; atrial and ventricular timing relationships; and left and right ventricular pace timing relationships in biventricular devices. Most devices also contain the ability to turn off atrial tracking should an SVT such as AF or AFL occur within a certain rate zone. Magnet application will inactivate tachycardia detection for most ICDs but will have no effect on the antibradycardia function of the pacemaker. ICDs have specific programming characteristics depending on the type, manufacturer, and model, and knowledge of the peculiarities of each device is mandatory to ensure proper understanding of device function and programming.

Implantable Cardioverter Defibrillator Indications

Indications for ICD implantation can be categorized into indications for primary versus secondary prevention of sudden cardiac death (SCD). Current guideline recommendations for ICD indications are summarized in Table 8.1 and Charts 8.1 to 8.5. An algorithm for primary prevention

TABLE 8.1

INDICATIONS FOR AN IMPLANTABLE CARDIOVERTER DEFIBRILLATOR

ICD recommended

- Cardiac arrest due to VF or hemodynamically destabilizing sustained VT after evaluation to define the cause of the event and to exclude any completely reversible causes
- Structural heart disease and spontaneous sustained VT, whether hemodynamically stable or unstable
- Syncope of undetermined origin with clinically relevant, hemodynamically significant sustained VT or VF induced at EP study
- LVEF ≤35% at least 40 days after MI in patients in NYHA functional class I–III
- Nonischemic cardiomyopathy with LVEF ≤35% in patients in NYHA functional class II or III
- Nonsustained VT in patients with prior MI, LVEF ≤40%, and inducible VF or sustained VT at EP study

Class IIa: ICD is reasonable

- Unexplained syncope, significant LV dysfunction, and nonischemic cardiomyopathy
- Sustained VT and normal or near-normal ventricular function
- Hypertrophic cardiomyopathy with one or more major risk factors for sudden death
- Arrhythmogenic RV cardiomyopathy (dysplasia) who have one or more risk factors for sudden cardiac death
- Long QT syndrome in patients with syncope and/or VT while receiving β-adrenergic blockers
- Patients awaiting heart transplant
- Brugada syndrome in patients who have had syncope
- Brugada syndrome in patients who have documented VT, but not cardiac arrest
- Catecholaminergic polymorphic VT who have syncope
- Cardiac sarcoidosis, giant cell myocarditis, or Chagas disease

Continued on following page

TABLE 8.1

INDICATIONS FOR AN IMPLANTABLE CARDIOVERTER DEFIBRILLATOR (Continued)

ICD may be considered

- Nonischemic heart disease in patients with LVEF ≤ 35% and NYHA functional class I
- LQTS and risk factors for SCD
- Syncope and advanced structural heart disease in patients in whom thorough invasive and noninvasive investigations have failed to define a cause
- Familial cardiomyopathy associated with sudden death
- LV noncompaction

ICD not indicated

- Patients with no reasonable expectation of survival with an acceptable functional status for at least 1 year
- Incessant VT or VF
- Significant psychiatric illnesses that may be aggravated by device implantation or preclude systematic follow-up
- Drug-refractory CHF in patients who are not candidates for cardiac transplantation or CRT-D
- No inducible ventricular tachyarrhythmias and no structural heart disease
- VF or VT amenable to surgical or catheter ablation (e.g., atrial arrhythmias associated with WPW syndrome, RV or LV outflow tract VT, idiopathic VT, fascicular VT) in the absence of structural heart disease
- VTs due to a completely reversible disorder in the absence of structural heart disease (e.g., electrolyte imbalance, drugs, or trauma)

CHF, Congestive heart failure; *CRT-D*, cardiac resynchronization therapy-defibrillator; *LQTS*, long QT interval syndrome; *LV*, left ventricle; *LVEF*, left ventricular ejection fraction; *MI*, myocardial infarction; *NYHA*, New York Heart Association; *RV*, right ventricle; *SCD*, sudden cardiac death; *VF*, ventricular fibrillation; *VT*, ventricular tachycardia.

of SCD is shown in Algorithm 8.1 and for secondary prevention of SCD in Algorithm 8.2. There are many patients who were not well represented in randomized clinical trials and who are thus not covered by guideline recommendations. These include patients within 40 days of myocardial infarction (Algorithm 8.3), 90 days of coronary revascularization (Algorithm 8.4), and 3 to 9 months of newly diagnosed cardiomyopathy (Algorithm 8.5).

All patients who are candidates for an ICD implant must first be treated with optimal medical therapy for a period realizing that improvement may occur with medical therapy so that an ICD may ultimately not be required to reduce the risk of SCD due to a ventricular arrhythmia. It is important to recognize that despite guidelines written by professional societies that provide reasonable recommendations for ICD implantation, in the United States, a physician and/or hospital system may be called to task if Centers for Medicare and Medicaid Services (CMS) indications for an ICD implant are not followed strictly.

Algorithms 8.6 to 8.11 review ICD implantation and other recommendations for specific ventricular arrhythmia syndromes,

Guidelines for ICD Implantation for Secondary prevention of SCD

ICD therapy is indicated:

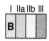

- Survivors of cardiac arrest due to VF or hemodynamically unstable sustained VT after evaluation of cause and exclusion of completely reversible causes.

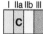

- SHD and spontaneous sustained VT, whether hemodynamically stable or unstable.
- Syncope of undetermined origin with clinically relevant, hemodynamically significant sustained VT or VF induced at EP study.

ICD implantation is reasonable:

- Sustained VT and normal or near-normal ventricular function.

Tracy et al. 2012 ACCF/AHA/HRS Focused Update of the 2008 Guidelines for Device-Based Therapy of Cardiac Rhythm Abnormalities.
JACC 2012;60;1297-1313.
Epstein et al. ACC/AHA/HRS 2008 Guidelines for Device-Based Therapy of Cardiac Rhythm Abnormalities.
Circulation 2008;117:e350-408.

CHART 8.1

Guidelines for ICD implantation for secondary prevention of SCD. *(From Tracy CM, Epstein AE, Darbar D, et al. 2012 ACCF/AHA/HRS focused update of the 2008 guidelines for device-based therapy of cardiac rhythm abnormalities. J Am Coll Cardiol 2012;60:1297-1313; Epstein AE, DiMarco JP, Ellenbogen KA, et al. ACC/AHA/HRS 2008 guidelines for device-based therapy of cardiac rhythm abnormalities. Circulation 2008;117:e350-408.)*

including hypertrophic cardiomyopathy (Algorithm 8.6), arrhythmogenic right ventricular cardiomyopathy (Algorithm 8.7), long QT syndrome (Algorithm 8.8), Brugada syndrome (Algorithm 8.9), catecholaminergic polymorphic VT (Algorithm 8.10), and sarcoidosis (Algorithm 8.11). For selected patients at risk for VT/VF in whom an ICD cannot be implanted or needs to be deferred, a wearable cardioverter defibrillator (WCD) could be considered. The WCD may also be used in patients at high risk for VT/VF as a bridge to definitive therapy with ICD implantation, transplantation, or improvement in LV function during a period of optimal medical management.

CARDIAC RESYNCHRONIZATION THERAPY

Systolic heart failure accompanied by prolonged ventricular conduction, manifested most commonly by a wide QRS complex, particularly with left branch bundle block (LBBB) conduction pattern, can produce dyssynchronous left ventricular contraction. Clinical trials have demonstrated functional and structural benefits, as well as improved survival, in such patients using biventricular pacing, or CRT. Delivery of CRT can be

Class I Indications for Primary Prevention of SCD

ICD therapy is indicated in patients with:

I	IIa IIb III	
A		• LVEF ≤35% due to prior MI, at least 40 days post-MI, NYHA FC II or III.

I	IIa IIb III	
B		• Nonischemic DCM with LVEF ≤35% and NYHA FC II or III.

I	IIa IIb III	
A		• LV dysfunction due to prior MI at least 40 days post-MI, LVEF ≤30%, NYHA FC I.

I	IIa IIb III	
B		• NSVT due to prior MI, LVEF <40%, inducible VF or sustained VT at EP study.

Tracy et al. 2012 ACCF/AHA/HRS Focused Update of the 2008 Guidelines for Device-Based Therapy of Cardiac Rhythm Abnormalities.
JACC 2012:60;1297-1313.
Epstein et al. ACC/AHA/HRS 2008 Guidelines for Device-Based Therapy of Cardiac Rhythm Abnormalities.
Circulation 2008;117:e350-408.

CHART 8.2

Class I indication for primary prevention of SCD. *(From Tracy CM, Epstein AE, Darbar D, et al. 2012 ACCF/AHA/HRS focused update of the 2008 guidelines for device-based therapy of cardiac rhythm abnormalities. J Am Coll Cardiol 2012;60:1297-1313; Epstein AE, DiMarco JP, Ellenbogen KA, et al. ACC/AHA/HRS 2008 guidelines for device-based therapy of cardiac rhythm abnormalities. Circulation 2008;117:e350-408.)*

incorporated into an implantable permanent pacemaker (CRT-P) or defibrillator (CRT-D) system and requires implantation of a pacing lead on the LV, either in a branch of the coronary sinus or on the epicardium. Response rates are dependent on patient selection, lead location, programming of appropriate intervals, ensuring a high percentage of biventricular pacing, and optimization of medical management. Patients who appear to respond best include those with very wide QRS complexes and LBBB.

Current CRT indications include the following:

- NYHA class III-IV heart failure symptoms receiving optimal medical therapy with left ventricular ejection fraction (LVEF) ≤35% and QRS duration ≥120 ms or frequent dependence on ventricular pacing.
- LBBB with QRS ≥130 ms, LVEF ≤30%, and NYHA class II ischemic or nonischemic heart failure or asymptomatic NYHA class I ischemic heart failure.
- Patients who are candidates for CRT-D devices must also meet criteria for an ICD, including long-standing (at least 3 to 9 months) impaired ventricular function with a left ventricular ejection fraction ≤0.35 despite optimal medical therapy for heart failure, at least 40 days after myocardial infarction, and at least 90 days after revascularization. In other words, patients must have a chronic long-standing risk for cardiac arrest despite all attempts at correcting the problems otherwise.

Primary Prevention Class IIa and IIb Indications for ICDs in Non-ischemic and Other Cardiomyopathies

Class IIa

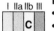

ICD implantation is reasonable for:

- Bridge to transplant:
  - Nonhospitalized patients awaiting transplantation
- HCM who have 1 or more major risk factors for SCD.
- ARVD/C who have 1 or more risk factors for SCD.
- Cardiac sarcoidosis
- Giant cell myocarditis
- Chagas disease

Class IIa

I	IIa	IIb	III
	C		

ICD therapy may he considered for:

- Nonischemic heart disease: LVEF 335% and NVHA FC I
- Familial cardiomyopathy associated with SD.
- LV noncompaction.

Tracy et al. 2012 ACCF/AHA/HRS Focused Update of the 2008 Guidelines for Device-Based Therapy of Cardiac Rhythm Abnormalities.
JACC 2012;60:1297-1313.
Epstein et al. ACC/AHA/HRS 2008 Guidelines for Device-Based Therapy of Cardiac Rhythm Abnormalities.
Circulation 2008;117:e350-408.

CHART 8.3

Primary prevention Class IIa and IIb indications for ICDs in nonischemic and other cardiomyopathies. *(From Tracy CM, Epstein AE, Darbar D, et al. 2012 ACCF/AHA/HRS focused update of the 2008 guidelines for device-based therapy of cardiac rhythm abnormalities. J Am Coll Cardiol 2012;60:1297-1313; Epstein AE, DiMarco JP, Ellenbogen KA, et al. ACC/AHA/HRS 2008 guidelines for device-based therapy of cardiac rhythm abnormalities. Circulation 2008;117:e350-408.)*

Primary Prevention Indications for ICDs in Unexplained Syncope

I	IIa	IIb	III
	C		

ICD implantation is reasonable for:

- Unexplained syncope, significant LV dysfunction, and NIDCM.

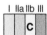

ICD Implantation may be considered for:

- Syncope and advanced SHD in whom thorough invasive and noninvasive invesligations have failed to define a cause.

Tracy et al. 2012 ACCF/AHA/HRS Focused Update of the 2008 Guidelines for Device-Based Therapy of Cardiac Rhythm Abnormalities.
JACC 2012;60:1297-1313.
Epstein et al. ACC/AHA/HRS 2008 Guidelines for Device-Based Therapy of Cardiac Rhythm Abnormalities.
Circulation 2008;117:e350-408.

CHART 8.4

Primary prevention indications for ICDs in unexplained syncope. *(From Tracy CM, Epstein AE, Darbar D, et al. 2012 ACCF/AHA/HRS focused update of the 2008 guidelines for device-based therapy of cardiac rhythm abnormalities. J Am Coll Cardiol 2012;60:1297-1313; Epstein AE, DiMarco JP, Ellenbogen KA, et al. ACC/AHA/HRS 2008 guidelines for device-based therapy of cardiac rhythm abnormalities. Circulation 2008;117:e350-408.)*

Class III Contraindications for ICDs

Class III

I IIa IIb III

C

ICD therapy is not indicated for:
- No reasonable expectation of survival with acceptable functional status for at least 1 year.
- Incessant VT or VF.
- Significant psychiatric illnesses that may be aggravated by a device or preclude systematic F/U.
- NVHA Class IV with drug-refractory CHF, not candidates for cardiac transplantation or CRT-D.
- Syncope of undetermined cause without inducible ventricular tachyarrhythmias and without SHD.
- VF or VT amenable to ablation
- Ventricular tachyarrhythmias due to a completely reversible disorder in the absence of SHD

Tracy et al. 2012 ACCF/AHA/HRS Focused Update of the 2008 Guidelines for Device-Based Therapy of Cardiac Rhythm Abnormalities.
JACC 2012;60;1297-1313.
Epstein et al. ACC/AHA/HRS 2008 Guidelines for Device-Based Therapy of Cardiac Rhythm Abnormalities.
Circulation 2008;117;e350-408.

CHART 8.5

Class III Contraindications for ICDs. *(From Tracy CM, Epstein AE, Darbar D, et al. 2012 ACCF/AHA/HRS focused update of the 2008 guidelines for device-based therapy of cardiac rhythm abnormalities. J Am Coll Cardiol 2012;60:1297-1313; Epstein AE, DiMarco JP, Ellenbogen KA, et al. ACC/AHA/HRS 2008 guidelines for device-based therapy of cardiac rhythm abnormalities. Circulation 2008;117:e350-408.)*

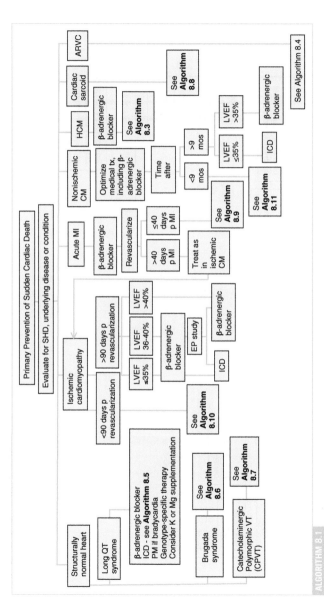

ALGORITHM 8.1
Primary prevention of sudden cardiac death.

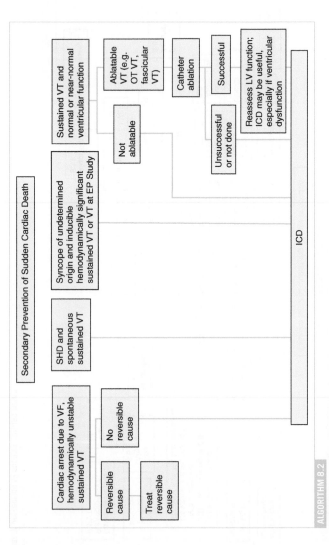

ALGORITHM 8.2

Secondary prevention of sudden cardiac death.

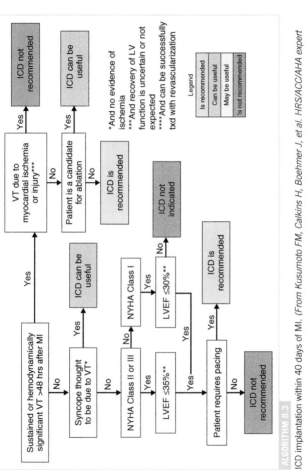

ALGORITHM 8.3

ICD implantation within 40 days of MI. *(From Kusumoto FM, Calkins H, Boehmer J, et al. HRS/ACC/AHA expert consensus statement on the use of implantable cardioverter-defibrillator therapy in patients who are not included or not well represented in clinical trials. Heart Rhythm 2014;11[7]:1271-1303.)*

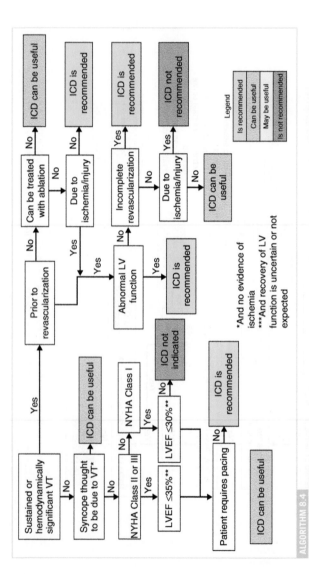

ALGORITHM 8.4

ICD implantation within 90 days of revascularization. *(From Kusumoto FM, Calkins H, Boehmer J, et al. HRS/ACC/AHA expert consensus statement on the use of implantable cardioverter-defibrillator therapy in patients who are not included or not well represented in clinical trials. Heart Rhythm 2014;11[7]:1271-1303.)*

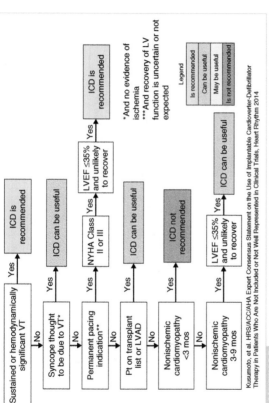

Kusumoto, et al. HRS/ACC/AHA Expert Consensus Statement on the Use of Implantable Cardioverter-Defibrillator Therapy in Patients Who Are Not Included or Not Well Represented in Clinical Trials, Heart Rhythm 2014

ALGORITHM 8.5

ICD implantation within 9 months of nonischemic cardiomyopathy diagnosis. (*From Kusumoto FM, Calkins H, Boehmer J, et al. HRS/ACC/AHA expert consensus statement on the use of implantable cardioverter-defibrillator therapy in patients who are not included or not well represented in clinical trials.* Heart Rhythm *2014;117):1271-1303.)*

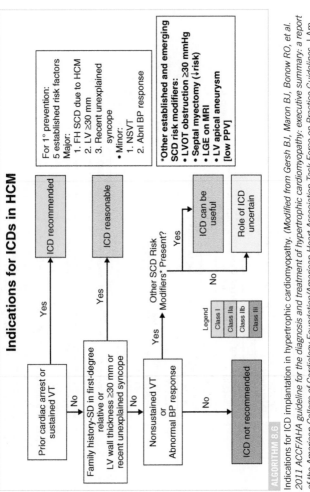

ALGORITHM 8.6

Indications for ICD implantation in hypertrophic cardiomyopathy. (Modified from Gersh BJ, Maron BJ, Bonow RO, et al. 2011 ACCF/AHA guideline for the diagnosis and treatment of hypertrophic cardiomyopathy: executive summary: a report of the American College of Cardiology Foundation/American Heart Association Task Force on Practice Guidelines. J Am Coll Cardiol 2011;58(25):2703-2738.)

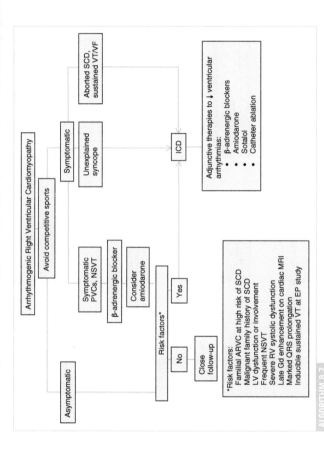

ALGORITHM 8.7

Arrhythmogenic right ventricular cardiomyopathy.

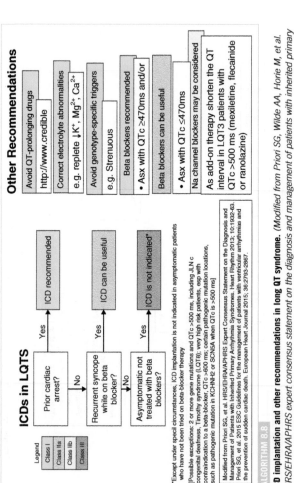

Other Recommendations

- Avoid QT-prolonging drugs
  http://www.credible
- Correct electrolyte abnormalities
  e.g. replete ↓K⁺, Mg²⁺, Ca²⁺
- Avoid genotype-specific triggers
  e.g. Strenuous
- Beta blockers recommended
  • Asx with QTc ≥470ms and/or
- Beta blockers can be useful
  • Asx with QTc ≤470ms
- Na channel blockers may be considered
  As add-on therapy shorten the QT interval in LQT3 patients with QTc >500 ms (mexiletine, flecainide or ranolazine)

ICDs in LQTS

Legend
Class I
Class IIa
Class IIb
Class III

Prior cardiac arrest? —Yes→ ICD recommended

No

Recurrent syncope while on beta blocker? —Yes→ ICD can be useful

No

Asymptomatic not treated with beta blockers? —Yes→ ICD is not indicated*

*Except under special circumstances, ICD implantation is not indicated in asymptomatic patients who have not been tried on beta-blocker therapy

[Possible exceptions: 2 or more gene mutations and QTc >500 ms, including JLN c congenital deafness, Timothy syndrome (LQT8); very high risk patients, esp with contraindication to a beta-blocker, QTc >600 ms; certain pathogenic mutation locations, such as pathogenic mutation in KCHNH2 or SCN5A when QTc is >500 ms]

Modified from Priori SG, et al. HRS/EHRA/APHRS Expert Consensus Statement on the Diagnosis and Management of Patients with Inherited Primary Arrhythmia Syndromes. Heart Rhythm 2013; 10:1932-63. Priori SG, et al. 2015 ESC Guidelines for the management of patients with ventricular arrhythmias and the prevention of sudden cardiac death. European Heart Journal 2015; 36:2793-2867.

ALGORITHM 8.8

ICD implantation and other recommendations in long QT syndrome. *(Modified from Priori SG, Wilde AA, Horie M, et al. HRS/EHRA/APHRS expert consensus statement on the diagnosis and management of patients with inherited primary arrhythmia syndromes. Heart Rhythm 2013; 10:1932-1963; Priori SG, Blomström-Lundqvist C, Mazzanti A, et al. 2015 ESC Guidelines for the management of patients with ventricular arrhythmias and the prevention of sudden cardiac death. Eur Heart J 2015;36:2793-2867.)*

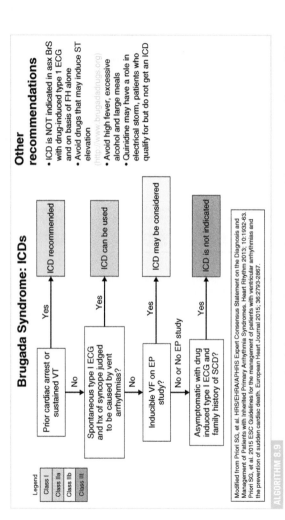

Brugada Syndrome: ICDs

Other recommendations

- ICD is NOT indicated in asx BrS with drug-induced type 1 ECG and on basis of FH alone
- Avoid drugs that may induce ST elevation (http://www.brugadadrugs.org)
- Avoid high fever, excessive alcohol and large meals
- Quinidine may have a role in electrical storm, patients who qualify for but do not get an ICD

Legend
- Class I
- Class IIa
- Class IIb
- Class III

Prior cardiac arrest or sustained VT → Yes → **ICD recommended**

↓ No

Spontaneous type I ECG and hx of syncope judged to be caused by vent arrhythmias? → Yes → **ICD can be used**

↓ No

Inducible VF on EP study? → Yes → **ICD may be considered**

↓ No or No EP study

Asymptomatic with drug induced type I ECG and family history of SCD? → Yes → **ICD is not indicated**

Modified from Priori SG, et al. HRS/EHRA/APHRS Expert Consensus Statement on the Diagnosis and Management of Patients with Inherited Primary Arrhythmia Syndromes. Heart Rhythm 2013; 10:1932-63. Priori SG, et al. 2015 ESC Guidelines for the management of patients with ventricular arrhythmias and the prevention of sudden cardiac death. European Heart Journal 2015; 36:2793-2867.

ALGORITHM 8.9

ICD implantation and recommendations in Brugada syndrome. *(Modified from Priori SG, Wilde AA, Horie M, et al. HRS/ EHRA/APHRS expert consensus statement on the diagnosis and management of patients with inherited primary arrhythmia syndromes. Heart Rhythm 2013;10(12):1932-1963. Additional reference: Priori SG, Blomström-Lundqvist C, Mazzanti A, et al. 2015 ESC Guidelines for the management of patients with ventricular arrhythmias and the prevention of sudden cardiac death. Eur Heart J 2015;36:2793-2867.)*

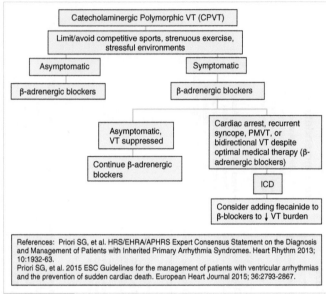

References: Priori SG, et al. HRS/EHRA/APHRS Expert Consensus Statement on the Diagnosis and Management of Patients with Inherited Primary Arrhythmia Syndromes. Heart Rhythm 2013; 10:1932-63.
Priori SG, et al. 2015 ESC Guidelines for the management of patients with ventricular arrhythmias and the prevention of sudden cardiac death. European Heart Journal 2015; 36:2793-2867.

ALGORITHM 8.10

Management of catecholaminergic polymorphic ventricular tachycardia. *(From Priori SG, Wilde AA, Horie M, et al. HRS/EHRA/APHRS expert consensus statement on the diagnosis and management of patients with inherited primary arrhythmia syndromes. Heart Rhythm 2013;10:1932-1963. Priori SG, Blomström-Lundqvist C, Mazzanti A, et al. 2015 ESC Guidelines for the management of patients with ventricular arrhythmias and the prevention of sudden cardiac death. Eur Heart J 2015;36:2793-2867.)*

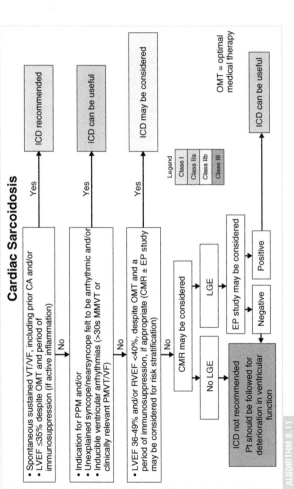

ALGORITHM 8.11

ICD implantation in cardiac sarcoidosis. *(Modified from Birnie DH, Sauer WH, Bogun F, et al. HRS expert consensus statement on the diagnosis and management of arrhythmias associated with cardiac sarcoidosis. Heart Rhythm 2014;11:1305-1323.)*

Chapter 9

Drug Effects and Electrolyte Disorders

ANTIARRHYTHMIC DRUGS

By several mechanisms, some drugs, particularly antiarrhythmic drugs, can cause serious rhythm disturbances in susceptible individuals. This is termed *proarrhythmia*. Proarrhythmia encompasses an extensive list of arrhythmia types, including increase in premature ventricular contractions (PVCs), nonsustained ventricular tachycardia, sustained monomorphic ventricular tachycardia, polymorphic ventricular tachycardia, and ventricular fibrillation. Some drugs increase the risk of bradycardia or atrioventricular (AV) block, another form of proarrhythmia.

Antiarrhythmic drugs that block sodium channels (class I drugs, including procainamide, quinidine, disopyramide, flecainide, and propafenone) prolong conduction in atrial and ventricular muscle and in the His Purkinje system. By so doing, they can cause QRS widening, AV block or monomorphic and/or polymorphic ventricular tachycardia in susceptible patients. Slowing of conduction in the atrium in patients treated for atrial fibrillation (AF) can result in organization to atrial flutter, which can be slow (<200 bpm) and conduct 1:1 through the atrioventricular node (AVN) at a paradoxically faster rate than typical faster (300 bpm) atrial flutter, which typically conducts through the AVN in 2:1 fashion at 150 bpm due to AV nodal refractoriness. The atrial proarrhythmia can occur with a narrow QRS complex or with a wide complex QRS due to concomitant slowing of conduction in the ventricles. At very high (toxic doses) of IC antiarrhythmic drugs, the electrocardiogram (ECG) can look like hyperkalemia or ventricular tachycardia.

Drugs that prolong repolarization (class IA antiarrhythmic drugs, such as procainamide and quinidine, and class III antiarrhythmic drugs, such as sotalol, dofetilide, and occasionally amiodarone) generally block the I_{Kr} channel, which can induce an acquired form of long QT syndrome (LQTS). Many noncardiac drugs can also prolong repolarization, prolong the QT interval, and predispose to torsades de pointes ventricular tachycardia (TdP VT) because of their effects on the I_{Kr} channel, the rapid component of the delayed rectifying potassium current. A partial list of drugs that prolong QT is provided in Table 6.2, and the reader is referred to the website https://www.crediblemeds.org for a more inclusive and up-to-date list of offending drugs. The most catastrophic effect of QT prolongation is the development of TdP with cardiac arrest and sudden death.

Antiarrhythmic drugs (class IC drugs, sotalol and amiodarone, in particular) can affect the sinus node and cause sinus bradycardia in susceptible patients.

DIGITALIS TOXICITY

Digitalis is used in the treatment of systolic heart failure and for ventricular rate control in AF. Digitalis has effects on the ECG, including depression of the PR and sagging of the ST segments, decrease in T-wave amplitude, shortening of the QT interval, and increase in U-wave amplitude. The therapeutic level of digitalis is typically 0.7 to 2.0 ng/mL, although toxicity can occur within this range, and worse survival has been associated with levels less than 0.9 ng/mL. Digitalis toxicity can be exacerbated by hypokalemia, hypomagnesemia, hypercalcemia, hypoxemia, hypothyroidism, renal insufficiency, and volume depletion. Drugs that interact with digitalis, that raise serum digitalis levels, and that could contribute to digitalis toxicity include certain antibiotics (e.g., tetracycline and erythromycin) and antiarrhythmics (quinidine, flecainide, amiodarone, and verapamil). Digitalis toxicity can lead to systemic symptoms, such as gastrointestinal symptoms (nausea, vomiting, diarrhea, anorexia), central nervous system abnormalities (headache, lethargy, seizures), and visual changes (scotoma, halos, color perception changes). In addition, digitalis toxicity can cause a wide range of arrhythmias and conduction disturbances. Some of the common digitalis toxicity rhythms include the following:

- Sinus bradycardia (see Fig. 1.4)
- Sinus pause (see Fig. 1.9)
- Mobitz type I second-degree AV block (see Fig. 2.3)
- High-grade AV block (see Fig. 2.8)
- Complete AV block (complete heart block [CHB]) with junctional or ventricular escape rhythms (see Fig. 2.12)
- Premature ventricular complexes (see Fig. 3.6)
- Accelerated junctional rhythm (see Fig. 3.15)
- Junctional tachycardia (JT) (see Fig. 5.23)
- Ventricular fibrillation (VF) (see Fig. 6.8 or 6.9)
- Ventricular tachycardia (VT) (see Fig. 4.2 or 6.2)
- Other rhythms that are associated more with digitalis toxicity than with other circumstances (although none are pathognomonic of digitalis toxicity) include the following:
  - AF with regular ventricular response (indicating CHB) (Fig. 9.1)
  - Atrial tachycardia (AT) with AV block, usually 2:1 (Fig. 9.2)
  - Fascicular tachycardia (Fig. 9.3)
  - Bidirectional tachycardia (Fig. 9.4)

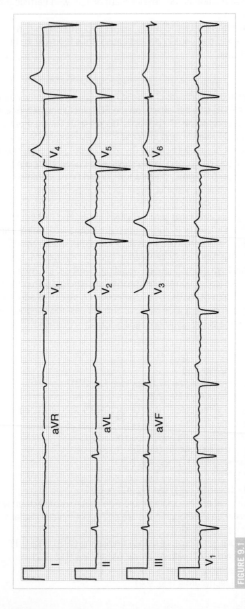

FIGURE 9.1

Atrial fibrillation with regular ventricular response. This 12-lead ECG and lead V_1 rhythm strip show atrial fibrillation (AF) with a regular ventricular response that is due to complete AV block with a junctional escape rhythm.

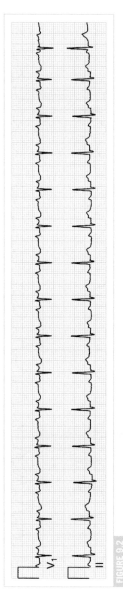

Atrial tachycardia with atrioventricular block. This lead V_1 and II rhythm strip shows atrial tachycardia (AT) with 2:1 atrioventricular (AV) block. The ventricular rate (90 bpm) is exactly half the atrial rate of 180 bpm, which helps to identify the presence of 2:1 AV block.

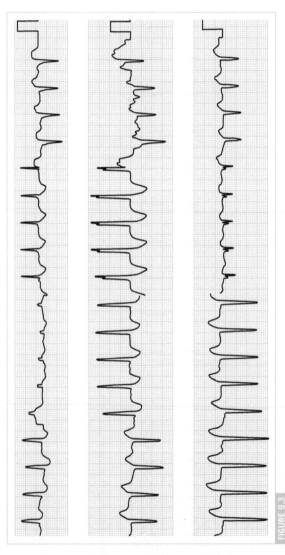

FIGURE 9.3

Fascicular tachycardia. This ECG tracing shows a fascicular tachycardia due to digitalis toxicity. This is a wide QRS complex with a right bundle branch block pattern and a leftward axis with a duration that is <0.12 s. It is an uncommon digitalis toxicity rhythm.

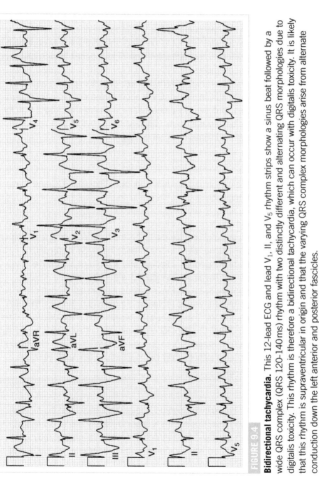

FIGURE 9.4

Bidirectional tachycardia. This 12-lead ECG and lead V₁, II, and V₅ rhythm strips show a sinus beat followed by a wide QRS complex (QRS 120–140 ms) rhythm with two distinctly different and alternating QRS morphologies due to digitalis toxicity. This rhythm is therefore a bidirectional tachycardia, which can occur with digitalis toxicity. It is likely that this rhythm is supraventricular in origin and that the varying QRS complex morphologies arise from alternate conduction down the left anterior and posterior fascicles.

Treatment of digitalis toxicity involves withdrawal of the drug and correction of any exacerbating electrolyte abnormalities; however, caution should be used with potassium administration, as it could cause or worsen AV block. For non–life-threatening arrhythmias, observe and monitor, if stable. For symptomatic bradycardias, atropine and/or temporary transvenous ventricular pacing may be needed. For VT, lidocaine or phenytoin can be tried. Electrical cardioversion should be used only if absolutely necessary in patients with digitalis toxicity because VT or VF can occur (which can then be very difficult to control).

For life-threatening ventricular arrhythmias, digitalis-specific antibody fragments should be administered. Clinical improvement typically occurs in 30 to 60 minutes, but it may be necessary to repeat the dose if toxicity does not reverse after several hours. Digitalis toxic rhythms can recur more than 24 hours later and require repeat dosing.

ELECTROLYTE DISORDERS

There are several electrolyte disorders that can affect the ECG and that could be arrhythmogenic.

Hypokalemia

Hypokalemia can cause characteristic ECG findings, including a prominent P wave ("pseudo-P-pulmonale") in the inferior leads, ST depression, flattened T waves, prolonged QT interval, and a prominent U wave (Figs. 9.5 and 9.6). Arrhythmias associated with hypokalemia include ventricular arrhythmias, such as PVCs and nonsustained VT (which is usually TdP). Treatment involves repletion of potassium through the oral and/or intravenous routes. Treatment with intravenous magnesium is often necessary to fully correct the hypokalemia, although the serum magnesium may be normal (serum magnesium represents only 1% to 2% of total body magnesium such that a patient may be magnesium depleted yet have a normal serum value).

Hyperkalemia

Hyperkalemia can be arrhythmogenic and at high levels can be rapidly fatal. Mildly elevated levels of serum K (approximately 5.5 to 6.5 mEq/L) are associated with narrow-based tented T waves that may or may not be tall (Fig. 9.7), and can be associated with QT-interval shortening and reversible left anterior or posterior fascicular block patterns. However, the correlation of these ECG findings with serum K^+ levels is not particularly strong. Higher levels of extracellular potassium (approximately 6.5 to 7.5 mEq/L) may be associated with first-degree AV block, flattening and widening of the P wave, QRS widening, and ST-segment depression. Even higher levels (>7.5 mEq/L) reduce the resting membrane potentials of atrial and ventricular myocytes, leading to inactivation of sodium channels and

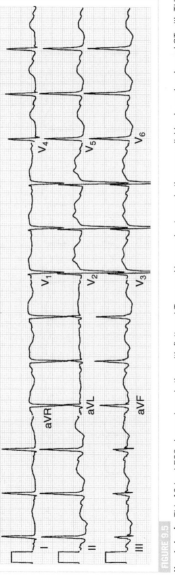

FIGURE 9.5

Hypokalemia. This 12-lead ECG shows sinus rhythm with flattened T waves, U waves best seen in the precordial leads, and prolonged QT with TU fusion. This patient had a potassium level of 2.5 mEq/L.

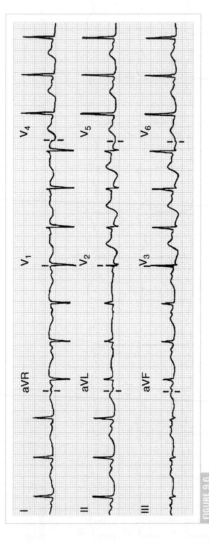

FIGURE 9.6

Hypokalemia. This 12-lead ECG shows the findings of hypokalemia, including ST depression (which can mimic myocardial ischemia), flattening of T waves, prolongation of the QT interval, and increased prominence of the U wave. The merging of the T and U waves makes distinguishing and measuring them more difficult. In this case the potassium level was 1.5 mEq/L.

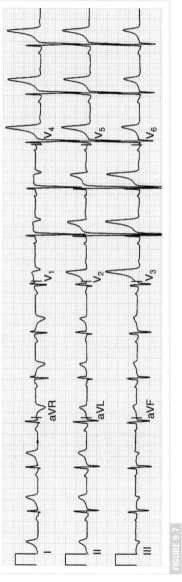

FIGURE 9.7

Tall peaked T waves with hyperkalemia. This 12-lead ECG shows the tented T waves that are commonly seen in mild to moderate degrees of hyperkalemia. Tented T waves of hyperkalemia need not be tall, although in this case they are.

slowing of conduction. This manifests as a decrease in P-wave amplitude or a disappearance of P wave; marked prolongation of the QRS interval (left bundle branch block [LBBB] or right bundle branch block [RBBB] patterns or nonspecific intraventricular conduction delay), which can lead to a sine-wave pattern in which there is no clear separation of the QRST waves (Figs 9.8 and 9.9); VT; VF; idioventricular rhythm; or asystole. These ECG changes are better correlated with high serum potassium levels than are tented T waves alone.

Treatment of Hyperkalemia

Treatment of hyperkalemia associated with ECG changes includes (1) calcium gluconate (10 mL of 10% solution intravenously over 2 to 3 minutes) to stabilize the heart against the depolarizing effects of hyperkalemia (but will not lower serum potassium levels) and (2) the combination of glucose (25 to 50 g intravenously) and insulin (10 to 20 units of regular insulin intravenously). Sodium bicarbonate (three ampules [150 mEq] added to 1 L of a 5% dextrose solution) can also shift potassium into cells, but should be used when there is concurrent metabolic acidosis. In addition, the resultant volume overload may be poorly tolerated in patients with end-stage renal failure. Longer-term treatment to rid the body of excessive potassium includes Kayexalate (25 to 50 g in 100 mL of 20% sorbitol given orally). Dialysis should be reserved for hyperkalemia that is unresponsive to these treatments.

CALCIUM DISORDERS

Hypocalcemia

Although hypocalcemia and hypercalcemia are rarely associated with arrhythmias, they produce characteristic ECG changes. The primary ECG manifestation of hypocalcemia is prolongation of the QT interval, which is due to ST segment prolongation without a change in the duration of the T wave (Fig. 9.10).

Hypercalcemia

The characteristic ECG findings of hypercalcemia are a shortened QT interval with a short ST segment and no change in the duration of the T wave (Fig. 9.11). There is typically no effect on the P, QRS, or T wave, but PR prolongation can occur.

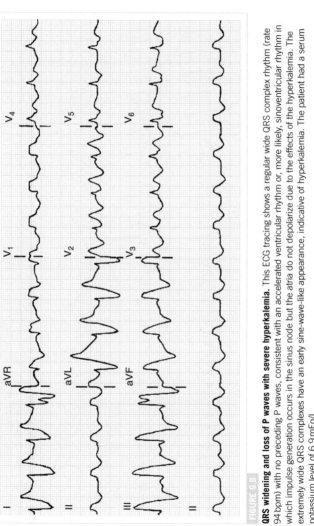

FIGURE 9.8

QRS widening and loss of P waves with severe hyperkalemia. This ECG tracing shows a regular wide QRS complex rhythm (rate 94 bpm) with no preceding P waves, consistent with an accelerated ventricular rhythm or, more likely, sinoventricular rhythm in which impulse generation occurs in the sinus node but the atria do not depolarize due to the effects of the hyperkalemia. The extremely wide QRS complexes have an early sine-wave-like appearance, indicative of hyperkalemia. The patient had a serum potassium level of 6.9 mEq/L.

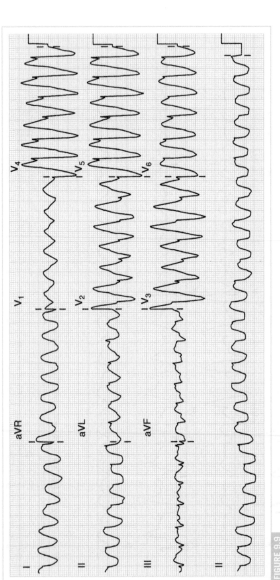

FIGURE 9.9

Ventricular tachycardia mimic: sine-wave pattern in severe hyperkalemia. This 12-lead ECG with lead II rhythm strip shows a rapid fairly regular wide QRS complex tachycardia (rate ~150 bpm) with a sine-wave pattern typical of severe hyperkalemia. When hyperkalemia is a consideration, such rhythms should not be mistaken for, and should not be treated as, ventricular tachycardia. The patient's serum potassium level was >7.5 mEq/L. Treatment included intravenous calcium, insulin, glucose, and sodium bicarbonate.

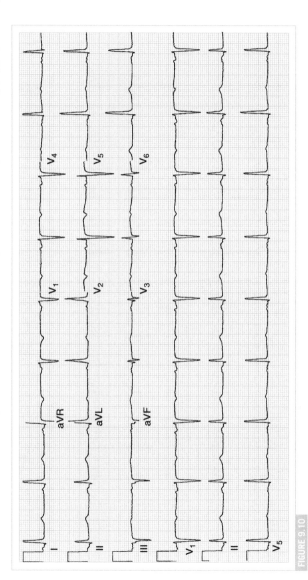

FIGURE 9.10

Hypocalcemia. This 12-lead ECG with V_1, II, and V_5 rhythm strips show normal sinus rhythm with prolongation of the QT interval (corrected QT interval of ~0.50s). The long QT interval is due to prolongation of the ST segment, which is typical of hypocalcemia. The patient had a serum calcium level of 7.9 mg/dL.

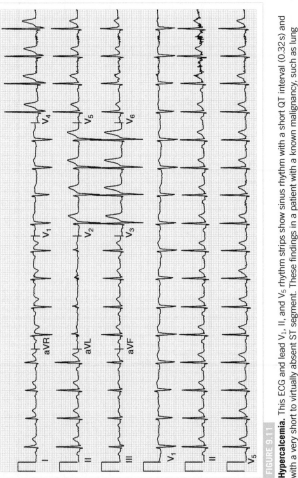

FIGURE 9.11

Hypercalcemia. This ECG and lead V_1, II, and V_5 rhythm strips show sinus rhythm with a short QT interval (0.32 s) and with a very short to virtually absent ST segment. These findings in a patient with a known malignancy, such as lung cancer, strongly suggest the presence of hypercalcemia. Short QT syndrome (not related to hypercalcemia) is in the differential diagnosis.

Athletes with arrhythmias constitute a potentially high-risk group that may need special attention and evaluation in addition to care that might be required for nonathletes, especially if these athletes have symptoms. Athletes with arrhythmias may have syncope, palpitations, or even cardiac arrest. Some athletes with arrhythmias require restriction of their athletic activities or at least aggressive therapy due to their underlying heart problems and/or their arrhythmias, but others can return to full activity if the arrhythmia is corrected (e.g., with ablation) and there are no other significant risks due to the presence of other heart disease.

Athletes are different from nonathletes because of their high visibility; their drive, which can push them beyond normal physiologic stresses; specific physiologic stresses that result in major changes in the sympathetic/parasympathetic innervation of the heart and vasculature; metabolic changes such as hypokalemia, hyponatremia, acidosis, and other electrolyte abnormalities; and alterations in carbon dioxide and oxygen saturation. There can be fluctuations in body temperature and other physical and psychological influences. There can be changes in circulating mediators such as angiotensin-converting enzymes, steroids, serotonin, and histamine. In addition, during sports activities, there can be extreme changes in heat and cold exposure, further stressing the physiologic milieu.

The type of exercise (static, dynamic, anaerobic, or aerobic) may have a significant impact on the outcome for that individual. Arrhythmias can start with extreme initial stress, during prolonged activity, and sometimes at abrupt termination of activity.

It can be difficult to determine if heart disease is present or if cardiac abnormalities represent adaptation to exercise; for example, increased left ventricular wall thickness may be due to "athlete's heart," and deconditioning might reverse the effects. This type of adaptation may be specific to both the type and amount of training. Furthermore, there can be bradycardia and other arrhythmias that are typical for a highly trained athlete. The difference between hypertrophic cardiomyopathy and athlete's heart may be related to the electrocardiographic patterns of left ventricular hypertrophy, the size of the left ventricular cavity, the presence or absence of left atrial enlargement, the presence or absence of bizarre electrocardiographic patterns, the change in wall thickness with deconditioning, a family history of channelopathies such as long QT interval syndrome (LQTS), hypertrophic cardiomyopathy, catecholaminergic polymorphic ventricular tachycardia (CPVT), or similar high-risk conditions.

Sudden death in the United States occurs only rarely in young athletes; the most common causes include hypertrophic cardiomyopathy, commotio cordis, coronary artery anomalies, ventricular hypertrophy from an undetermined cause, myocarditis, ruptured aortic aneurysm, arrhythmogenic right ventricular cardiomyopathy, coronary artery obstruction or anomalies, aortic valve stenosis, atherosclerotic coronary disease, dilated cardiomyopathy, myxomatous mitral valve degeneration, asthma and other lung conditions, heatstroke, drug abuse, and cardiac channelopathies.

The most common sports in which sudden death tends to occur are basketball, football, track, soccer, and swimming.

There are now new recommendations and guidelines on eligibility for competitive athletics and sports based on underlying cardiovascular conditions. Additionally, there have been revisions in evaluation, management, and restriction of athletes at risk for arrhythmias.

Evaluation of the athlete with palpitations or syncope is a challenge because athletes tend to have conditions that do not necessarily lend themselves to easy testing and testing tends to have a low sensitivity and specificity. Neurocardiogenic syncope is the diagnosis of exclusion.

Supplements of concern regarding induction of arrhythmias and even sudden death include stimulants such as amphetamines and cocaine, androstenedione, dehydroepiandrosterone (DHEA), growth hormone, erythropoietin, alcohol, narcotics, ephedra, and many other drugs. Drug testing may be required.

The electrocardiogram is often abnormal in trained athletes and therefore is not predictive of development of arrhythmias. These abnormalities include prominent QRS voltage, tall T waves, and early repolarization waves. Early repolarization is a notch on the down stroke of the R wave and is actually a prominent J wave (Fig. 10.1). It can occur several millimeters above the isoelectric line and may be mistaken for ST elevation, as in myocardial infarction or pericarditis. Recently, a form of early repolarization unassociated with high QRS voltage, and especially prominent in the inferior leads, has been associated with sudden death due to primary ventricular fibrillation (VF) but its occurrence is thought to be rare. Other ECG abnormalities include ECGs suggesting right ventricular cardiomyopathy, LQTS, Brugada syndrome, and hypertrophic cardiomyopathy.

Regarding restrictions, emerging data indicate that it may be safe for some athletes to participate in competitive sports even with an implantable cardioverter defibrillator (ICD), but recommendations vary and are, in part, dependent on the underlying condition (e.g., hypertrophic cardiomyopathy). For athletes with isolated premature ventricular depolarizations or nonsustained ventricular tachycardia (VT), no restriction is required as long as structural heart disease is not present. For sustained VT,

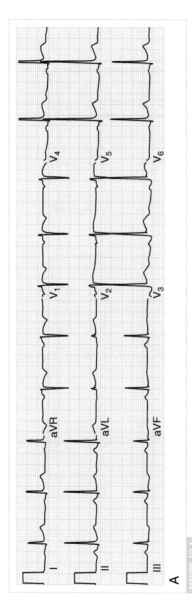

FIGURE 10.1

Spectrum of early repolarization. (A–C) This 12-lead electrocardiogram (ECG) shows sinus rhythm with differing degrees of notching of the J point, concave upward ST segment elevation, and tall upright T waves. This pattern is consistent with early repolarization abnormality.

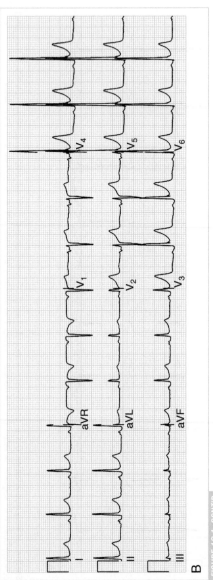

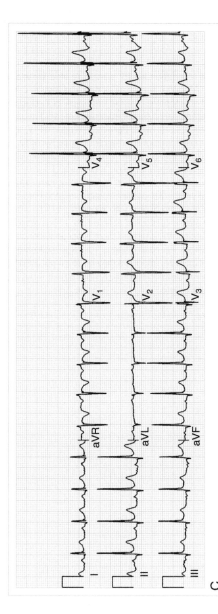

FIGURE 10.1. CONT'D

if there is no structural heart disease, ablation is recommended, and if there is structural heart disease, the patient requires evaluation for the use of antiarrhythmic drugs and an ICD. If the patient has a history of cardiac arrest, an ICD is generally recommended as long as there is a risk of recurrence.

No restrictions are recommended for premature atrial depolarizations. For atrial fibrillation (AF)/atrial flutter (AFL), rate and rhythm control, anticoagulation, and ablation are possible therapies, but ablation has become first-line therapy particularly if episodes are rapid and/or symptomatic. For patients with Wolff-Parkinson-White (WPW) syndrome, AV node reentry, or other forms of supraventricular tachycardia (SVT), catheter ablation is recommended, and a return to sports activity can be fairly quick as long as successful ablation is performed.

Restriction is in order for patients with hypertrophic cardiomyopathy, arrhythmogenic right ventricular cardiomyopathy, dilated cardiomyopathy, and Brugada syndrome. For patients with idiopathic VT, the athlete can return to full activity after a successful ablation. An ICD is recommended for patients with idiopathic VF, although there is some evidence now that ablation of VF is possible. For other channelopathies, including LQTS and CPVT, restriction, β-blockade, and ICDs may be required. Restriction after ICD implant is not necessarily a reason to restrict athletics but individual athletes need to be considered on a case by case basis.

Proper and effective monitoring is required to assess and manage arrhythmias and to document and diagnose the etiology of the problem. Many individuals have symptoms that might appear to be arrhythmic in origin but are not. Many arrhythmias may be of prognostic importance but are not easily diagnosed by symptoms alone. It is not uncommon for individuals to be completely asymptomatic during serious and potentially life-threatening arrhythmias; therefore, proper selection of monitoring techniques is crucial to secure the rhythm diagnosis and develop a management strategy.

There have been important advancements in the technology for monitoring arrhythmias. The 24- to 48-hour Holter monitor provides complete disclosure of rhythm disturbances, but only during a short window of time. These multilead monitors (from which a 12-lead electrocardiogram [ECG] can be constructed to analyze QRS morphology during arrhythmias) can provide information on minimum, maximum, and mean heart rates, all types of arrhythmias, diurnal changes in arrhythmia frequency and duration, heart rate variability, abnormalities in the ST segments and their relationship to rhythm disturbances or heart rate, changes in the QRS and QT intervals, and presence or absence of normal pacing system function. They can also disclose symptoms that occur during recordings, directly by patient triggering or by written diary entries, allowing for rhythm-symptom correlation. They can further determine the "burden" of a specific arrhythmia over time.

If, however, a patient has intermittent symptoms, Holter monitor recordings, performed at a specific point in time, will be of no use. For example, if a patient has syncope and has a Holter recording that does not show any episodes of arrhythmia and the patient does not record an episode of syncope, the monitor is of no use. Furthermore, nonspecific arrhythmias such as atrial and ventricular premature complexes recorded in patients with serious symptoms such as syncope will have little, if any, meaning. For example, recording of a sinus pause in the middle of the night, which is likely vagally mediated, in a patient with syncope has neither specific meaning nor prognostic significance regarding the type of evaluation and management that needs to be performed.

There are other ways to monitor arrhythmias. Event monitors now available are more advanced than in years past. Multilead recordings can be provided with full disclosure over a 24-hour period. Furthermore, the information can be downloaded and sent transtelephonically to a monitoring center; this can be accomplished during symptoms or periodically in patients with previously defined severe arrhythmias. Recordings can be triggered manually or automatically. These monitors can act as real-time or endless loop recorders with memory capability and therefore can provide continuous monitoring and playback should a patient have a symptom that occurred minutes before the device was manually activated and marked. Monitors can be worn for 30 to 60 days. They can also be used intermittently and applied as required in patients with long-standing symptoms. They can provide ample leeway for a patient to apply and then remove the monitor so that the patient does not need to wear the device all the time.

In addition to these noninvasive monitoring techniques, there are now implantable loop recorders (ILRs). These small leadless devices are implanted or injected subcutaneously as a minor operation and provide real-time and endless loop recordings that are stored in the device for a period of up to 3 years. The ILR can transmit information transtelephonically and then send information over the Internet to the physician. Stored data can be interrogated in the same way as pacemakers are interrogated, and the information can be printed. These devices are currently indicated for patients with occasional syncopal spells that are infrequent enough that they cannot be recorded on a Holter monitor or an external loop recorder. The ILR can also be used for diagnosis of the cause of palpitations and other nonspecific but arrhythmia-related symptoms. Ultimately, as this technology advances, these devices may be able to store in memory episodes of asymptomatic atrial fibrillation (AF) and determine its burden.

ILRs are not the only implanted method to record rhythm disturbances. Permanent pacemakers and implantable cardioverter defibrillators (ICDs) can store rhythm disturbances in memory, allowing for diagnosis. Specific criteria for such stored data must be programmed into these devices; otherwise they will not be recognized. Arrhythmia storage capability is not as great as that for the ILR.

Other forms of monitoring are also available, such as treadmill exercise testing. In patients with exercise-induced arrhythmias, a treadmill test may be used to document the rhythm and assess effects of therapy; correlation with myocardial ischemia can also be made, although this is unusual. Development of atrioventricular (AV) block during treadmill testing helps to localize the site of AV block and will aid in the decision to implant a permanent pacemaker. Appropriate shortening of the QT interval with increasing heart rate during exercise can be documented. Ventricular rate in patients with AF can be assessed. Finally, for athletes in whom extreme exertion is the only way to trigger an arrhythmia, monitors can be used during this type of exercise if it is deemed safe enough to measure and diagnose a rhythm disturbance that cannot be found any other way.

CAROTID SINUS MASSAGE

Carotid sinus massage (CSM) is performed to terminate some supraventricular tachycardias (SVTs), such as AV node reentry and AV reentry SVTs. It may also be useful for sinoatrial (SA) reentrant SVT. CSM can be helpful to diagnose the atrial rhythm during a tachycardia by producing AV block. For example, CSM-induced AV block can allow atrial flutter (AFL) waves to be seen. CSM may also be helpful to cause ventriculoatrial conduction block when there is a wide QRS complex tachycardia. CSM may also be useful to determine whether carotid sinus syndrome is present in syncopal patients.

The proper way to perform CSM is to make sure that the carotid pulse is felt directly under the fingertips. Two or three fingertips placed on the carotid artery are important to make sure that a vagal reflex is initiated. It can be performed on the right or the left side, but the left side is more likely to act on the AV node, whereas the right side acts on the sinus node. When performing CSM, it is important to realize that there is a small risk of stroke if there is carotid artery plaque; thus, it is important to check for carotid bruits before performing this procedure. The carotid sinus area should be massaged for about 5 seconds, beginning gently and progressing more rapidly to heavier pressure. Monitoring the patient for signs of cerebral hypoperfusion such as weakness, paresthesias, and numbness are important in avoiding transient ischemic attacks.

The head is turned away from the carotid sinus area to be massaged. For example, if right-sided CSM is to be performed, the head is turned to the left. The patient should be supine or even in a Trendelenburg position to maximize intravascular volume. To terminate tachycardias, it may be useful in some cases to combine CSM with Trendelenburg positioning and with a Valsalva or handgrip maneuver.

ELECTROPHYSIOLOGY STUDIES

Electrophysiology testing is invasive testing in which electrical catheters are placed inside the heart in an attempt to understand the mechanisms responsible for arrhythmias, to help map and localize an arrhythmia for curative procedures, to assess risk of sudden cardiac death and/or arrhythmia recurrence, to determine the need for other therapies such as a pacemaker or defibrillator, to better understand symptoms such as syncope, to determine the effectiveness of a specific drug to treat an arrhythmia, and to determine hemodynamic effects of pacing from various sites. Over the years, the indications and utility of electrophysiology studies have evolved, and many of the hoped-for predictive benefits of electrophysiologic testing have not turned out to be as useful as was initially thought.

An electrophysiology study can be used to assess sinus node dysfunction, AV node and His-Purkinje system conduction disturbances, the possible etiology of syncope, the risk for out-of-hospital cardiac arrest, the presence or absence of accessory pathways, and by induction of SVTs and ventricular tachycardias (VTs), localization and understanding of the mechanisms responsible for specific arrhythmias. Today, electrophysiology studies are mostly used in conjunction with mapping and ablation procedures directed toward potential cure of selected arrhythmias.

Electrophysiology studies can be performed noninvasively, through ICDs or pacemakers, or can be invasive. The invasive studies use 1 to 6 electrical wires with 2 to 20 poles (electrodes) for recording signals inside the heart and for induction of arrhythmias in the atria and ventricles. It can include use of a transseptal catheter for mapping and ablation of AF originating from the left atrium, for localizing left-sided accessory pathways, and for inducing and mapping VTs originating in the left ventricle. There are now new electroanatomical mapping systems that include methodologies to evaluate the cardiac chamber itself, the electrical signals generated in the cardiac chamber, and the activation sequences within different cardiac chambers. For this type of mapping system, there can be noncontact balloon-type mapping systems or contact mapping systems that involve point-by-point or large activation sequences.

The catheters used can have 2, 4, 6, 8, 10, 12, or 20 poles, depending on the purpose of the study. Ablation catheters can have 4-, 6-, 8-, or 10-mm tips.

Attempted induction of arrhythmias can include one or two atrial extrastimuli delivered at one or two fixed cycle lengths using a variety of protocols. Atrial pacing can also be used to determine sinus node function, AV node function, and His refractoriness. In the ventricles, one, two, or three premature ventricular extrastimuli delivered at one to three cycle lengths, and in some cases ventricular burst pacing, can be used to attempt to induce VTs. Often, extrastimulus testing is performed from more than one site.

Occasionally, the infusion of isoproterenol or an antiarrhythmic drug is part of the electrophysiologic test. These tests tend to be performed under some degree of conscious sedation, but it is realized that the conscious sedation itself may affect induction of some tachyarrhythmias, as they may suppress catecholamine effects on various tissues and pathways.

Although electrophysiology testing can be used for the evaluation of sinus node dysfunction, the sensitivity and specificity are relatively modest, if not poor; the same is true for investigation of AV nodal function. On the other hand, the evaluation of presence or absence of His-Purkinje conduction disease is quite accurate. The test is very good for induction of SVTs when they are documented to be present, but it is not good for prediction of who will or will not develop AF. The test is very good for determining the presence or absence and properties of an accessory pathway.

The electrophysiologic test has varying degrees of sensitivity and specificity regarding the induction of VTs, depending on the clinical characteristics of the patients and the arrhythmia. For example, the test has a relatively high sensitivity and specificity for induction of VT when a monomorphic VT is present in a patient with underlying ventricular dysfunction and coronary artery disease (CAD). On the other hand, sensitivity and specificity are not as good for patients with nonischemic dilated cardiomyopathy and are even worse, and therefore not indicated, for patients who have long QT interval syndrome (LQTS), who may be at risk for torsades de pointes (TdP) or sudden death. Occasionally, the test is used to diagnose rhythm disorders that are potential etiologies for syncope; its use in documenting the cause of palpitations is questionable. The electrophysiologic test is not used routinely as a prognostic marker in patients who are at risk for sudden cardiac death and who are already known to have other risk factors that are accepted indications for implantation of an ICD.

PALPITATIONS

Palpitations are a common complaint, occurring in up to 10% to 20% of patient evaluations. The symptom of palpitations is an uncomfortable, often anxiety-provoking awareness of the heart beating, and therefore does not necessarily signify the presence of an arrhythmia. The awareness of heart action can be described as a "pounding" that can be felt in the chest and/or neck. It can be perceived as an irregular, rapid, or forceful heartbeat, which can be intermittent or sustained; episodic palpitations are commonly described as "skipped beats." Most palpitations are caused by normal sinus rhythm, although depending on the population, can be a result of cardiovascular causes in up to 40% of patients; in many cases, because of their episodic nature, the exact cause remains undefined.

Associated Causes and Conditions

Several cardiac causes can be responsible for palpitations, including arrhythmias, CAD (in which they can be an anginal equivalent), high catecholamine states, or valvular disease causing a sensation of increased contractility.

Psychological causes, which can be present in up to 20% of patients, are often related to anxiety. Sometimes it is uncertain whether the anxiety represents the cause or the effect of palpitations. Miscellaneous causes for palpitations are fairly extensive. In addition to anxiety, infections and hormonal changes have been associated with palpitations. Several commonly used stimulants, such as caffeine, theophylline, decongestants such as pseudoephedrine, or components of diet or stimulant supplements, can be associated with palpitations. Alcohol can trigger palpitations, as can several herbal supplements, such as ginkgo biloba, ginseng, guarana, yohimbine, and ephedra (*ma huang*). Stress, changes in sleeping habits, anemia, and hyperthyroidism can cause palpitations.

The major issue in evaluating palpitations is a relationship to cardiac rhythm. Although there is an extensive differential diagnosis, palpitations can be a somatic manifestation of a psychiatric disorder, including depression and panic disorder. These patients are often young and more susceptible to hypochondriacal concerns. However, attributing palpitations to a supratentorial disorder is a diagnosis of exclusion.

Palpitations can be caused by a sustained or nonsustained rapid or irregular arrhythmia. When there is a sensation of pulsation in the neck and large neck veins (AV or cannon waves) or a sensation of pulsation in the throat, AV node reentry tachycardia should be considered. In patients with intermittent cannon A waves during sustained palpitations, AV dissociation is present, and VT should be considered. Atrial tachycardias (ATs), SA reentry, and AV reentry tachycardia (AVRT) tend to occur as rapid regular palpitations without an abnormal sensation in the neck. Short-duration, regular palpitations can be a result of nonsustained VT or nonsustained SVT. An irregular sensation that is sustained or nonsustained is often found to be AF or AFL with variable AV conduction. Patients who have any of these identified arrhythmias become very good at recognizing that rhythm disturbance.

It is important to recognize that palpitations can occur in patients with documented arrhythmias, but may not be caused by those arrhythmias, and correlation can be difficult. This becomes crucial in patients who have multiple arrhythmias, such as AF or SVT and atrial ectopy. Ablation of AF or the SVT may cure the tachycardia but not the atrial ectopy, and if the palpitations are not caused by the arrhythmia, they will continue to be felt.

Approach to Evaluation

The history can provide important clues concerning the presence or absence of a cardiac arrhythmia and can often suggest a rhythm diagnosis. Occasional "skipped" beats are likely ectopic activity. Prolonged rapid rates that begin suddenly and stop suddenly with a Valsalva maneuver, cough, or other vagal maneuver are likely to be a supraventricular reentry tachycardia. Irregular and rapid heart rates that begin abruptly are likely to represent AF. A slow pounding sensation can represent an accelerated junctional or ventricular rhythm or ventricular bigeminy, in which the "pounding" sensation is caused by the postextrasystolic beat.

If there are concomitant medical conditions or complaints, these should be explored. In some cases, palpitations are associated with acute onset of dyspnea or chest discomfort. These may provide clues to the diagnosis of heart failure or myocardial ischemia.

The evaluation of patients with palpitations depends on the degree to which the palpitations cause symptoms and impair quality of life; the type of rhythm diagnosed, if abnormal (rapid and irregular palpitations, such as those as a result of AF), which can be of significant consequence; and the underlying cardiovascular conditions that may be present.

An ECG should be performed. Although it may be normal, this is a cost-effective approach to determine the presence of myocardial ischemia or past myocardial infarction (MI) (substrate for VT), ventricular and atrial hypertrophy, long QT interval, Brugada pattern, Wolff-Parkinson-White (WPW) conduction, ventricular arrhythmias, AV dissociation, and any other potential arrhythmic or ischemic causes for the sensation of palpitations.

The type of approach used to evaluate the cause of the symptoms depends on their frequency. For an individual who is having daily palpitations, it makes most sense to perform a 24- to 48-hour Holter monitor with the patient recording in a diary when symptoms occur. For the patient who is having occasional palpitations that occur only every several days, an event monitor or a memory loop event recorder makes the most sense to record and document the rhythm disturbance during the palpitations. For patients who have serious or severe symptoms associated with the palpitations, such as syncope, longer-term event monitoring may be achieved by an ILR, which can activate automatically for serious rhythm disturbances or can be triggered by the patient. The ILR can remain implanted for more than 1.5 years and can be used to diagnose arrhythmias that occur with a low frequency or that may not have been captured with an event recorder that has been worn for a few weeks. The rhythms stored in the memory of the device are downloaded in a manner similar to cardiac pacemaker interrogation.

An echocardiogram should be performed in patients with palpitations that result from ventricular arrhythmias if there are abnormalities on the physical examination consistent with underlying structural heart disease, in older individuals, and in patients with abnormal ECGs.

In older individuals, especially in the presence of underlying structural heart disease, palpitations can be a premonitory sign for sudden cardiac death. If the symptoms are of new onset, careful and complete evaluation should be undertaken. If there are new premature ventricular contraction (PVCs), although they may turn out be benign and the ventricular function may be normal, it is important to assess the patient carefully to determine the presence of a progressive underlying cardiac diagnosis, such as CAD or valvular heart disease.

Approach to Management

In some cases, palpitations are a result of nonsustained ventricular or atrial tachyarrhythmias. Treatments for these problems may reduce arrhythmia recurrence or duration and thus reduce symptoms. Although antiarrhythmic drugs may be effective, the risk of proarrhythmia should always be considered.

Although PVCs, couplets, and triplets may be benign causes for palpitations in patients with no heart disease, long-standing ventricular bigeminy or very frequent PVCs, especially if originating in the right ventricle, leading to functional left bundle branch block (LBBB), can lead to a tachycardia-induced cardiomyopathy; in these cases, suppression with antiarrhythmic drugs or ablation in refractory cases can improve ventricular function.

Summary

Palpitations are a common, potentially debilitating symptom that may be related to an arrhythmia or a serious underlying clinical condition. Ablation can cure many SVTs and some VTs. It may also be used to treat AF, a common cause of irregular palpitations. Palpitations are sometimes not a result of an arrhythmic cause, and the relationship between the arrhythmia and the palpitations is not always clear.

SYNCOPE

Syncope is a transient loss of consciousness with or without a prodrome, with rapid, usually complete, recovery. It is a nonspecific but alarming and potentially debilitating symptom with diverse causes. The cumulative incidence of syncope in the general population is as high as 35%, with peaks in the late teenage years, especially for women, and in the older population, especially for those over the age of 80 years. Syncope can be a premonitory sign for sudden cardiac death or total mortality when it is ascribed to a cardiovascular cause or cardiac disease is present.

The symptom of syncope can be confusing. Some patients have neurocardiogenic episodes but do not completely pass out. Syncope can be associated with or related to other nonspecific symptoms such as dizziness, lightheadedness, near syncope, fatigue, nausea, and diaphoresis. Alternatively, patients can be found on the ground because they tripped or were in a confusional state and yet they did not have syncope. Syncope is a short-lived phenomenon. It can be confused with loss of consciousness, which is prolonged and may be a result of various toxic/metabolic causes or head trauma. Hypoglycemia and other abnormal metabolic states can cloud consciousness but do not necessarily or routinely cause syncope. Stroke tends to present with transient or persistent neurologic abnormalities but not with transient loss of consciousness alone. A seizure disorder tends to be associated with movement disorder and a postictal state.

Etiologies

The causes of syncope are diverse. The most common cause is neurocardiogenic, but orthostatic hypotension, cardiac arrhythmias, and psychiatric syncope must be considered. In older patients, orthostatic hypotension, drug-induced syncope, and syncope with multifactorial contributing causes are more common.

In neurocardiogenic syncope, there is usually associated relative bradycardia and hypotension. Neurocardiogenic syncope tends to be benign, although in some patients substantial disability may result. Life-threatening causes for syncope tend to be related to malignant cardiac arrhythmias. Several conditions in particular raise levels of concern when syncope is present. These include syncope during athletics and syncope in patients with heart failure, underlying structural heart disease, prior MI, or bundle branch block (BBB).

In older patients, a neurally mediated cause for syncope is, in a sense, a neurocardiogenic cause with a specific trigger. In the older population, common reflexes that cause syncope include defecation, micturition, deglutition, and other vagally mediated triggers. Older persons are often injured when they pass out, have heart disease, and need medical attention and hospitalization.

In younger individuals, emotion, pain, or anxiety can cause neutrally mediated syncope. Although most syncope in younger individuals is a result of a neurocardiogenic or situational cause, it is important to recognize the possibility that syncope can be psychiatric in origin. Cough, acute inferior wall MI, and pulmonary embolism are potential neurally mediated triggers for syncope. To confound the assessment of the cause or trigger, 50% of individuals are amnestic for the episode, and most episodes are unwitnessed.

There are a variety of potential life-threatening arrhythmic causes for syncope. These include LQTS, Brugada syndrome, arrhythmogenic right ventricular cardiomyopathy (ARVC) (dysplasia), hypertrophic cardiomyopathy, and WPW syndrome.

Approach to Evaluation and Management

The initial approach to the patient with syncope is to obtain a careful and complete history and perform a thorough physical examination. It is important to obtain old medical records and a history not only from the patient but also from witnesses. Important components of the history include patient age; a description of any prodromal symptoms; speed of recovery from symptoms; the circumstances surrounding the event, such as eating or exercise; the symptom type, frequency, and length; any associated cardiovascular or other medical conditions that may be present, medications, family history of syncope, and sudden death; and the presence of injury. On physical examination, orthostatic blood pressures and carotid massage are often of use, especially in patients with a history consistent with orthostatic hypotension or carotid sinus hypersensitivity.

The diagnostic evaluation of syncope is not standardized. Although guidelines have been published, syncope evaluation depends on the acuteness of the presentation, the location of the evaluation (emergency department, clinic, inpatient), the presence of comorbidities, the age of the patient, the number of episodes of syncope, the presence of cardiovascular disease, and the medications that the patient has been taking. There is no single diagnostic battery of tests that is useful in patients with syncope. Potentially useful tests include the ECG; the echocardiogram; varying types of monitoring systems to attempt to link a rhythm disturbance, if it exists, to syncope; a treadmill test, especially for patients with exercise-induced syncope; a tilt-table test; and an electrophysiology test. A head/brain computed tomography (CT) or magnetic resonance imaging (MRI) scan, electroencephalogram (EEG), carotid Dopplers, neurology consult, assessment for MI, and assessment for pulmonary emboli may be pursued in patients with suggestive neurologic or cardiopulmonary causes, but as a routine, these are not helpful. Unless a direct rhythm correlation is made with a typical syncopal episode, all etiologic diagnoses are inferred and presumptive. Although a diagnosis of the cause of syncope may remain unclear in up to one-third of patients, approximately 85% of these patients will remain undiagnosed. An ILR is useful for episodes of recurrent syncope that occur only occasionally; the loop recorder has reduced the number of patients with syncope of uncertain etiology by up to 25%. The ILR has its best use in patients with relatively normal ventricular function in whom the risk of sudden death is low.

Even when an etiologic diagnosis is presumptively made, the patient should continue to be followed on medical therapy to determine recurrence of syncope and effectiveness of therapy. The natural history of syncope is uncertain, and it appears to occur in a sporadic fashion despite the cause. The treatments for syncope are complex with several goals. For example, an ICD is usually indicated in patients with syncope, heart failure, and poor left ventricular ejection fraction (LVEF). On the other hand, an ICD may not reduce the risk of recurrent syncope as much as it will reduce the risk of sudden cardiac death. Indeed, patients who have an ICD for recurrent syncope caused by left ventricular dysfunction, heart failure, and presumed ventricular arrhythmias may continue to have syncope, depending on the underlying cause and time to ICD therapy delivery.

Adenosine

Adenosine is an intravenous (IV) purinergic blocker that inhibits sinus node and atrioventricular (AV) node automaticity and conduction, similar to high parasympathetic activity. Adenosine binds to the adenosine A1 receptor and activates a potassium current in the atrium (I_{KAdo}) with clinical transient effects of sinus node slowing, AV node block, and atrial refractory period shortening.

INDICATIONS. Termination of AV node– and sinus node–dependent tachycardias, such as AV node reentry tachycardia (AVNRT), reentrant tachycardias using an accessory pathway and the AV node, and sinus node reentrant tachycardia. Adenosine may also terminate some atrial tachycardias (ATs) and idiopathic ventricular tachycardias (VTs), particularly those that originate from the right ventricular outflow tract.

DOSAGE. Because adenosine has a very short half-life of about 10 seconds, it should be given as a rapid 6-mg IV bolus followed by a bolus of saline. If needed, a 12- to 18-mg IV bolus can be given 1 to 2 minutes later, followed by another 12- to 18-mg IV bolus 1 to 2 minutes after the second dose. Each IV dose should be followed with a rapid saline flush (20cc).

CONTRAINDICATIONS. Avoid in drug-induced tachycardias, wide QRS tachycardias of unknown origin, heart transplant patients (it may cause prolonged asystole), patients taking dipyridamole (it may cause prolonged asystole), and in those in whom severe bronchospasm can be produced. It will be ineffective if the patient is taking theophylline and will be less effective if the patient has just consumed large amounts of caffeine-containing substances.

COMMENTS. Does not terminate AV node–independent tachycardias such as atrial fibrillation (AF), atrial flutter (AFL), and multifocal AT, although the AV block produced can allow the atrial rhythm to be more easily diagnosed. Transient side effects include flushing, chest pain, dyspnea, bronchospasm, brief asystole, bradycardia, and premature ventricular contractions (PVCs). Patients should be forewarned that such marked discomfort may occur, but reassured that the sensation should pass after a few seconds. Transient sinus bradycardia (SB) and PVCs are common after conversion to sinus rhythm. Large doses can initiate AF. If used to diagnose the presence of AFL, the hypotension resulting from the drug can (rarely) facilitate AV conduction and produce 1:1 AV conduction.

Amiodarone

Amiodarone is a class I, II, III, and IV antiarrhythmic drug with a large volume of distribution, a long loading phase, and a long half-life. As a β-adrenergic blocker, it is noncompetitive.

INDICATIONS. Amiodarone is a complex drug with many potential arrhythmia indications. It is currently the most used antiarrhythmic drug despite the fact that it has only one U.S. Food and Drug Administration (FDA)-approved indication, which is for potentially life-threatening ventricular arrhythmias. It is the most versatile antiarrhythmic drug and can be used for virtually all ATs and VTs. Although it may be FDA approved specifically for potentially life-threatening VTs, amiodarone has not been shown to reduce the risk of death or sudden cardiac death in patients with cardiovascular disease or arrhythmias, although in patients with out-of-hospital cardiac arrest due to refractory VT/ventricular fibrillation (VF), IV amiodarone has been shown to improve survival to hospital admission. Nevertheless, the drug is excellent in reducing episodes of AF and VT. It is important to recognize that IV amiodarone has different electrophysiological effects from oral amiodarone. IV amiodarone loading does not provide the same electrophysiological benefit as oral drug therapy, and for reasons that are not entirely clear, it takes some time for IV amiodarone to be effective even if drug levels are high. IV amiodarone has a greater effect on blocking conduction through the AV node and has less effect on refractoriness. IV amiodarone can cause vasodilation and reflex sympathetic effects. The indications for IV amiodarone include cardiac arrest caused by VF or pulseless VT, VT that is hemodynamically better tolerated and has a monomorphic or polymorphic morphology with normal QT interval (and is not torsades de pointes ventricular tachycardia [TdP VT]), nonsustained VTs that are symptomatic, VTs that cause implantable cardioverter defibrillator (ICD) shocks, and atrial arrhythmias, including AT, AF, and AFL. It is useful for prevention of atrial arrhythmias after sinus rhythm has been restored and for prophylaxis of AF after open heart surgery.

DOSAGE

Intravenous Use. In the setting of a cardiac arrest, the initial IV bolus is 300 mg. Repeat 150- to 300-mg bolus doses can be given as needed up to a total maximum dose of 2.1 g in 24 hours. If there is restoration of sinus rhythm, large doses of IV amiodarone can cause hypotension and bradycardia.

For recurrent or refractory VF or VT, hemodynamically unstable VT, or stable wide QRS complex tachycardia of unknown origin, begin with IV infusion of 150 mg over no less than 10 minutes, followed by an infusion of

1 mg/minute for 6 hours, then a maintenance infusion of 0.5 mg/minute for 18 hours or until the switch to oral amiodarone is made. Additional bolus infusions of 150 mg over no less than 10 minutes can be administered for breakthrough arrhythmias.

For patients with acute-onset AF, such as in the postoperative setting, and for patients who cannot take oral drugs, IV amiodarone may be a quick way to load patients and to help control the ventricular response rate. The half-life of amiodarone given intravenously is less than it is after the patient is fully loaded and is 24 to 48 hours.

For treatment of AFL and AF, IV amiodarone can be used to rapidly obtain clinically effective levels of the drug and to help control the ventricular rate, if not restore the rhythm to normal, but it is important to recognize that IV amiodarone levels do not necessarily provide the same electrophysiological effects as does long-term use of the drug. IV amiodarone slows AV conduction, thus reducing the ventricular rate in AFL and AF. IV amiodarone is used in the setting of perioperative AFL and AF and in conditions in which paroxysmal arrhythmias have rapid rates that are hemodynamically decompensating, such as in hypertrophic cardiomyopathy.

The drug may also help block conduction through accessory pathways and the AV node. IV dosing is much the same as it is for VT, but the speed at which the infusion is given can often be reduced because the rhythm disturbance is usually better tolerated than VTs. As such, there is less risk of hypotension.

Oral Use. Oral dosing for recurrent VF or hemodynamically unstable VT and for prevention of ICD shocks: Loading dose of 800 to 1600 mg per day for 5 to 7 days (occasionally longer) until the arrhythmia is controlled or significant side effects occur. These large doses are preferably initiated in the hospital. The dose should then be reduced to 400 to 800 mg/day for 1 month, followed by the usual maintenance dose of 200 to 400 mg/day. Maintenance doses should be administered once daily (or in divided doses with meals for total daily doses that can be as low as 100 mg/day). Use lowest clinically effective doses because plasma levels do not reflect tissue levels and are therefore not useful. The half-life of oral amiodarone is approximately 40 to 45 days.

Typical oral dosing can be initiated in the hospital at up to 1200 mg/day for 3 to 5 days, with a decrease to 800 mg/day for 1 week, then 600 mg/day for 1 week, then 400 mg/day for several weeks, and finally 100 to 200 mg/day. Alternatively, the drug can be started more slowly in the outpatient setting at 600 or 400 mg/day for 3 to 4 weeks. Amiodarone is unlikely to convert AFL and AF to sinus rhythm acutely and should not be used for this purpose.

CONTRAINDICATIONS. Severe sinus node dysfunction causing marked SB, second-degree or third-degree AV block (AVB), and symptomatic bradyarrhythmias, unless rate support is provided by a pacemaker. Although the drug is best avoided in patients with interstitial lung disease, it can be used with caution in patients with chronic obstructive pulmonary disease (COPD). Although the incidence of proarrhythmia is low using amiodarone alone, caution should be used if given with other drugs that prolong the QT interval. Avoid this in patients with hepatic dysfunction. Amiodarone is absolutely contraindicated in pregnant women because of neonatal hypothyroidism, prematurity, bradycardia, and congenital abnormalities. Statin dosing may need to be reduced.

COMMENTS. The most common serious side effects of IV amiodarone include hypotension, bradycardia, AV block, TdP VT (<2%), interstitial pulmonary fibrosis, an acute respiratory distress syndrome (ARDS)-like condition if used acutely (2%), and liver toxicity. Thyroid dysfunction and central nervous system (CNS) side effects are not rare.

Side effects of oral amiodarone include hypothyroidism, hyperthyroidism, photosensitivity, blue discoloration of the skin, corneal deposits that can cause halos around lights, liver function abnormalities, nausea, tremor, neuropathy, or difficulty with gait due to neurotoxicity, pulmonary fibrosis, and bradycardia. Although the QT interval can lengthen significantly with oral amiodarone, TdP VT is rare. Optic neuritis has been rarely reported.

When given for high-risk ventricular arrhythmias or poorly controlled atrial arrhythmias, therapy should be initiated in the hospital after withdrawal of other antiarrhythmic drugs. Liver, lung (chest x-ray at minimum and pulmonary function tests with diffusing capacity of the lung for carbon monoxide [DLCO] in selected patients), and thyroid function should be evaluated at baseline and periodically thereafter. Plasma concentrations (normal, 1 to 2.5 mcg/mL) may be helpful in evaluating nonresponsiveness or unexpected severe toxicity but do not reflect tissue levels of the drug. Patients should be monitored closely after dose adjustments because of the drug's long half-life. Amiodarone can increase serum levels of digoxin, quinidine, procainamide flecainide, cyclosporine, and warfarin (prothrombin times must be followed closely, and dosage of warfarin may need to be reduced). Because of increased risk of rhabdomyolysis, concomitant doses of simvastatin greater than 20mg should be avoided. Phenytoin and cholestyramine can reduce amiodarone levels. Amiodarone generally does not increase myocardial stimulation threshold in patients with pacemakers but will elevate the defibrillation threshold in patients with ICDs. It may also slow VT below the programmed detection interval in patients with ICDs.

Atropine

Atropine is an IV antimuscarinic drug.

INDICATIONS AND DOSAGE. Ventricular asystole, pulseless electrical activity, bradycardia associated with hypotension: 1-mg IV push (may repeat).

Symptomatic SB or intranodal (Mobitz type I) AV block; nausea and vomiting caused by morphine: 0.5 to 1.0 mg. This may be repeated up to a total dose of 3 mg. Tracheal dose/route: 1 to 2.5 mg in 10 to 25 cc normal saline.

CONTRAINDICATIONS. Use with caution in acute coronary syndromes (increased heart rate can provoke myocardial ischemia, acute myocardial infarction [MI], and rarely VT or VF). Avoid in patients with cardiac denervation (e.g., transplant patients) and those taking dipyridamole. This can have antimuscarinic effects, including urinary retention in patients with prostate disease. Use caution if there is glaucoma. This can cause constipation and blurred vision.

COMMENTS. Atropine can worsen infranodal (Mobitz type II) second-degree AVB, due to an increase in sinus rate and enhanced AV nodal conduction, resulting in the atrial impulses encountering refractoriness in the His-fascicular system.

β-Adrenergic Blockers

This class of drugs (class II antiarrhythmics) blocks the β-sympathetic nervous system at the receptor level.

ARRHYTHMIC INDICATIONS. β-adrenergic blockers may be used acutely for patients with AFL and AF with a rapid ventricular response rate, although adequate rate control in flutter is not likely to be achieved. β-adrenergic blockers can be used chronically for rate control in AFL and AF and to prevent some recurrences of AF. β-adrenergic blockers can also be used for prevention of catecholamine-related VTs. β-adrenergic blockers reduce the risk of total mortality and sudden cardiac death in patients with underlying coronary artery disease (CAD), especially after MI. β-adrenergic blockers also reduce the risk of death in patients with cardiomyopathy and congestive heart failure (CHF) due to systolic left ventricular dysfunction.

β-adrenergic blockers may also help to prevent recurrences of ATs and other supraventricular tachycardias (SVTs) after conversion to sinus rhythm, although it is uncertain if β-adrenergic blockade alone actually helps to achieve the conversion to sinus rhythm. IV β-adrenergic blockade may also be used for VT and VF storm and for prevention of recurrent catecholaminergic-dependent VT.

The types of β-adrenergic blockers that are useful in treating arrhythmias include metoprolol, esmolol (acutely), carvedilol, and acebutolol. Metoprolol is longer acting than esmolol (half-life of approximately 9 minutes) but is more cardioselective. Propranolol and long-acting propranolol are useful because they cross the blood-brain barrier; they may have greater effects in neurocardiogenic syncope, although β-adrenergic blockade does not appear to be very effective to treat this disorder. Propranolol is no more effective than any other β-adrenergic blocker for any antiarrhythmic effects.

Atenolol is relatively short acting. It is best to use one or two β-adrenergic blockers and become familiar with them. Nadolol has been used particularly for long QT syndrome and some arrhythmias. It has a longer half-life and is a nonselective β blocker. Acebutolol and pindolol have some sympathomimetic effects. Acebutolol appears to be well tolerated in young individuals with palpitations and SVTs.

Acute Use

Indications and Dose. Start oral therapy unless there is a compelling reason to give IV (e.g., ventricular arrhythmias or significant hypertension). Metoprolol: Begin with 12.5 or 25 mg by mouth (PO) every 12 hours × 1, 50 mg every 12 hours × 2, then 100 mg PO every 12 hours, as tolerated. If IV metoprolol is indicated, 2.5 to 5 mg over 1 to 2 minutes, repeated every 5 minutes to a total dose of 15 mg before transitioning to oral therapy. Initial doses can be reduced to 1 to 2 mg if a conservative regimen is desired.

Esmolol may be preferred because of its brief half-life: 0.1 mg/kg per minute (IV) infusion, titrated in increments of 0.05 mg/kg per minute every 5 to 15 minutes (as tolerated by blood pressure [BP]) until the desired therapeutic response is achieved, limiting symptoms develop, or a dose of 0.25 mg/kg per minute is reached. For more rapid onset of action, a loading dose of 0.5 mg/kg can be given IV over 2 to 5 minutes followed by the usual maintenance dose.

For patients with left ventricular ejection fraction (LVEF) less than or equal to 0.40 post-MI, carvedilol (starting dose 3.125 to 6.25 mg twice per day [BID], titrated over 4 to 6 weeks to 25 mg BID as tolerated) is reasonable. For hospitalized patients unable to tolerate β-adrenergic blockers, attempts to reinitiate therapy after 1 to 2 weeks of clinical stability are recommended.

Atenolol is not particularly good for treating arrhythmias because the half-life is relatively short. The dose starts at 25 mg twice a day and goes up to 100 mg twice a day. For atenolol to be used for arrhythmias, it should be given BID.

Contraindications (Relative). Systolic BP less than 90 mm Hg; sinus rate less than 50 bpm; initiation during severe, decompensated heart failure (although patients already receiving these drugs may be continued on them); PR interval greater than 0.24 seconds, or higher degrees of AV block or sinus node dysfunction unless rate support is provided by a permanent pacemaker; history of clinically important bronchospasm. Concurrent use with verapamil or diltiazem can result in severe hypotension, heart failure, or cardiac arrest.

Comments. Monitor heart rate, BP, echocardiogram (ECG); evaluate lungs for rales and wheezing. For mild wheezing or COPD, consider using low doses of a β₁-selective drug (e.g., metoprolol). Patients with a contraindication to β-adrenergic blockers in the first 24 hours should be reevaluated for candidacy later in the hospital course.

Chronic Use

Indications. Long-term treatment of SVT, AFL, and AF to control the ventricular response rate, VTs to prevent recurrence, and premature ventricular beats if highly symptomatic; inappropriate sinus tachycardia and palpitations if treatment is deemed necessary. It is for any catecholamine-dependent arrhythmia.

Dose. Metoprolol 50 to 200 mg PO every 12 hours. Acebutolol 200 to 800 mg/day. Carvedilol 3.125 to 25 mg BID. Atenolol 50 to 200 mg PO every 12 hours. Propranolol short-acting 40 to 80 mg four times a day or its long-acting equivalent. Nadolol 10 to 80 mg daily (preferable β-blocker for LQTS), although higher doses to 240 to 320 mg have been used for angina or hypertension. Atenolol is generally not recommended for treatment of arrhythmias, but does have cardioselectivity. Atenolol is contraindicated in the pregnant patient. There has been no evidence of risk in humans using acebutolol and pindolol in pregnancy; the chance of fetal harm is felt to be remote with these agents. The use of other β-adrenergic blockers in pregnancy is likely safe, although risk to the fetus cannot be ruled out.

Calcium Antagonists

This class of drugs (class IV antiarrhythmics) can suppress triggered activity, slow or block AV nodal conduction, and slow sinus rates. These include diltiazem and verapamil.

INDICATIONS. Calcium antagonists are used to treat ventricular ectopy and to control rate during SVTs such as AFL, AF, and reentrant SVT (especially those that use the AV node as part of the circuit). Calcium antagonists should not be used with AF that is associated with ventricular preexcitation because AV nodal blockade can facilitate AV conduction over the accessory pathway. IV verapamil is often used in patients with AV node reentry and orthodromic AV reciprocating tachycardias if the arrhythmia recurs after adenosine or if the tachycardia is adenosine unresponsive. IV diltiazem can also be used to control the ventricular rate in AFL and AF.

DOSE. Verapamil 120 to 480 mg/day PO in single or divided doses, depending on the preparation. Diltiazem: Initial IV bolus of 0.25 mg/kg (approximately 20 mg) over 2 minutes. If response is inadequate, a second bolus of 0.35 mg/kg (approximately 25 mg) can be given 15 minutes later. For continued reduction of ventricular rate (up to 24 hours), an IV infusion of 5 to 15 mg/hour can be started immediately after the bolus and titrated to heart rate. Infusion rates of more than 15 mg/hour are not recommended. IV verapamil: Initial IV bolus of 2.5 to 5.0 mg over 1 to 2 minutes (3 minutes in older patients). The peak effect should be seen in 3 to 5 minutes. If required, a second 5- to 10-mg bolus can be given 15 to 30 minutes later; alternatively, 5-mg IV boluses can be given every 15 minutes to a cumulative dose of 30 mg.

To terminate paroxysmal SVT in patients with adequate BP and preserve left ventricle (LV) function in lieu of adenosine or if adenosine terminates SVT only temporarily: Diltiazem or verapamil IV can be given in doses as described previously.

CONTRAINDICATIONS. Diltiazem and verapamil should be used with extreme caution, if at all, with IV β-adrenergic blockers or in patients with heart failure, significant LV dysfunction, or sick sinus syndrome or greater than first-degree AVB without a functioning pacemaker. Neither drug should be used IV to slow the ventricular response to AF or AFL in Wolff-Parkinson-White (WPW) syndrome, due to an increased risk of one-to-one conduction and subsequent VF, or to treat VT (increased risk of fatal hypotension).

COMMENT. The risk to the fetus from the use of most calcium channel blocking drugs has not been excluded.

Digoxin

Digoxin enhances vagal activation of the heart to specifically slow AV nodal conduction and to have a mild effect on the sinus node function.

INDICATIONS. The main use for digoxin is to control the ventricular response rate to AF. It can also be effective in prevention of AV node–dependent SVTs. Furthermore, it can help to control the ventricular response rate to ATs and AFL.

DOSING. Digoxin is available intravenously and orally. Potassium levels should be in the therapeutic range when using digoxin. The loading dose is 1 mg over 24 hours in divided doses. It is not clear that patients need to be loaded unless they have an uncontrolled ventricular response rate to AF. The maintenance dose is usually between 0.125 and 0.25 mg. In patients with renal insufficiency and in older patients, smaller doses are recommended. For patients with renal failure, the dose may have to be much smaller and given only several times a week. Propafenone, verapamil, and amiodarone will increase digoxin levels. The Digitalis Investigation Group (DIG) trial showed that serum levels less than 0.9 ng/mL were associated with lower mortality than higher levels, and so dosing should aim at such lower levels.

COMMENTS. Used separately, in younger active individuals, digoxin is not particularly effective in controlling the ventricular response rate to AF because it is not a direct-acting AV node-blocking drug, but acts through vagal mechanisms. Its main use is in older patients and in the pediatric age range where it can have a more potent effect. The risk is that the toxic-to-therapeutic ratio is higher than for many modern drugs. Alternatively, it has important synergistic effects with β-adrenergic blockers and calcium channel antagonists. The combination of β-adrenergic blockers and digoxin can be very effective in controlling the ventricular response rate to AF. Digoxin toxicity is often associated with evidence of high-grade AV block in the presence of triggered arrhythmias such as AT (classically with 2:1 AV conduction ratio) or frequent ventricular ectopy. It can cause VT or VF at high levels. Adverse noncardiac effects include anorexia, nausea, vomiting, and change in color perception. Treatment of digoxin toxicity or refractory proarrhythmia may include use of antidigoxin Fab antibody fragments.

Disopyramide

Disopyramide is a class IA antiarrhythmic drug that is similar to procainamide and quinidine but with greater negative inotropic and more anticholinergic effects. It should be used in individuals who are not at risk for urinary retention and should not be used in older men with known prostatic hypertrophy or patients with glaucoma.

INDICATIONS. This drug may be useful in vagally mediated AF. The main use now for disopyramide is AF with or without preexcitation. When used in patients with AF, it should be used with AV nodal blocking drugs, because it is vagolytic and can increase conduction through the AV node. Some early data suggested that it is valuable for neurocardiogenic syncope, but it now appears to be of little use. Disopyramide has been used for its negative inotropic effect in patients with hypertrophic obstructive cardiomyopathy and in neurocardiogenic syncope (with little firm evidence as to effectiveness).

DOSING. The dose is 400 to 600 mg in divided doses. With controlled-release disopyramide formulation, the dose can be given twice daily. Otherwise, it should be given three to four times daily.

COMMENTS. Disopyramide is rarely used due to its adverse effects, including TdP VT (perhaps less likely than quinidine or procainamide), negative inotropic effect, which can trigger CHF, and anticholinergic effects. It is a third-line antiarrhythmic drug but may be useful for vagally mediated AF.

Dofetilide

Dofetilide is a pure class III antiarrhythmic (I_{Kr} blocker).

INDICATIONS. It is used to treat persistent AF. It is also effective for AFL. In some instances, dofetilide will terminate persistent AF and AFL, and in other cases, it will prevent its recurrence. As with amiodarone, dofetilide is useful regardless of ventricular function and does not appear to increase the risk of death when ventricular function is poor or when there has been a recent MI. The drug is perhaps less used because of the complexity of its initiation, which requires hospitalization and a physician who is approved for its use. However, despite the 3-day observation period required to initiate the drug in the hospital, it is one of the most effective antiarrhythmic drugs for AF.

DOSE. Initiate the dose in the hospital in a monitored setting (125 to 500 mcg twice daily). The higher dose is for patients with normal renal function. The initial dose must be adjusted in patients with calculated creatinine clearance (CrCl) of less than 60 mL/minute (250 mcg twice daily if CrCl is 40 to 60 mL/minute or 125 mcg twice daily if CrCl is 20 to 40 mL/minute). Electrocardiographic monitoring must be performed for a minimum of 3 days in the hospital. ECGs must be obtained 2 to 3 hours after giving each of the first five doses of the drug. If the QTc increases more than 15% of baseline or if the QTc is more than 500 ms (550 ms in patients with abnormal ventricular conduction), the dose should be reduced. The patient must be compliant with taking the medications, because missing one or two doses means starting the dosing process over again. Medication must be given by an individual considered qualified to use the drug. The QTc interval should not exceed 500 ms.

CONTRAINDICATIONS. Patients with a long QT interval (QTc >440 ms, or if intraventricular conduction abnormality, >500 ms), severe renal dysfunction (CrCl <20 mL/minute).

COMMENTS. Dofetilide should not be used with verapamil, cimetidine, trimethoprim, and ketoconazole, because these can cause significant increases in dofetilide concentration. Other known renal cation transport system inhibitors, such as prochlorperazine and megestrol, should also not be used with dofetilide. Hydrochlorothiazide has also been shown to increase dofetilide concentrations and should not be used concurrently. Dofetilide is generally well tolerated. It has no negative inotropic effects. It does not facilitate conduction through the AV node. It must be given with adequate maintenance of potassium levels. Adherence to the hospital initiation guidelines appears to reduce the risk of TdP VT.

Dronedarone

Dronedarone is an oral antiarrhythmic drug with an uncertain mechanism of action. It has a formula similar to amiodarone except without the iodine. It appears to be less toxic than amiodarone but it is also less effective as an antiarrhythmic drug.

Dronedarone was given a class I indication to maintain sinus rhythm and to decrease cardiovascular events in patients with paroxysmal AF or after conversion of persistent atrial ablation and to control the ventricular response during AF. It was also given a class III indication; that is, there is no benefit to those patients with NYHA FC IV CHF or those patients who have had recent decompensated heart failure and for those with permanent AF, due to higher mortality with dronedarone observed in these groups in clinical trials.

INDICATIONS. For long-term use, to reduce the risk of hospitalization in patients with AFL or AF and cardiovascular risk factors (age >70 years, hypertension, diabetes, prior stroke, left atrial diameter >50 mm, or LVEF <40%), who are in sinus rhythm or who will be cardioverted. The drug may not only reduce the incidence of AF but also slow the ventricular response rate.

DOSE. Dosage of 400 mg BID with morning and evening meals. Dronedarone should be discontinued if the QTc interval increases to 500 ms or more.

CONTRAINDICATIONS. Dronedarone is contraindicated in patients with New York Heart Association (NYHA) FC IV heart failure or NYHA FC II-III heart failure with recent decompensation requiring hospitalization or referral to a specialized heart failure clinic. Dronedarone is also contraindicated in second-degree or third-degree AVB or sick sinus syndrome unless rate support is provided by a pacemaker, bradycardia less than 50 bpm, QTc greater than or equal to 500 ms, and severe hepatic dysfunction.

COMMENTS. The drug can increase serum creatinine by about 0.1 mg/dL due to an inhibition of the tubular secretion of creatinine, but with no effect on the glomerular filtration rate; it is thus not nephrotoxic and the effect on serum creatinine is reversible after drug discontinuation. The drug can be initiated in the outpatient setting. The risk of TdP VT is low. It does not have pulmonary toxicity. The most common adverse reactions ($\geq$2%) are diarrhea, nausea, abdominal pain, vomiting, and asthenia. Dronedarone may increase mortality in patients with acute CHF and LVEF of less than 35%. It should not be administered together with strong cytochrome P450 3A (CYP3A) inhibitors (e.g., ketoconazole), grapefruit juice, or other QT-prolonging drugs or herbals. Simvastatin exposure is increased by dronedarone, and adjustment of statin dose may be necessary. Discontinuation or halving of the dose of digoxin should be considered and concomitant β-adrenergic blockers and calcium channel blockers used with ECG verification of tolerability. Normal potassium and magnesium levels should be maintained. Rare, but potentially severe, liver injury has been reported. Monitoring of liver enzymes would be prudent, especially during the first 6 months of therapy. If heart failure develops or worsens, suspension or discontinuation of dronedarone should be considered. Higher mortality was reported in one study of patients with severe heart failure requiring recent hospitalization or referral to a specialized heart failure clinic for worsening symptoms. Dronedarone is a teratogen and is contraindicated in pregnancy or nursing mothers. Women of childbearing potential should use appropriate contraception.

Droxidopa

Droxidopa, L-threo-dihydroxyphenylserine, is a norepinephrine precursor, that has been recently approved in the United States as an "orphan" drug for treatment of symptoms in patients who have neurogenic orthostatic hypotension; that is, symptomatic orthostatic hypotension as a result of a neurologic deficiency as can occur in multiple-system atrophy, Parkinson disease, and pure autonomic failure. It has been used in dopamine β-hydroxylase deficiency and nondiabetic autonomic neuropathy. It can treat dizziness, lightheadedness, syncope, and falls related to changes in BP.

INDICATIONS. Droxidopa is indicated for neurogenic orthostatic hypotension. Although potentially an off-label use, some have considered using this drug in patients (younger individuals as well) with postural orthostatic tachycardia syndrome and those with a transient orthostatic drop in BP not associated with extreme elevation in heart rate but also not due to an explainable cause.

DOSE. The initial recommended dose is 100 mg PO TID with titration in increments of 100 mg TID every 24 to 48 hours, not to exceed 600 mg TID based on symptoms.

COMMENTS. Droxidopa has been used and approved for short-term use. There have been some long-term follow-up data but because it is not completely certain that the long-term efficacy is as good as the short-term efficacy, patients should be watched carefully for recurrence of symptoms. Droxidopa may cause hypertension and may exacerbate supine hypertension in patients who have severe orthostatic hypotension but have baseline supine hypertension. Droxidopa has not been tested rigorously in patients with underlying ischemic heart disease or structural heart disease with regard to safety. The drug is not been tested in patients with diabetes. For patients who have supine hypertension but have severe orthostatic hypotension, there are no specific drugs that have been used to treat both the hypertension in the supine position in combination with droxidopa, but if an antihypertensive medication is required, an angiotensin-converting enzyme inhibitor may be the best drug to consider.

Epinephrine

Epinephrine is a catecholamine that activates α- and β-receptors.

INDICATIONS. Asystole; pulseless electrical activity; VF or pulseless VT resistant to electrical defibrillation; severe hypotension; anaphylactic shock; symptomatic bradycardia after atropine.

DOSE. Cardiac arrest: 1 mg (10 cc of 1:10,000 solution) IV bolus or 2 mg (diluted in 10 cc normal saline) if given via endotracheal tube. This may be repeated every 3 to 5 minutes. Higher doses (up to 0.2 mg/kg) are not recommended. Each IV bolus should be followed by a saline flush (20 cc). Profound bradycardia or hypotension: 2 to 10 mcg/minute IV infusion.

COMMENTS. Epinephrine can precipitate myocardial ischemia even at low doses, and it may be proarrhythmic. Epinephrine may be inactivated if mixed in the same solution as bicarbonate. If subcutaneous extravasation occurs, tissue necrosis can develop. Inadvertent overdose can be counteracted by phentolamine. Discontinue if paradoxical worsening of respiratory function occurs in sulfite-allergic patients (epinephrine contains sulfite).

Flecainide

Flecainide is a class IC antiarrhythmic drug.

INDICATION. Most commonly, flecainide is used to treat paroxysmal AF. It is highly effective at suppressing ectopy and an excellent antiarrhythmic drug to use in patients without ischemic heart disease and without structural heart disease. It also has indications for prevention of ventricular ectopy, nonsustained VT, and sustained VT, but only when there is no evidence of structural heart disease.

DOSE. It has been used as a "pill in the pocket," given acutely to terminate AF or BID given chronically to suppress AF. The dosing is 100 to 300 for "pill in the pocket" and 50 to 200 mg BID chronically. Drug levels can be measured and may be useful to determine effects.

COMMENTS. Can be started as an outpatient. Check for QRS widening of more than 20%, because this can be a toxic effect. It should be used with caution if there is evidence of His-Purkinje system disease. It can have noncardiac side effects, such as dizziness, visual disturbances, or headache, but it is generally well tolerated. It can have a negative inotropic effect. It can cause a proarrhythmic effect of sustained monomorphic VT. It can "organize" AF into a slow AFL and allow 1:1 AV conduction. It can increase pacing and defibrillation thresholds, and if initiated in these patients, thresholds should be checked. It should be avoided in patients with CAD or prior MI with LV dysfunction.

Fludrocortisone

Fludrocortisone is a mineralocorticoid that can cause sodium and thus water resorption for patients who have orthostatic hypotension, including neurogenic orthostatic hypotension. It has also been considered useful in some instances of vasovagal syncope and, perhaps, postural orthostatic tachycardia syndrome. The drug has not been rigorously tested for the latter conditions. Nevertheless, because there are few drugs that are effective for these particular conditions, fludrocortisone may be tried when other drugs have not been effective or even as an initial therapy.

INDICATIONS. Orthostatic hypotension not due to fluid depletion (e.g., neurogenic orthostatic hypotension). Fludrocortisone has also been used for postural orthostatic tachycardia syndrome and in patients with recurrent and neurocardiogenic syncope alone and in combination with other medications, such as droxidopa or midodrine.

DOSE. The dose is often initiated 0.1 mg PO per day and has been used in doses up to 0.4 mg per day. If the medication is not effective at these doses, it is not clear that a higher dose would be effective.

COMMENTS. The long-term side effects of fludrocortisone are uncertain. In diabetics, fludrocortisone may increase blood sugar levels. For the most part, the side effects are generally minor, although fluid retention and weight gain are possible. Difficulty sleeping, dizziness or lightheadedness, increased appetite, increased sweating, and nervousness may occur. Hypokalemia is a possibility. Methotrexate may increase the effectiveness of fludrocortisone, whereas phenytoin, barbiturates, estrogens, and rifampin can decrease fludrocortisone's effectiveness. Warfarin dosing may need to be adjusted. Occasionally, low blood sugar may occur.

Ibutilide

Ibutilide is an IV class III antiarrhythmic drug.

INDICATIONS. Ibutilide is used to terminate AF and AFL. It is modestly effective to terminate AF, especially if the episode of AF is relatively short lived. It is effective to treat AFL. Although there is no efficacy advantage over DC cardioversion and there is a potential risk of TdP VT that can be as high as 8% depending on the population to which it is given, ibutilide can be used in patients who require urgent cardioversion who have recently eaten, in contrast to electrical cardioversion. It is also useful in those individuals who prefer not to have an external shock. It can be used in patients with left ventricular dysfunction, although extremely low LVEF (<20%) may increase the risk of proarrhythmia.

DOSE. The dose of ibutilide is 1 mg IV given over 10 minutes. It is given in 0.1-mg aliquots or 1 cc every minute over a period of 10 minutes, observing the QT interval. If the QT interval increases to greater than 500 ms, the drug needs to be stopped. When the drug is given, there should be a defibrillator at the bedside. After the drug is given over a 10-minute period, there is a 20-minute waiting period, at which time conversion of the AFL or AF is assessed. If conversion has not occurred, the drug dosing can be repeated, but no more than 2 mg total should be given. Some advocate the use of IV magnesium (1 to 3 g) as a prophylaxis against TdP VT before giving ibutilide, but there is some controversy as to whether it is protective; it may also have an effect that counteracts the antiarrhythmic effect of the drug. Nevertheless, IV magnesium sulfate administration makes sense prior to initiation of ibutilide.

COMMENTS. Ibutilide needs to be used with caution in patients with acute heart failure or ongoing myocardial ischemia. It should not be used in patients with a long QT interval. After the dose, the patient needs to be observed for approximately 4 hours before discharge from the hospital because of the risk of TdP VT, although the risk is greatest immediately after giving the drug. The drug has limited use for treatment of AFL and AF. It may have use also for early or immediate return of AF after DC cardioversion.

Ivabradine

Ivabradine blocks the hyperpolarization-activated cyclic nucleotide-gated channel current (I_f) in the sinus node, which can slow the sinus rate. It shows promise in several small studies for treatment of inappropriate sinus tachycardia (IST), although its approved indication is for heart failure.

INDICATIONS AND DOSAGE. Reduction of the risk of hospitalization for worsening heart failure in patients with stable symptomatic chronic heart failure, LVEF of 35% or less with resting heart rate of 70 bpm or greater on maximally tolerated doses of β-adrenergic blockers or who have a contraindication to β-adrenergic blockers. It has been used off-label for IST. Initial dose is 2.5 to 5 mg twice daily, titrating at 2- to 4-week intervals in increments of 2.5 mg for heart rate response. The maximum dose is 7.5 mg twice daily. Heart rate should be monitored, including with dose adjustments.

COMMENTS. Ivabradine can cause bradycardia, GI side effects, headache, or dizziness. It can also cause phosphenes, which are luminous visual phenomena thought to be mediated through effects on retinal photoreceptors. Ivabradine may cause bradycardia, including conduction disturbances. Contraindications include a resting heart rate less than 60 bpm prior to treatment, severe hepatic impairment, sinus node dysfunction, sinoatrial block, second- or third-degree AV block unless a pacemaker is present, acute decompensated heart failure, and hypotension. CYP3A4 inhibitors increase and inducers decrease ivabradine concentrations. Concomitant use with strong CYP3A4 inhibitors (e.g., azole antifungals, macrolide antibiotics, HIV protease inhibitors, and nefazodone) are contraindicated. Concomitant use with moderate CYP3A4 inhibitors (e.g., diltiazem, verapamil, grapefruit juice) should be avoided. Females should use effective contraception due to fetal toxicity.

Lidocaine

Lidocaine is a class IB IV antiarrhythmic drug that slows phase 0 of the action potential in the ventricles but does not lengthen refractoriness. More potent effects exist in ischemic myocardium, although it has not been shown to improve mortality after MI. The drug is metabolized by the liver.

INDICATIONS AND DOSE. Used to treat and suppress VF or pulseless VT resistant to defibrillation and epinephrine, hemodynamically stable VT, and hemodynamically unstable PVCs (e.g., nonperfusing PVCs occurring frequently or in bigeminy). Normal LV function and no hepatic impairment: loading dose of 75 to 100 mg IV (1 to 1.5 mg/kg) followed by 50 mg IV

(0.5 to 0.75 mg/kg) in 5 to 10 minutes (up to a total dose of 3 mg/kg). For VF or pulseless VT (after defibrillation), may give repeat 0.5- to 0.75-mg doses every 5 to 10 minutes after the initial dose for a maximum of 3 doses. Give a maintenance infusion of 1 to 4 mg/minute. Dosage should be reduced in older patients, CHF, shock, or hepatic disease, including congestive hepatopathy. For moderate decrease in LV function, give a loading dose of 75 mg IV followed by one 50-mg IV after 5 minutes (total dose 125 mg); maintenance infusion of 1 mg/minute.

Severe decrease in LV function or significant hepatic impairment: one loading dose of 50 to 75 mg IV; maintenance infusion of 0.5 mg/minute. A single IV bolus of 1.5 mg/kg is acceptable for cardiac arrest. Tracheal administration is 2 to 4 mg/kg.

COMMENTS. Monitor for lidocaine toxicity: confusion, acute psychosis, drowsiness, respiratory depression, perioral numbness, and seizures. It may cause bradycardia due to sinus arrest or AV block. Do not give for ventricular escape beats or escape rhythms (increased risk of asystole). Use in pregnancy appears to be safe. Lidocaine levels should be monitored 4 to 6 hours after the boluses and at least daily while on the drug.

Magnesium Sulfate

Magnesium sulfate may block triggered activity that can lead to TdP VT.

INDICATIONS AND DOSE. Cardiac arrest due to TdP VT: 2 to 5 g IV push over 1 to 2 minutes in 10 cc D_5W. TdP VT without cardiac arrest: 1 to 2 g in 50 to 100 cc D_5W IV over 5 to 60 minutes. Consider an additional 2 g IV over the next several hours. Regimens vary.

Follow for reduction in QT interval and reduction in amplitude of the U wave as part of the therapeutic effect. It can be given without measuring magnesium levels, because they do not reflect total body magnesium stores.

COMMENTS. Magnesium is a coronary vasodilator, has antiplatelet and antiarrhythmic effects, and can prevent calcium overload of reperfused myocytes. Magnesium may be of benefit for refractory VT after lidocaine and amiodarone and for life-threatening ventricular arrhythmias caused by digitalis toxicity. It is not routinely recommended for acute MI unless magnesium deficiency is documented.

Mexiletine

Mexiletine is an oral class IB antiarrhythmic drug.

INDICATION. Mexiletine can suppress VT and ventricular ectopy. Mexiletine is indicated for symptomatic ventricular arrhythmias, although success in VT is relatively low. Generally, it is considered for use if a patient has multiple ICD shocks and appears to respond to lidocaine. It may be particularly useful in patients with LQT3 syndrome.

Dose. 150 to 300 mg three times a day. Some side effects (e.g., gastrointestinal [GI]) may be minimized if given with meals. In the absence of an ICD, initiation in the hospital is recommended.

Comments. Does not appear to increase the risk of TdP VT, but there are other potential side effects, including ataxia, dizziness, tremor, slurred speech, abdominal discomfort, anorexia, nausea, vomiting, and diarrhea. There is a risk of proarrhythmia as well as CHF, hypotension, and bradycardia. It does not cause TdP VT or affect atrial arrhythmias. Mexiletine has been used in the past in combination with quinidine, and the combination was considered relatively potent; however, there are possible proarrhythmia and side effects associated with this combination. It is now used in combination with amiodarone if amiodarone alone is ineffective in suppressing recurrent VT in patients who have ICDs. It has little effect on the sinus node, AV node, or His-Purkinje system. It does not affect atrial refractoriness. It can increase defibrillation thresholds but does not markedly slow VTs.

Midodrine

Midodrine is prodrug of desglymidodrine that is an α_1 adrenergic receptor stimulant (agonist) that has been used to treat hypotension, and in particular, orthostatic hypotension. Its effect is on venous and arteriolar vascular tone. It does not cross the blood-brain barrier well. Standing BP is elevated approximately 15 to 30 mmHg 1 hour after a 10-mg dose.

Indications. While midodrine is indicated to treat symptomatic orthostatic hypotension, the drug is also been used to treat patients who have neurocardiogenic syncope and postural orthostatic tachycardia syndrome.

Dose. The usual dose of midodrine is 2.5 mg three times a day with increments to 10 mg PO four times per day.

Comments. Midodrine can cause a sensation of "gooseflesh" and can cause hypertension. It would not make sense to use midodrine with an antihypertensive medication. The drug has a relatively short half-life of about 3 to 4 hours. Midodrine can potentially cause severe supine hypertension. It can potentially cause urinary retention by affecting the α-adrenergic receptors of the bladder neck. Midodrine should be used with caution in diabetic patients and in those people taking fludrocortisone, because it is known to increase intraocular pressure and potentially cause glaucoma. When used concomitantly with digoxin, it may precipitate bradycardia or AV block. α-Adrenergic blocking drugs, such as terazosin, can antagonize the effects of midodrine.

Procainamide

Procainamide is a class IA antiarrhythmic drug with active metabolites, including N-acetyl-procainamide, which is a class III antiarrhythmic drug.

The drug lengthens refractoriness, lengthens the QT interval, and slows atrial and ventricular conduction. The drug is metabolized in the liver and excreted by the kidneys.

INDICATIONS AND DOSE. For refractory VF or VT, especially if ischemic, 100-mg IV bolus doses repeated every 5 minutes. A loading dose of 10 to 15 mg/kg can be given up to 50 mg/minute IV with reduction of the rate of infusion if hypotension results. Procainamide may also be effective for treatment of AFL and AF acutely and chronically. For other indications (stable wide QRS complex tachycardia, reentrant SVT resistant to adenosine and vagal maneuvers, and rate control of AF in the WPW syndrome due to block in the accessory pathway), treatment of AF: 20 to 50 mg/minute IV infusion until the arrhythmia is suppressed, hypotension develops, QRS widens by 50%, or a total dose of 15 mg/kg is given, followed by an IV maintenance infusion of 1 to 4 mg/minute. Oral dosing is 500 to 1000 mg four times daily (but it is not readily available in this form anymore).

CONTRAINDICATIONS. Avoid in patients with a prolonged QT interval or TdP VT. Use with caution in conjunction with other drugs that prolong the QT interval. Do not use in patients with CrCl of less than 20 mL/minute.

COMMENTS. Can induce TdP VT, especially in patients with renal insufficiency, hypokalemia, or hypomagnesemia. For patients with heart failure or renal insufficiency, the loading dose should be reduced to 10 to 12 mg/kg, and the maintenance dose reduced to 1 to 2 mg/minute. BP and ECG should be monitored continuously during IV administration, because sharp drops in BP can occur with rapid infusion, especially in patients with LV dysfunction. Follow blood levels and renal function of procainamide and N-acetylprocainamide in renal failure and during prolonged IV use. Procainamide has been associated with a lupus-like syndrome and has several other important, although rare, side effects, including CNS effects and agranulocytosis. Procainamide can cause SB or sinus arrest in patients with sick sinus syndrome. Procainamide can cause AV block in patients with conduction system disease, including intraventricular conduction delays. Procainamide should probably not be used in pregnancy.

Its use has been superseded in most cases by IV amiodarone. The long-acting oral drug is no longer on the market.

Propafenone

Propafenone is a class IC antiarrhythmic drug that possesses some mild β-blocking properties.

INDICATION. It is mainly used to suppress or terminate paroxysmal AF. Although it may suppress ventricular ectopy, it is potentially proarrhythmic and should not be used when there is ventricular dysfunction or CAD.

It may be used to suppress some VTs, such as nonsustained idiopathic VT. It is not particularly useful for AFL, because it slows the rate of AFL and allows for 1:1 AV conduction.

Dose. The dosage is 150 to 300 mg three times a day, although there is a long-acting form that allows twice-a-day dosing.

Comment. Propafenone has been used as the "pill in the pocket" technique to suppress or terminate AF after its onset. The dose is 150 to 450 mg at one time. The drug is similar to flecainide, although the metabolism is more complex. Seven percent are slow metabolizers and exhibit significant β-blocking activity. Proarrhythmia is about the same as it is for flecainide. Check for QRS widening of more than 20%, because this can be a toxic effect. The drug can be started as an outpatient. It should be used with caution if there is evidence for His-Purkinje system disease. It can have some noncardiac side effects, such as metallic taste, neutropenia, and other vague, nonspecific symptoms such as nausea, vomiting, constipation, and dizziness. It is generally well tolerated. It can have a negative inotropic effect. It can cause a proarrhythmic effect of sustained monomorphic VT as well as organization of AF to slow AFL with 1:1 AV conduction. It can increase pacing thresholds, although generally not to a clinically relevant degree.

Pyridostigmine

Pyridostigmine is an acetylcholinesterase inhibitor that can treat myasthenia gravis by increasing acetylcholine at the postsynaptic motor endplate. It can also affect ganglionic neurotransmission and enhance sympathetic activation in the standing position. It may thus improve orthostatic hypotension but not affect supine hypertension to the same extent as midodrine or droxidopa. It has been used off label for the treatment of postural orthostatic tachycardia syndrome. The drug has also been effective in combination with other therapies for the same problem.

Indications. Although pyridostigmine may be used for myasthenia gravis, it may improve orthostatic hypotension. It has been used in combination with midodrine and fludrocortisone to treat patients with orthostatic hypotension and postural orthostatic tachycardia syndrome. These indications are off label.

Dose. For orthostatic hypotension and postural orthostatic tachycardia syndrome, low-dose therapy is generally recommended at a dose of 60 mg PO twice a day.

Comments. Common side effects include GI side effects, such as diarrhea and abdominal cramping. The effects of pyridostigmine may be reduced when using quinidine.

Quinidine

Quinidine is a class IA antiarrhythmic drug with electrophysiological effects similar to procainamide. Quinidine is more vagolytic than procainamide.

INDICATIONS. Quinidine is an old, yet versatile, multipurpose antiarrhythmic drug with class IA antiarrhythmic properties. It can suppress atrial and ventricular ectopy, nonsustained AT and VT, AF and AFL, sustained VT, and accessory pathway conduction in the WPW syndrome. It is less effective than more modern antiarrhythmic drugs, and there are substantial side effects. The drug is rarely used now due to the increased risk of toxicity, GI side effects, and proarrhythmia (TdP VT); thus, it is considered a third-line antiarrhythmic drug.

Potential side effects of quinidine include thrombocytopenia, diarrhea, anticholinergic effects, and most importantly, TdP VT.

DOSE. The oral dosing of quinidine sulfate is 200 to 400 mg four times a day but it is rarely used anymore. There are long-acting (slow absorbing) preparations that can be given every 8 hours or even every 12 hours. IV quinidine can produce marked hypotension and is rarely used anymore. The dose is up to 1 g IV.

COMMENTS. Quinidine increases digoxin levels. Hypotension during IV use is due to an α-adrenergic blocking effect. Quinidine can also cause cinchonism, psychosis, depression, and agranulocytosis. Quinidine lengthens the QT interval. Prolongation of the QT interval on quinidine is associated with TdP VT. Quinidine can increase the ventricular response rate to AF. It should be started in the hospital. Because quinidine can block Ito current, it may have some use in the Brugada syndrome and in individuals with idiopathic VF.

Sotalol

Sotalol is a class III and class II antiarrhythmic drug. There are two stereoisomers to make the racemic mixture of D, L-sotalol. The L stereoisomer is a β-adrenergic blocker that is not selective and water soluble, and the D stereoisomer has class III properties.

INDICATIONS. To treat persistent and paroxysmal AF with or without the presence of structural heart disease. Sotalol is a versatile antiarrhythmic drug and can also be used to suppress nonsustained VT in patients with idiopathic VT; sustained VT in patients with structural heart disease, including arrhythmogenic right ventricular cardiomyopathy; VT; and VF in patients in whom ICDs are implanted but who have relatively intact ventricular function.

DOSE. Although the starting dose is 80 mg BID, at this low dose, the drug mainly has a β-blocking effect. The recommended starting dose is

120 mg twice a day. For most, if not all, patients, in the absence of an ICD, especially for patients with structural heart disease, for older women, for patients with mild renal insufficiency, and for patients in AF, it is advisable to start sotalol in the hospital and observe until a steady state is achieved. The QTc interval should be less than 500 ms.

COMMENTS. To achieve the class III antiarrhythmic effect, the dose must be at least 120 mg BID for patients with normal renal function. Caution is advised for mild renal insufficiency, and use of the drug should be avoided in patients with moderate renal insufficiency. Care must be taken for patients with poor ventricular function. As a rule, sotalol should be given to patients with an LVEF of 30% or more and/or NYHA FC I and II. Sotalol should be avoided in patients with acute hemodynamic decompensation or impaired baseline hemodynamic state. Sotalol can have a potent effect on the sinus node and can exacerbate sinus node dysfunction. It can encourage serious bradycardia in select individuals. There are no active metabolites or serious interactions with other drugs. Sotalol does not increase the pacing threshold, and it may decrease the defibrillation threshold. When using sotalol, TdP VT risk is greatest at doses of greater than 320 mg BID.

Vernakalant

Vernakalant is a novel I_{KUR} blocker.

INDICATIONS. Vernakalant is a new IV and oral antiarrhythmic drug that is an I_{KUR} blocker. It is used to terminate AF acutely and perhaps prevent its return. The advantage of this drug given intravenously is that it may have a lower risk of causing TdP VT than ibutilide or procainamide. Ultimately, after IV use of the drug to terminate AF, it may be continued orally, but the drug has not yet been approved for use.

DOSE. Oral doses tested include 150-, 300-, or 500-mg doses twice a day. The IV dose is 2 to 5 mg/kg.

CONTRAINDICATIONS. These are uncertain.

COMMENTS. Vernakalant may be more effective and safe than ibutilide to terminate AF, but this is not yet clear. It is also not yet clear that TdP VT will not occur with this drug.

Further Comments About Antiarrhythmic Drugs

The concept of proarrhythmia has developed over the years, because it has been shown that antiarrhythmic drugs can not only suppress arrhythmias, but under certain conditions, can actually increase the risk of specific arrhythmias and may even increase the risk of sudden cardiac death. There are various forms of proarrhythmic reactions, and these can include an increased number of premature atrial or ventricular depolarizations, an increase in the ventricular response rate in AF or AFL, a slowing in tachycardia rate that can make it undetectable as an arrhythmia to be terminated by an implanted cardioverter defibrillator, an increased risk of a monomorphic VT, conversion of a nonsustained tachycardia into a sustained tachycardia, and increased risk of polymorphic VT or TdP VT. In some instances, a drug may have antiarrhythmic and proarrhythmic effects. Patients who are acutely ill, have acute exacerbations of heart failure, have recent ischemia or MI, or are older with renal and liver dysfunction are at greatest risk for developing proarrhythmic effects.

Several drugs have recently been removed from the U.S. market. These include tocainide, bretylium, some forms of long-acting procainamide, and moricizine.

ORAL ANTICOAGULANTS

For patients with AF/AFL who are at risk for thromboembolic complications, including stroke, chronic anticoagulation is often recommended (see Chapter 5).

Warfarin

Warfarin is a vitamin K antagonist and inhibits synthesis of vitamin K–dependent clotting factors (II, VII, IX, X) and proteins C and S.

Indications

Prophylaxis and treatment of thromboembolic disorders and complications (e.g., from AF, valve replacement, LV thrombus, prolonged immobilization, low cardiac output).

Dosage

Initial dose of 2 to 10 mg PO daily for 2 to 4 days, then titrated to maintain the prothrombin time/international normalized ratio (PT/INR) target (for AF 2.0 to 3.0). Dosage should be individualized.

PRIOR TO INVASIVE OR SURGICAL PROCEDURES REQUIRING HOLDING OF ANTICOAGULANTS. Warfarin is typically held 4 to 5 days before the procedure with need for bridging dependent upon the risk of thromboembolism versus bleeding. Warfarin can often be started 12 to 24 hours, again depending upon these risks.

Contraindications

Active bleeding; when risk of bleeding exceeds the benefit of anticoagulation; pregnancy; surgery of the CNS or eye; malignant hypertension; lack of patient cooperation. Use with caution in renal or hepatic dysfunction.

Reversal

Warfarin's anticoagulant effects can be reversed by vitamin K, fresh whole blood, fresh frozen plasma (200 to 2000 mL), or prothrombin complex concentrates (PCC).

Comments

Warfarin has no direct effect on existing thrombus but can prevent propagation and embolism of clot. Numerous factors including medications and vitamin K–containing foods, especially green leafy vegetables, can influence the response to therapy. Studies have shown that systematic follow-up of patients through anticoagulation clinics results in better compliance and control. Pharmacogenomics can also play a role in dose prediction and adjustment. Specific genetic variations in CYP2C9 and VKORC1 have been associated with decreased dose requirement and increased bleeding risk. Warfarin remains the anticoagulant of choice for patients with a mechanical valve prosthesis or end-stage kidney disease (CrCl <15 mL/minute). Advantages include proven efficacy and the ability to check the level of anticoagulation by measurement of PT/INRs and the availability of reversal agents (vitamin K, fresh frozen plasma). Disadvantages include variable dosing, need for PT/INR monitoring, delayed onset and offset of effect, and interaction with common vitamin K–containing foods.

NON-VITAMIN K ORAL ANTICOAGULANTS

Because of the limitations of vitamin K antagonists, such as warfarin, novel oral anticoagulants that act via direct inhibition of thrombin or inhibition of factor Xa have been developed. The four agents currently approved in the United States have each been directly compared to adjusted-dose warfarin in randomized controlled trials (Table 12.1). *Advantages* include removal of the need for frequent PT/INR monitoring and avoidance of vitamin K–containing foods. All have shown comparable or lower risk of stroke or systemic embolism or death. Moreover, all four have shown lower rates of intracranial hemorrhage compared to warfarin. *Disadvantages* include lack of a readily available reversing agent or antidote, although one specific antidote for dabigatran has been approved; several nonspecific hemostatic agents are being studied, including recombinant factor VIIa and prothrombin complex concentrates; and specific antidotes for factor Xa inhibitors are also under study, including andexanet alfa. Dabigatran can also be removed at least partially with hemodialysis. There has also been concern about possible increased risk of thromboembolism when these agents are held, based on data during transitions back to warfarin from rivaroxaban and apixaban, although there was no increase with a transition protocol used for edoxaban. A further disadvantage to edoxaban is reduced efficacy with CrCl greater than 95 mL/minute with a higher rate of ischemic stroke in patients with CrCl greater than 95 mL/minute treated with the lower dose of 60 mg daily compared to warfarin. This is believed to be related to lower plasma edoxaban levels in these groups. Reversal, monitoring, and perioperative management are summarized in Table 12.2. Drug interactions with non-vitamin K oral anticoagulants (NOACs) are reviewed in Table 12.3.

TABLE 12.1

COMPARISON OF NOVEL ORAL ANTICOAGULANTS

	Dabigatran	Rivaroxaban	Apixaban	Edoxaban
Mechanism	Direct thrombin inhibitor	Factor Xa inhibitor	Factor Xa inhibitor	Factor Xa inhibitor
Metabolism	Renal (~80%)[†]	Hepatic (~60%)[*] Renal (~30%)[†]	Hepatic (~25%)[*] Biliary & renal (~75%)[†]	Renal (~50%)
Plasma $t_{1/2}$	12-17 h	5-9 h (11-13 h in the elderly)	9-14 h	10-14 h
Dosage for AF	150 mg BID (CrCl >30 mL/min) 75 mg BID (CrCl 15-30 mL/min) Not recommended for CrCl <15 mL/min or on dialysis	20 mg daily with evening meal (CrCl >50 mL/min) 15 mg daily with evening meal (CrCl 15-50 mL/min) Not recommended for CrCl <15 mL/min or on dialysis in patients with AF and <30 mL/min in patients with DVT or PE	5 mg BID If 2 of 3 factors (Cr 1.5, age 80, weight <60 kg), then 2.5 mg BID	60 mg daily (CrCl 50-95 mL/min) 30 mg daily (CrCl 15-50 mL/min, weight ≤60 kg Not recommended for CrCl >95 mL/min
Pivotal trial	*RE-LY*	*ROCKET-AF*	*ARISTOTLE*	*ENGAGE AF-TIMI 48*
Dose in trial	150, 110 mg BID PO (blinded dabigatran dose vs. open label adjusted dose warfarin)	20 mg QDay PO; 15 mg if CKD (double blinded)	5 mg BID PO; 2.5 mg BID if 2 of 3 factors (Cr 1.5, weight <60 kg) (double blinded)	60, 30 mg QDay PO; half dose if CrCl 30-50 mL/min, weight ≤60 kg or concomitant verapamil, quinidine or dronedarone (p-GP inhibitors) (double blinded)
CHADS$_2$, mean	2.1	3.5	2.1	2.8
TTR	64%	55%	62%	65%

Stroke, systemic embolism, RR (95% Cl)	150 mg: 0.65 (0.52-0.81) p=0.001 p(non-inf) <0.001 p(sup) <0.001	0.88 (0.74-1.03) p(non-inf) <0.001 p(sup) =0.12	0.79 (0.66-0.95) p(non-inf) <0.001 p(sup) =0.01	High dose: 0.79 (97.5% CI 0.63-0.99) p(non-inf) <0.001 p(sup) =0.02 ITT 0.87 (0.73-1.04) p(sup) =0.08 Low dose: 1.07 (97.5%CI 0.87-1.31) p(noninf) =0.005 p(sup) =0.44 ITT 1.13 (0.96-1.34) p(sup) =0.10
Death, RR	150 mg: 0.88 p=0.051 110 mg: 0.91 p=0.13	0.85 p=0.07	0.89 p=0.047	High dose: 0.92 (0.83-1.01) p=0.08 Low dose: 0.87 (0.79-0.96) p=0.006
Adverse Effects	Dyspepsia; GI bleeding; MI risk? 150 mg: RR 1.38 p=0.048	GI bleeding; possible increase in thromboembolism when held		Higher risk of ischemic stroke with low dose (HR 1.41 p <0.001)
Advantages	<ul><li>60% removable by dialysis</li><li>Not metabolized by the cytochrome P450 system</li><li><u>Compared to warfarin:</u></li><li>↓Stroke and systemic embolism (150 mg dose)</li><li>↓ Ischemic stroke</li><li>Trend toward ↓ mortality</li><li>↓ Intracranial bleeding</li><li>↓ Major or minor bleeding</li></ul>	<ul><li>Once daily dosing</li><li><u>Compared to warfarin:</u></li><li>Trend toward ↓mortality</li><li>↓ Intracranial bleeding</li><li>↓ Fatal bleeding</li></ul>	<ul><li><u>Compared to warfarin:</u></li><li>↓Stroke and systemic embolism</li><li>↓ Mortality</li><li>↓ Major bleeding</li><li>↓ Major and non-major clinically significant bleeding</li><li>↓ Intracranial bleeding</li></ul>	<ul><li>Once daily dosing</li><li><u>Compared to warfarin:</u></li><li>↓Stroke and systemic embolism (high dose)</li><li>↓ CV deaths both doses; ↓ overall deaths with low dose, trend toward ↓ deaths with high dose</li><li>↓ Risk of major bleeding (except higher GI bleeding with high dose)</li><li>↓ Intracranial bleeding</li></ul>

Continued on following page

TABLE 12.1

COMPARISON OF NOVEL ORAL ANTICOAGULANTS (Continued)

	Dabigatran	Rivaroxaban	Apixaban	Edoxaban
Disadvantages	• Dyspepsia • ↑ GI bleeding with 150 mg dose • Possible MI risk • Twice daily dosing • No readily available reversing agent, but 60% removed by dialysis	• Possible ↑ risk of thromboembolism when held • No readily available reversing agent; possible use of prothrombin complex concentrate	• Possible ↑ risk of thromboembolism when held • Twice daily dosing • No readily available reversing agent; possible use of prothrombin complex concentrate, activated prothrombin complex	• Possible ↑ risk of thromboembolism when held (transition protocol to warfarin without ↑ risk) • ↓ Efficacy with CrCl >95 mL/min • Low dose with ↑ risk of ischemic stroke • No readily available reversing agent; possible use of prothrombin complex concentrate

AF, Atrial fibrillation; *BID*, twice per day; *CI*, confidence interval; *CKD*, chronic kidney disease; *CrCl*, creatinine clearance; *CV*, cardiovascular; *DVT*, deep venous thrombosis; *GI*, gastrointestinal; *HR*, hazard ratio; *MI*, myocardial infarction; *non-inf*, non-inferiority; *PE*, pulmonary embolism; *PO*, by mouth; *RR*, relative risk, *sup*, superiority; *TTR*, % time in therapeutic range (international normalized ratio [INR] ≥2).

*Drug metabolized to inactive moiety.

†Active drug excreted.

TABLE 12.2

PERIOPERATIVE MANAGEMENT, REVERSAL, AND MONITORING OF ANTICOAGULANTS

	Warfarin	Dabigatran	Rivaroxaban	Apixaban	Edoxaban
Perioperative management for procedures requiring holding of anticoagulants	• Hold at least 4-5 days before • If urgent, consider reversal with low-dose IV or with oral vitamin K • Bridging dependent on risk of TE vs. bleeding • Resume 12-24 h after procedure, dependent on risks	• CrCl ≥50 mL/min: hold 1-2 days • CrCl <50 mL/min: hold 3-5 days • Consider >5 days for major surgeries or spinal/epidural procedures	• Hold at least 24 h • Some recommend: • CrCl ≥ 50 mL/min: 3 days • CrCl <50 mL/min: 5 days	• Low bleeding risk procedures: hold at least 24 h • Moderate-high bleeding risk procedures: hold at least 48 h	• Hold at least 24 h
Reversing agents	• Vitamin K • FFP • PCC	• Specific antidote: idarucizumab • 60% dialyzable • Consider PCC, recombinant factor VIIa • Consider activated charcoal if recent ingestion	• No specific antidote • Consider PCC, activated PCC, recombinant factor VII • Consider activated charcoal if recent ingestion	• No specific antidote • Consider PCC, recombinant factor VIIa • Consider activated charcoal if recent ingestion	• No specific antidote • Consider PCC, recombinant factor VIIa • Consider activated charcoal if recent ingestion
Lab monitoring	PT/INR	• Routine not required • To detect presence: aPTT, ECT (if available), TT • Renal function	• Routine not required • To detect presence: PT • Renal function	• Routine not required • To detect presence: PT, INR, aPTT • Renal function	• Routine not required • Renal function

aPTT, Activated partial thromboplastin time; *CrCl,* creatinine clearance; *ECT,* ecarin clotting time; *FFP,* fresh frozen plasma; *INR,* international normalized ratio; *PCC,* prothrombin complex concentrate; *PT,* prothrombin time; *TE,* thromboembolic; *TT,* thrombin time.

TABLE 12.3

DRUG INTERACTIONS WITH NOVEL ORAL ANTICOAGULANTS

A. DRUG INTERACTIONS WITH DABIGATRAN ETEXILATE

Mechanism of Interaction	Specific Agents	Effect	Recommendation
P-gp inducers	Rifampin	↓ Dabigatran	Avoid concomitant use
P-gp inhibitors & CrCl 30-50 mL/min	Ketoconazole, dronedarone	↑ Dabigatran	Consider reducing the dose to 75 mg twice daily or changing to an alternative anticoagulant
P-gp inhibitors & CrCl 15-30 mL/min	Ketoconazole, dronedarone, Amiodarone, verapamil, diltiazem, clarithromycin	↑ Dabigatran	Avoid concomitant use

B. DRUG INTERACTIONS WITH RIVAROXABAN

Mechanism of Interaction	Specific Agents	Effect	Recommendation
Strong dual CYP3A4 & P-gp inducers	Rifampin, carbamazepine, phenytoin, St. John's wort	↓ Rivaroxaban	Avoid concomitant use
Strong dual CYP3A4 & P-gp inhibitors	Ketoconazole, itraconazole, HIV protease inhibitors, conivaptan	↑ Rivaroxaban	Avoid concomitant use
Weak or moderate dual CYP3A4 & P-gp inhibitors & CrCl 15-50 mL/min	Amiodarone, verapamil, diltiazem, erythromycin, chloramphenicol, cimetidine	↑ Rivaroxaban	Consider alternative anticoagulant

C. DRUG INTERACTIONS WITH APIXABAN

Mechanism of Interaction	Specific Agents	Effect	Recommendation
Strong dual cccYP3A4 & P-gp inducers	Rifampin, carbemazepine, phenytoin, St. John's wort	↓ Apixaban	Avoid concomitant use
Strong dual CYP3A4 & P-gp inhibitors	Ketoconazole, itraconazole, HIV protease inhibitors, clarithromycin, ritonavir	↑ Apixaban	If on >2.5 mg BID (e.g., on 5 mg BID), reduce dose by half (e.g., to 2.5 mg) or if already on 2.5 mg BID, avoid or consider alternative anticoagulant

D. DRUG INTERACTIONS WITH EDOXABAN

Mechanism of Interaction	Specific Agents	Effect	Recommendation
P-gp inducers	Rifampin	↓ Edoxaban	Avoid concomitant use; consider alternative anticoagulant
P-gp inhibitors	Verapamil, quinidine, dronedarone	↑ Edoxaban	In ENGAGE AF-TIMI 48, dose reduction resulted in lower blood levels than patients on full dose; dose reduction is not recommended for AF. However, for DVT/PE, reduce dosage to 30 mg daily
	Ketoconazole, itraconazole, HIV protease inhibitors, clarithromycin		

AF, Atrial fibrillation; *BID,* twice per day; *CrCl,* creatinine clearance, *CYP3A4,* cytochrome P450 3A4; *DVT,* deep venous thrombosis; *HIV,* human immunodeficiency virus; *NOAC,* non-vitamin K oral anticoagulants; *PE,* pulmonary embolism; *P-gp,* permeability glycoprotein-1, P-glycoprotein;

Modified with permission from Tanaka-Esposito C and Chung MK. Selection of antithrombotic therapy for risk management of thromboembolism in patients with atrial fibrillation. Cleve Clin J Med 2015; 82: 49-63.

Dabigatran

Dabigatran etexilate mesylate is a competitive, direct thrombin inhibitor. Thrombin enables conversion of fibrinogen into fibrin and activation of factors V, VIII, XI, and XIII; inhibition prevents development of a thrombus. Both free and clot-bound thrombin and thrombin-induced platelet aggregation are inhibited.

Indications

For reduction of the risk of stroke and systemic embolism in patients with nonvalvular AF. For treatment of deep venous thrombosis (DVT) and pulmonary embolism (PE) after 5 to 10 days of parenteral anticoagulation, or to reduce the risk of recurrence in previously treated patients with DVT or PE. In Canada, approved for postoperative thromboprophylaxis after total hip or knee replacement.

Dosage

For AF patients with CrCl greater than 30 mL/minute, the recommended dose is 150 mg PO BID. For patients with CrCl 15 to 30 mL/minute, the recommended dose is 75 mg BID. If available and approved, 110 mg BID may be considered for patients at high risk for bleeding and CrCl greater than 30 mL. Maximal plasma concentrations are achieved 1 to 3 hours after administration. Dabigatran may be taken with or without food. Dabigatran is not recommended for patients with CrCl less than 15 mL/minute or on dialysis.

CONVERTING FROM WARFARIN OR PARENTERAL ANTICOAGULANTS. Discontinue warfarin and start dabigatran when INR is less than 2.0. For parenteral anticoagulants, start dabigatran 0 to 2 hours before the next dose of parenteral drug or at the time of discontinuation of a continuous IV parenteral drug.

CONVERTING TO WARFARIN OR PARENTERAL ANTICOAGULANTS. Start warfarin 3 days (CrCl ≥ 50 mL/minute), 2 days (CrCl 31 to 50 mL/minute), or 1 day (CrCl 15 to 30 mL/minute) before stopping dabigatran. The INR may or may not be elevated on dabigatran, but when converting from dabigatran to warfarin, INR is unlikely to be useful until at least 2 days after discontinuation of dabigatran.

Wait 12 hours (CrCl ≥30 mL/minute) or 24 hours (CrCl <30 mL/minute) after the last dose of dabigatran before starting a parenteral anticoagulant.

ADJUSTMENT WITH CONCOMITANT MEDICATIONS (SEE TABLE 12.3A). Dabigatran is not metabolized by the cytochrome P450 system. Dabigatran should be avoided with use of any P-glycoprotein inducer (e.g., rifampin), which may reduce dabigatran exposure. With renal insufficiency and concomitant use of P-glycoprotein inhibitors, exposure of dabigatran may be increased. Dabigatran should be avoided in patients with CrCl less than 30 mL/minute and concomitant use of any P-glycoprotein inhibitor (e.g., amiodarone, clarithromycin, dronedarone, quinidine, verapamil, and others). For dronedarone or ketoconazole with CrCl 30 to 50 mL/minute, dose reduction to 75 mg BID or an alternative anticoagulant should be considered.

PRIOR TO INVASIVE OR SURGICAL PROCEDURES REQUIRING HOLDING OF ANTICOAGULANTS.
Dabigatran should be discontinued 1 to 2 days (CrCl ≥ 50 mL/minute) or 3 to 5 days (CrCl < 50 mL/minute) prior to the procedure. Longer times should be considered for major surgeries or spinal or epidural procedures.

Contraindications

Active pathological bleeding, history of serious hypersensitivity to dabigatran or any component of the formulation; mechanical prosthetic heart valves.

Advantages

In RE-LY, compared to warfarin, dabigatran was associated with a significant reduction in ischemic stroke, a reduction in intracerebral hemorrhage, and a trend toward reduction in mortality. Dabigatran is not metabolized by the CYP450 system.

Disadvantages

Side effects include dyspepsia and for the 150-mg BID dosing, a higher risk of GI bleeding. There was a possible MI risk seen in initial analyses that was not reported in a subsequent analysis. There is no readily available specific reversing agent, but 60% can be removed by hemodialysis. Activated prothrombin complex concentrates (aPCCs, such as factor eight inhibitor bypassing activity [FEIBA]), recombinant factor VIIa, or concentrates of coagulation factors II, IX, or X may be considered.

Comments

Use with caution and reduce dosage in severe renal impairment (CrCl 15 to 30 mL/minute); not recommended with CrCl less than 15 mL/minute due to insufficient evidence to support use. Bleeding risk can be assessed by ecarin clotting time (ECT). If ECT is not available, activated partial thromboplastin time (aPTT) provides an approximation of anticoagulant activity. Dabigatran can be dialyzed with removal of approximately 60% of the drug over 2 to 3 hours. Potential adverse reactions include bleeding and GI side effects (dyspepsia and gastritis-like symptoms). Dabigatran is available in bottles and blister packs. Patients should not put dabigatran in pill boxes. Patients should also open only one bottle at a time, keep the bottle tightly closed, and use the supply within 4 months of opening.

Reversing Agent

Idarucizumab is the first approved reversal agent for dabigatran. Idarucizumab is a humanized monoclonal antibody fragment (Fab) indicated when reversal of dabigatran is needed for emergency surgery/urgent procedures or life-threatening or uncontrolled bleeding.

The recommended dose is 5 g, provided as two vials each containing 2.5 g/50 mL, given as two consecutive infusions or IV bolus injections.

Rivaroxaban

Rivaroxaban is a factor Xa inhibitor, which blocks conversion of prothrombin to thrombin. Thrombin activates platelets and catalyzes the conversion of fibrinogen to fibrin. An advantage of rivaroxaban is its once-daily dosing regimen.

Indications

Nonvalvular AF for prevention of stroke and systemic embolism; DVT or PE treatment; secondary prevention of recurrent DVT/PE after an initial 6 months of treatment; postoperative DVT prophylaxis after knee or hip replacement.

Dosage

For patients with AF, rivaroxaban is given as a single daily dose with the evening meal. Oral bioavailability is greater than 80% when taken with food (66% without food) with maximal anticoagulant effect at 2 to 4 hours. For CrCl greater than 50 mL/minute, the recommended dose is 20 mg once daily. If CrCl is 15 to 50 mL/minute, the dose should be reduced to 15 mg daily. Rivaroxaban is contraindicated in patients with CrCl less than 15 mL/minute.

CONVERTING FROM WARFARIN OR PARENTERAL ANTICOAGULANTS. Discontinue warfarin and start rivaroxaban when the INR is less than 3.0. From IV unfractionated heparin (UFH), start rivaroxaban after the IV UFH is discontinued. From low-molecular-weight heparin (LMWH), rivaroxaban can be started when the next dose would have been taken.

CONVERTING TO WARFARIN OR PARENTERAL ANTICOAGULANTS. For warfarin: discontinue rivaroxaban and initiate warfarin and a parenteral anticoagulant when the next dose of rivaroxaban would have been taken and continue until therapeutic warfarin is achieved. For parenteral anticoagulants: discontinue rivaroxaban and start the parenteral anticoagulant at the time when the next dose of rivaroxaban would have been taken.

ADJUSTMENT WITH CONCOMITANT MEDICATIONS (SEE TABLE 12.3B). Rivaroxaban is a substrate of CYP3A4/5, CYP2J2, and the P-glycoprotein and ATP-binding cassette G2 (ABCG2) transporters. Concomitant use should be avoided and alternative anticoagulants considered for strong dual CYP3A4 and P-glycoprotein inducers (rifampin, carbamazepine, phenytoin, St. John's wort), which can decrease rivaroxaban. Due to the potential for an increase in rivaroxaban effect, concomitant use should also be avoided and alternate anticoagulants considered when strong dual CYP3A4 and P-glycoprotein inhibitors (ketoconazole, itraconazole, HIV protease inhibitors, conivaptan) are used. For use of weak or moderate dual CYP3A4 and

P-glycoprotein inhibitors (amiodarone, verapamil, diltiazem, erythromycin, chloramphenicol, cimetidine) in the presence of CrCl 15 to 80 mL/minute, consider alternative anticoagulant use.

PRIOR TO INVASIVE OR SURGICAL PROCEDURES REQUIRING HOLDING OF ANTICOAGULANTS. Rivaroxaban should be discontinued at least 24 hours prior to the procedure. Some recommend discontinuation 3 days prior to a procedure in patients with CrCl greater than or equal to 50 mL/minute or 5 days with CrCl of less than 50 mL/minute.

Contraindications

Active pathologic bleeding or history of severe hypersensitivity to rivaroxaban or any component of the formulation.

Advantages

Once daily dosing. In the ROCKET-AF trial, compared to warfarin, there was a reduction in intracerebral hemorrhage and a trend toward reduction in mortality.

Disadvantages

There was a possible increased risk of thromboembolism when rivaroxaban was transitioned to warfarin in clinical trials. There is no readily available reversing agent, although prothrombin complex concentrate could possibly be used.

Comments

Two-thirds is metabolized by CYP450-dependent (CYP3A4, 212) or CYP-independent mechanisms; the inactive drug is then excreted via renal and fecal routes. One-third is removed using the P-glycoprotein transporter via the kidneys.

Due to the possible increased risk of thromboembolism (including stroke) when rivaroxaban was transitioned to warfarin in clinical trials of AF patients, alternate anticoagulation therapy should be considered when holding rivaroxaban for reasons other than pathologic bleeding or completion of therapy.

Apixaban

Apixaban is a selective factor Xa inhibitor that does not require antithrombin III for antithrombotic activity. It inhibits free and clot-bound factor Xa and prothrombinase activity. It indirectly inhibits platelet aggregation induced by thrombin. Apixaban inhibits free and clot-bound factor Xa, blocking the conversion of prothrombin to thrombin, decreasing thrombus development.

Indications

Nonvalvular AF for prevention of stroke and systemic embolism; DVT or PE treatment or reduction in risk of recurrence; prophylaxis of DVT after hip or knee replacement surgery.

Dosage

Oral bioavailability is 50% with maximum blood concentration achieved at 3 to 4 hours. For patients with AF, the recommended dose for apixaban is 5 mg BID, but should be reduced to 2.5 mg BID if the patient has any two of the following three factors: is age 80 years or older, weight of 60 kg or less, and serum Cr of 1.5 mg/dL or more. Use in end-stage renal disease (ESRD) or on hemodialysis has not been studied in efficacy and safety studies. Based on pharmacokinetic and pharmacodynamics data, the dose for ESRD patients on hemodialysis is 5 mg BID, reduced to 2.5 mg BID if the patient is 80 years of age or older or weighs 60 kg or less.

CONVERTING FROM WARFARIN OR PARENTERAL ANTICOAGULANTS. Discontinue warfarin and start apixaban when the INR is less than 2.0. From IV UFH, start apixaban once the IV UFH is discontinued. From LMWH, apixaban can be started when the next dose would have been taken.

CONVERTING TO WARFARIN OR PARENTERAL ANTICOAGULANTS. For warfarin: discontinue apixaban and initiate warfarin and a parenteral anticoagulant when the next dose of apixaban would have been taken and continue until therapeutic warfarin is achieved. For parenteral anticoagulants: discontinue apixaban and start the parenteral anticoagulant at the time when the next dose of apixaban would have been taken.

ADJUSTMENT WITH CONCOMITANT MEDICATIONS. Apixaban is a substrate of CYP3A4 and P-glycoprotein. One-quarter is metabolized via CYP3A4 and the remaining active drug is excreted using the P-glycoprotein transporter via the kidneys and biliary and intestinal system. Inhibitors of CYP3A4 and P-glycoprotein increase apixaban exposure, increasing the risk of bleed. Inducers of CYP3A4 and P-glycoprotein decrease apixaban exposure and may reduce its efficacy in reducing the risk of stroke and thromboembolic events. For patients on dual strong CYP3A4 and P-glycoprotein inhibitors (e.g., ketoconazole, itraconazole, clarithromycin, HIV protease inhibitors, ritonavir) and on apixaban greater than 2.5 mg BID (e.g., on 5 mg BID), apixaban dosage should be reduced by 50%; if the patient is on 2.5 mg BID, then apixaban should be avoided and alternative anticoagulants considered. For strong dual CYP3A4 and P-glycoprotein inducers (rifampin, carbamazepine, phenytoin, St. John's wort), which can decrease apixaban effect, concomitant use with apixaban should be avoided and alternative anticoagulants considered.

PRIOR TO INVASIVE OR SURGICAL PROCEDURES REQUIRING HOLDING OF ANTICOAGULANTS. Apixaban should be discontinued at least 48 hours prior to procedures with a moderate-to-high risk of unacceptable or significant bleeding and at least 24 hours prior to procedures with a low risk of bleeding and where bleeding could be easily controlled and not in a critical location. Bridging during this 24 to 48 hours is generally not required. Apixaban can be resumed after adequate hemostasis is achieved.

Contraindications

Active pathologic bleeding or history of severe hypersensitivity to apixaban or any component of the formulation.

Advantages

In ARISTOTLE, compared to warfarin, there was a significant reduction in stroke and systemic embolism, a reduction in intracerebral hemorrhage, and significant reduction in mortality.

Disadvantages

There was a possible increased risk of thromboembolism when apixaban was transitioned to warfarin in clinical trials. There is no readily available reversing agent, although prothrombin complex concentrates could possibly be used.

Comments

Due to the possible increased risk of thromboembolism (including stroke) when apixaban was transitioned to warfarin in clinical trials of AF patients, alternate anticoagulation therapy should be considered when holding rivaroxaban for reasons other than pathologic bleeding or completion of therapy.

Edoxaban

Edoxaban is a selective inhibitor of factor Xa that does not require antithrombin III for antithrombotic activity. Edoxaban inhibits free factor Xa and prothrombinase activity, inhibiting thrombin-induced platelet aggregation, and reducing thrombin generation and thrombus formation.

Indications

Nonvalvular AF to reduce the risk of stroke and systemic embolism. For nonvalvular AF, edoxaban should not be used in patients with CrCl greater than 95 mL/minute due to an increased risk of ischemic stroke compared to warfarin at 60 mg. DVT or PE treatment after 5 to 10 days of initial parenteral anticoagulant.

Dosage

Oral bioavailability is 62% with maximum blood concentration achieved at 1.5 hours. Renal clearance accounts for approximately 50% of edoxaban clearance and metabolism and biliary/intestinal excretion for the remaining. For patients with AF, the recommended dose for edoxaban is 60 mg once daily in patients with CrCl greater than 50 but less than 95 mL/minute and 30 mg once daily for CrCl 15 to 50 mL/minute. Use is not recommended in AF patients with CrCl greater than 95 mL/minute due to decreased efficacy.

With only limited data on use in patients with CrCl less than 15 mL/minute, edoxaban is not recommended in these patients. Dose is different for DVT/PE indications.

CONVERTING FROM WARFARIN OR PARENTERAL ANTICOAGULANTS. Discontinue warfarin and start edoxaban when INR is less than or equal to 2.5. From LMWH, discontinue the LMWH and start edoxaban at the time of the next scheduled dose. From IV UFH, start edoxaban 4 hours after discontinuation of the infusion.

CONVERTING TO WARFARIN OR PARENTERAL ANTICOAGULANTS. For warfarin: take a half dose of edoxaban while initiating warfarin until stable therapeutic warfarin (INR ≥2.0) is achieved. An alternative parenteral option is to discontinue edoxaban, administer a parenteral anticoagulant and warfarin at the next scheduled edoxaban dose, and discontinue the parenteral anticoagulant once a stable INR greater than or equal to 2.0 is achieved. For parenteral anticoagulants: discontinue edoxaban and start the parenteral anticoagulant at the time when the next dose of edoxaban would have been taken.

ADJUSTMENT WITH CONCOMITANT MEDICATIONS. Edoxaban does not inhibit the major cytochrome P450 enzymes, nor does it induce the CYP1A2, CYP3A4, or the P-glycoprotein transporter. Edoxaban is a substrate of the P-glycoprotein transporter. Concomitant use should be avoided with P-glycoprotein inducers (rifampin). Dose reduction is not recommended for concomitant use with P-glycoprotein inhibitors, because dose reduction resulted in lower edoxaban blood levels than in patients on the full dose.

PRIOR TO INVASIVE OR SURGICAL PROCEDURES REQUIRING HOLDING OF ANTICOAGULANTS. Edoxaban should be discontinued at least 24 hours prior to invasive or surgical procedures. Edoxaban can be resumed after adequate hemostasis is achieved, noting that the time to onset of effect is 1 to 2 hours. There may be an increased risk of bleeding with spinal/epidural anesthesia, puncture, or procedures. These should not be performed earlier than 12 hours after the last dose of edoxaban. After epidural or intrathecal catheter removal, edoxaban should not be given earlier than 2 hours afterward.

Contraindications

Active pathologic bleeding.

Advantages

Once daily dosing. In ENGAGE AF–TIMI 48, compared to warfarin, there was a significant reduction in stroke and systemic embolism and a trend toward reduction in overall death with the higher dose of edoxaban. For both doses there was a reduction in intracerebral hemorrhage and lower cardiovascular deaths. There was a reduction in risk of major bleeding (except for a higher risk of GI bleeding with the high dose).

Disadvantages

There is no readily available reversing agent, although prothrombin complex concentrate could possibly be used.

There is a decrease in efficacy with increased rate of ischemic stroke compared to warfarin in nonvalvular AF patients with normal renal function (CrCl >95 mL/minute). Edoxaban is not recommended for patients with CrCl greater than 95 mL/minute. A lower dose of edoxaban was associated with a higher risk of ischemic stroke.

Comments

There is a possible increased risk of thromboembolism or ischemic events when edoxaban is prematurely discontinued, but a transition protocol using half dosing of edoxaban upon transition to warfarin in ENGAGE AF–TIMI 48 did not show an increase in thromboembolism. When edoxaban is discontinued for a reason other than pathological bleeding or completion of a course of therapy, coverage with another anticoagulant as described in the transition guidance is recommended. Use has not been studied and is not recommended for mechanical heart valves or moderate to severe mitral stenosis. Edoxaban is not recommended for patients with moderate or severe hepatic impairment, because these patients may have intrinsic coagulation abnormalities and there is no clinical experience with edoxaban in severe hepatic impairment.

NONPHARMACOLOGIC THERAPY

Cardioversion

Cardioversion is a method to terminate specific reentrant and triggered automatic arrhythmias. Cardioversion can be accomplished electrically or pharmacologically. Most cardioversions are electrical.

Rhythm disturbances that can respond to cardioversion include (1) AF, (2) AFL, (3) AT, (4) sinoatrial (SA) reentrant tachycardia, (5) VT, (6) AV nodal reentrant SVT, (7) AV reciprocating tachycardia due to an accessory pathway, and (8) VF.

The effectiveness of electrical cardioversion depends on the vector of the electrical energy delivered, the strength of the energy, the rhythm disturbance, the underlying cardiovascular condition, and other factors such as body habitus.

Electrical cardioversion for AT, AFL, and AF is highly effective, with a greater than 90% efficacy for the short-term return of sinus rhythm.

Cardioversion should only be undertaken if the risk for thromboemboli is small. Thromboemboli can occur not only with the conversion to normal sinus rhythm but also as mechanical remodeling increases the strength of atrial contraction over the subsequent several days to weeks after cardioversion. Therefore, it is essential that adequate anticoagulation be undertaken, beginning prior to (unless the cardioversion is emergent) and for 4 to 6 weeks after the procedure.

New-onset AF (<48 hours) can be cardioverted without anticoagulation if the exact time of onset can be determined. Otherwise, cardioversion should be performed only after 3 to 4 weeks of adequate anticoagulation (INR consistently >2.0 on warfarin or on dabigatran for 3 to 4 weeks) or after a transesophageal echocardiogram that shows no left atrial clots (and with adequate anticoagulation).

Electrical cardioversion for AV node reentry SVT, AV reentry SVT, and SA reentry SVT is rarely necessary, because these rhythm disturbances often stop with autonomic maneuvers or adenosine.

Electrical cardioversion for VT can terminate a sustained VT, but if the tachycardia causes hemodynamic instability or cardiac arrest, or is of an irregular polymorphic form or VF, the procedure is considered to be defibrillation rather than cardioversion.

The procedure is performed under general anesthesia with propofol, methohexital, etomidate, or other general anesthetic and should be administered and monitored by personnel who are certified in deep sedation. Use of a sedative, such as midazolam, may be acceptable. The goal is to ensure that the patient is not aware of the shock and/or has retrograde amnesia.

The electrical shock is delivered through patches or paddles, which must be placed properly. One is placed over the apex of the heart and the other in the upper right scapular region or anterior chest, generally below the right clavicle. An anterior-posterior approach is generally preferred because it is likely to cardiovert the patient from AF; however, for an individual patient, one approach may be more effective than another.

Biphasic shock cardioverter-defibrillators are more effective than monophasic ones. Generally, for AF, 100 to 360 J is required. For AFL, 50 to 360 J is required.

Generally, there is no harm in starting at the low end of energy with 100 or 200 J in all cases. If this is ineffective, an increase to 360 J may be required or repositioning of the paddles or patches. If patches are used, switching to paddles may be more effective; efficacy increases with firm pressure on the chest, which decreases impedance. It is crucial that the patches or paddles are not placed in locations that are unlikely to cardiovert, such as the spleen or below.

In cardioverting patients with implanted cardiac pacemakers and/or defibrillators, ensuring that the vector of delivered energy is perpendicular to the axis formed by the pulse generator and leads will avoid interference with, or damage to, the implanted device. All pacemakers and ICDs today have some shielding from the effects of cardioversion, and permanent damage to or unwanted reprogramming of the devices is not expected to occur. Nonetheless, device interrogation after the procedure is prudent.

After some cardioversions, even if successful, there is early return of the arrhythmia. This is most common in patients who have AF for long periods of time. So-called early return of atrial fibrillation (ERAF) or immediate return of atrial fibrillation (IRAF) may occur. IV verapamil or IV ibutilide may prevent this from happening. Alternatively, repeating cardioversion after a specific antiarrhythmic drug is given may be required.

Electrical cardioversion can be performed as an outpatient for many individuals. Proper use of anticoagulation is essential for maintaining low risk for thromboembolic events.

Ablation

Ablation is a method used to cure specific rhythm disturbances. Most ablations use radiofrequency energy and heating of the catheter tip; cryo or freezing ablation has been used for some rhythm disturbances.

Radiofrequency ablation is generally safe and effective but requires invasive intracardiac testing. During radiofrequency ablation, alternating current between 370 and 50 kHz is used to achieve the tissue heating temperature of between 45°C and 100°C. The lesion diameter created by the catheter is 5 to 6 mm, and the depth is 2 to 3 mm. For some specific rhythm disturbances, such as VT or AF, deeper and larger lesions are created using an "irrigated tip" or a larger-tip catheter. Ablation methodology now includes use of highly sophisticated technology, such as three-dimensional electroanatomic mapping systems.

The typical ablation procedure involves conscious sedation with insertion of three to five venous catheters and sometimes a transseptal catheter, depending on the type of rhythm problem being evaluated and treated. The arrhythmia is usually induced and then mapped. The ablation site is then targeted and the patient tested by attempting to reinduce the arrhythmia after the ablation procedure to determine whether there has been complete cure of the arrhythmia.

Ablation has replaced antiarrhythmic drug therapy for treatment of many arrhythmias because it can be curative. For example, for the typical form of AVNRT, the procedure in experienced hands has a success rate of greater than 95%, with a complication rate of less than 1%. In this procedure, during which the slow AV node pathway is being targeted for ablation, the main risk is AV block due to the proximity of the slow pathway to the fast pathway of the AV node. Each arrhythmia has its own success rate and ascribed complication rate; this is, in part, related to the experience and expertise of the operator. Rhythm disturbances that have a high success rate of complete cure include typical AF, atrioventricular reentrant tachycardia (AVRT), WPW syndrome, idiopathic right ventricular outflow tract VT, idiopathic left VT, and bundle branch reentry VT. Arrhythmias that have a modest cure rate include atrial arrhythmias caused by congenital heart disease, atypical AFL, AF, VT occurring in the presence of structural heart disease, and premature atrial and ventricular depolarizations. Arrhythmias with relatively low rates of success include inappropriate sinus tachycardia and automatic JT. Radiofrequency ablation is rarely used for polymorphic VT or VF as identification and mapping of the involved sites are not possible; however, recent work suggests that ablation of specific triggers in the His-Purkinje system may be useful to eliminate some forms of VF that initiate with a predominant PVC trigger.

Ablation may be used to eliminate AV conduction entirely, by creating complete AV block in patients with ATs that result in rapid ventricular rates that cannot be controlled with AV nodal blocking drugs or other treatments. When ablation of the AV node is performed, the patient will require a pacemaker. Patients with chronic AF and uncontrolled ventricular rates may benefit hemodynamically and clinically from AV node ablation and permanent cardiac pacing; however, this renders the patient pacemaker dependent, and some patients may develop cardiac dysfunction long term because of desynchronization of left ventricular contractility. In such patients, biventricular pacing (cardiac resynchronization therapy) may improve ventricular function. Recent studies suggest some potential benefit from biventricular pacing as the preferred method of permanent pacing at the onset of AV junction ablation.

Complications of radiofrequency ablation are rare but include death in approximately 0.1%, cardiac tamponade, AV block, pericarditis, thromboembolic events, hematomas, and AV fistulae. Other complications of AF ablation, which targets pulmonary vein isolation typically using RF energy or cryoablation, include pulmonary vein stenosis or occlusion, which may require balloon dilatation or stenting, rarely atrioesophageal fistula, which can be fatal, or phrenic nerve paralysis, which is usually reversible.

The best candidates for radiofrequency ablation as primary therapy include patients with SVTs, especially if severe symptoms are associated with the tachycardia or it is unresponsive to tolerated drug therapy. It is also very effective for typical AFL, atypical AFL is more challenging. Although some cases of AF result from a flutter mechanism, cure of the AFL may not affect the AF, which will recur. Ablation is also effective for symptomatic idiopathic VT and, in certain specific patient groups, for AF, which remains symptomatic despite antiarrhythmic drug therapy.

Recent American guideline updates moved catheter ablation from a class II to a class I indication with the level of evidence A for those patients with symptomatic paroxysmal AF who failed treatment with an antiarrhythmic drug. In addition, catheter ablation is now considered reasonable to treat symptomatic persistent AF or symptomatic paroxysmal AF in patients with significant left atrial dilatation.

Ablation tends to improve quality of life by decreasing symptoms and decreasing arrhythmias and is generally cost effective except perhaps for AF, in which the actual efficacy and benefits over the long term are not known.

Patients should be fully informed of the risks and benefits of the procedure and understand the procedure.

During pregnancy, preexisting arrhythmias may or may not increase. Hemodynamic changes, particularly during the third trimester, may predispose to some arrhythmias. Palpitations due to higher plasma volumes or ectopy are common and benign; noninvasive ambulatory monitoring may be considered if symptoms suggest sustained or symptomatic tachyarrhythmias. Compression of abdominal venous or arterial vessels can cause supine hypotension, associated symptoms, and exacerbation of neurocardiogenic syncope. Management includes nonpharmacologic measures, such as maintaining good hydration, support stockings, avoidance of supine positioning, and possibly higher salt intake. Some forms of long QT syndrome (LQTS), especially LQTS 2, are associated with higher risk for ventricular arrhythmias during pregnancy or in the postpartum period. β-blocker therapy can often be continued. For those individuals who develop a cardiomyopathy or who are at risk for life-threatening ventricular arrhythmias, a wearable cardioverter defibrillator may be considered.

ANTIARRHYTHMIC AND ANTICOAGULANT MEDICATIONS DURING PREGNANCY

Risks of antiarrhythmic medications to the mother and fetus should be considered. Medications may affect the fetus if they cross the placenta. Fetal arrhythmias can potentially be treated by medications that cross the placenta. Dosing may be complicated by the higher volume status, increase in renal and hepatic blood flow, lower plasma protein concentration, and hormonal changes that can affect drug levels and efficacy. Safety of drugs to the child during breast feeding should also be considered.

Table 13.1 summarizes U.S. Food and Drug Administration (FDA) pregnancy categories for common antiarrhythmic and anticoagulant medications. However, classification is not provided for drugs approved after June 30, 2015, when the FDA removed common antiarrhythmic and anticoagulant medications from the Physician Labeling Rule format, requiring information to assist in counseling for pregnancy, lactation, and females and males of reproductive potential.

Table 13.2 summarizes pregnancy categories for commonly used drugs in arrhythmia management. Few drugs are in category B, where there is no evidence of harm in humans and risk to the fetus is assessed to be rare, but these drugs include lidocaine, pindolol, and sotalol. The most common

U.S. FOOD AND DRUG ADMINISTRATION PREGNANCY CATEGORIES

A	No risk in controlled human studies: Adequate and well-controlled human studies have failed to demonstrate a risk to the fetus in the first trimester of pregnancy (and there is no evidence of risk in later trimesters).
B	No risk in other studies: Animal reproduction studies have failed to demonstrate a risk to the fetus and there are no adequate and well-controlled studies in pregnant women *or* animal studies have shown an adverse effect, but adequate and well-controlled studies in pregnant women have failed to demonstrate a risk to the fetus in any trimester.
C	Risk not ruled out: Animal reproduction studies have shown an adverse effect on the fetus and there are no adequate and well-controlled studies in humans, but potential benefits may outweigh potential risks.
D	Positive evidence of risk: Positive evidence of human fetal risk based on adverse reaction data from investigational or marketing experience or studies in humans, but potential benefits may outweigh potential risks.
X	Contraindicated in pregnancy: Studies in animals or humans have demonstrated fetal abnormalities and/or there is positive evidence of human fetal risk based on adverse reaction data from investigational or marketing experience. Risks in pregnant women clearly outweigh potential benefits.
N	The FDA has not classified the drug.

FDA, U.S. Food and Drug Administration.

category is C, for which there is a lack of adequate studies. Older drugs, with which there is more experience, may be preferable to newer drugs, with which there is less experience. Drugs that should be avoided include those in category D, for which there is evidence of risk, and category X, which includes contraindicated drugs. These drugs to be avoided include phenytoin (fetal hydantoin syndrome and bleeding risk), amiodarone (fetal thyroid abnormality), dronedarone (teratogenicity), warfarin (see below), and atenolol (evidence of fetal risk). Risks and benefits of drug therapy before, during, and after pregnancy should be discussed in detail with patients.

Anticoagulant drugs have potential risks for bleeding in the mother, but because some may also be potentially less effective due to lower drug concentrations with higher plasma volume, if continued anticoagulation is required, it may be preferable to use a drug for which anticoagulant effects can be monitored. In addition, it is not known for all agents whether they cross the placenta, and there may be bleeding risks for the fetus.

Warfarin crosses the placenta and is contraindicated in the first trimester because of the risks of teratogenic congenital defect, spontaneous abortion, fetal hemorrhage, and death. It is contraindicated during pregnancy except in patients with high-risk mechanical heart valves (e.g., older mechanical mitral valves or history of thromboembolism). In such patients, low-molecular-weight heparin (LMWH) can be used for bridging during the first trimester, but anticoagulant effect should be monitored.

TABLE 13.2

COMMON DRUGS USED TO TREAT ARRHYTHMIAS AND THEIR SAFETY IN PREGNANCY AND LACTATION

Class	Drug	FDA Category	Crosses Placenta	Pregnancy Comments	Crosses to Breast Milk	Breast-feeding Comments
Class IA						
	Quinidine	C	Yes	Relatively low risk for fetus; neonatal thrombocytopenia reported. Has been used to treat fetal arrhythmias.	Yes	Limited data in humans. Probably low risk.
	Procainamide	C	Yes	Limited data in humans. Has been used to treat fetal arrhythmias.	Yes	Limited data in humans. Probably low risk.
	Disopyramide	C	Yes	Risk in third trimester. Oxytocic effect: may cause contractions; adverse effects at high doses in animals.	Yes	Limited data in humans. Probably low risk.
Class IB						
	Mexiletine	C	Probably	Limited data in humans. Low risk suggested by animal studies.	Yes	Limited data in humans. Probably low risk.
	Lidocaine	B	Yes	Human experience suggests low risk.	Yes	Limited data in humans. Probably low risk.
	Phenytoin	D	Yes	Avoid use for arrhythmias. Congenital abnormalities, fetal hydantoin syndrome, malignancies, hemorrhage in the newborn.	Yes	Expected to be low risk.

Continued on following page

TABLE 13.2

COMMON DRUGS USED TO TREAT ARRHYTHMIAS AND THEIR SAFETY IN PREGNANCY AND LACTATION (Continued)

Class	Drug	FDA Category	Crosses Placenta	Pregnancy Comments	Crosses to Breast Milk	Breast-feeding Comments
Class IC						
	Flecainide	C	Yes	Limited data in humans. Animal studies suggest risk at higher doses. Used to treat fetal arrhythmias.	Yes	Limited data in humans. Probably low risk.
	Propafenone	C	Yes	Limited human data; animal data suggest risk at higher doses. Until more information, generally reserve use for when other agents are not effective.	Yes	Limited data in humans. Probably low risk.
	Propranolol	C	Yes	Risk in second/third trimester.	Yes	Limited data in humans. Possible clinically significant risk. Breast feeding not recommended.
	Atenolol	D	Yes	Risk in second/third trimester.	Yes	Limited data in humans. Possible clinically significant risk. Breast feeding not recommended. With availability of other agents, avoid renally excreted β-blockers, such as atenolol.
	Metoprolol	C	Yes	Risk in second/third trimester. Only limited experience in first trimester.	Yes	Limited data in humans. Possible clinically significant risk. Breast feeding not recommended.
	Carvedilol	C	Yes	Risk in second/third trimester.	Unknown/ probably	No data in humans. Might be low risk.

Pindolol	B	Yes	Risk in second/third trimester.	Yes	No data in humans. Possible clinically significant risk. Breast feeding not recommended.
Acebutolol	B	Yes	Limited data in humans. Low risk suggested by animal studies.	Yes	Limited data in humans. Possible clinically significant risk. Breast feeding not recommended.
Bisoprolol	C	Probably	Risk in second/third trimester.	Unknown/probably	No data in humans. Possible clinically significant risk. Breast feeding not recommended.
Class III					
Ibutilide	C	Unknown/Possibly	Limited data in humans. Animal studies suggest risk at higher doses.	Unknown	No data in humans. Might be low risk. Probably can be used.
Amiodarone	D	Yes	Significant risk suggested by human and animal studies. Should avoid, if possible.	Yes	Contraindicated.
Sotalol	B	Yes	Risk in second/third trimester.	Yes	Limited data in humans. Possible clinically significant risk. Breast feeding not recommended.
Dofetilide	C	Unknown/probably	No data in humans. Animal studies suggest risk at higher doses with possible teratogenicity and toxicity.	Unknown/probably	No data in humans. Possible clinically significant risk. Breast feeding not recommended.
Dronedarone	X	Unknown/probably	No data in humans. Animal studies suggest risk at higher doses. Contraindicated, especially in first trimester, no data later in pregnancy; fetal abnormalities in animals.	Unknown/probably	No data in humans. Possible clinically significant risk. Breast feeding not recommended.

Continued on following page

TABLE 13.2

COMMON DRUGS USED TO TREAT ARRHYTHMIAS AND THEIR SAFETY IN PREGNANCY AND LACTATION (Continued)

Class	Drug	FDA Category	Crosses Placenta	Pregnancy Comments	Crosses to Breast Milk	Breast-feeding Comments
Class IV: Calcium Channel Blockers						
	Diltiazem	C	Yes	Limited experience, but low risk suggested.	Yes	Limited data in humans suggest low risk. Probably can be used.
	Verapamil	C	Yes	Human experience suggests very low risk. Can be used.	Yes	Limited data in humans suggest low risk. Probably can be used.
Miscellaneous						
	Adenosine	C	Unknown	Human experience suggests very low risk. Can be used when maternal benefit greatly exceeds embryo–fetal risk.	Unknown	No data in humans. Might be low risk. Probably can be used.
	Digoxin	C	Yes	Human experience suggests very low risk. Can be used.	Yes	Not expected to cause significant infant toxicity. Can be used.
	Ivabradine	N	Unknown	Fetal toxicity and teratogenesis in animals.	Unknown/Probably	Not recommended.
	Fludrocortisone	C	Unknown	Adverse events observed with corticosteroids in animal studies.	Yes	—
	Midodrine	C	Unknown/probably	Limited information; adverse events in animal studies.	Unknown/probably	—

Anticoagulants

Warfarin	D (mechanical heart valves) X (other indications)	Yes	Contraindicated in first trimester. Teratogenic with coumarin embryopathy in first trimester; CNS abnormalities in any trimester; spontaneous abortion, fetal hemorrhage, fetal death. Contraindicated in pregnancy except with mechanical heart valves at high risk for thromboembolism.	No	Expected to be low risk for infant. May be used in breast-feeding women.
Apixaban	B	Yes in animals	No data in humans. Low risk suggested by animal studies. Avoid use in pregnancy; data insufficient.	Unknown/ probably	No data in humans. Possible clinically significant risk. Breast feeding not recommended; use of alternative anticoagulation preferred.
Dabigatran	C	Yes	No data in humans. Animal studies suggest risk at higher doses. Avoid use in pregnancy.	Unknown	No data in humans. Possible clinically significant risk. Breast feeding not recommended; use of alternative anticoagulation preferred. Canadian labeling contraindicates.
Edoxaban	C	Unknown	Avoid use in pregnancy.	Unknown/ Probably	Use of alternative anticoagulation recommended.
Rivaroxaban	C	Yes	No data in humans. Animal studies suggest risk at higher doses. Avoid use in pregnancy.	Unknown	No data in humans. Possible clinically significant risk. Breast feeding not recommended; use of alternative anticoagulation preferred. Canadian labeling contraindicates.

Class II β-Adrenergic Blockers: Risks of intrauterine growth restriction (IUGR), reduction in placental perfusion, small placentas, fetal/neonatal bradycardia, hypoglycemia, respiratory depression, premature labor; in general, risk suggested in second/third trimester.

CNS, Central nervous system; *FDA,* U.S. Food and Drug Administration.

In patients on chronic anticoagulation with warfarin who are planning to become pregnant, substitution with LMWH should ideally be done prior to conception. Although warfarin can be resumed after the first trimester, LMWH or heparin can be substituted near term. Ideally, warfarin does not appear to pass into breast milk and so can be used in lactating women. The non-vitamin K oral anticoagulants (NOACs) should probably be avoided.

Dabigatran and rivaroxaban probably cross the placenta, but it is not known if apixaban and edoxaban cross the placenta. Anticoagulant effects may not be easily monitored or readily reversed, especially in the fetus. Risks and benefits should be carefully weighed, including risks of thromboembolism in the mother, bleeding risks, and adverse effects in the mother and fetus.

CARDIAC ARREST, DEFIBRILLATION, AND CARDIOVERSION

Fortunately rare in pregnant women, cardiac arrest is managed according to standard basic and advanced cardiac life support guidelines. Later in pregnancy, when the uterus is at or above the umbilicus, manual left uterine displacement (LUD) can be helpful during cardiopulmonary resuscitation (CPR) to reduce aortocaval compression. This is performed by using one or two hands to push or cup the gravid abdomen, lifting the uterus upward and leftward off the mother's vessels. LUD allows CPR to be performed with the patient remaining supine.

Defibrillation for ventricular fibrillation or pulseless ventricular tachycardia is vital for survival in the pregnant and nonpregnant patient and should be performed promptly when indicated. The risk to the fetus is low, and restoration of maternal blood flow is critical. For cardioversion, risk to the fetus is also small. For elective cardioversion, fetal monitoring should be performed during and after the cardioversion.

Preparation for urgent delivery of the fetus by cesarean delivery should be initiated in critically ill or arresting pregnant women and in some circumstances may increase the survival rate of the mother. Decisions should ideally be made in conjunction with the family and medical team, which includes an obstetrician and a pediatrician/neonatologist.

ABLATION, PACEMAKERS, AND DEFIBRILLATORS

Because of the typical use of fluoroscopy to guide ablation and implantation of cardiac electrical devices, elective procedures should generally be performed prior to pregnancy or after delivery. Rarely, urgent device implantation or ablation may need to be considered, but ideally should be at least deferred until after the first trimester.

In patients at risk for life-threatening ventricular arrhythmias without pacing indications, a wearable cardioverter defibrillator may be considered to avoid radiation from implantation of a defibrillator. Recently pacemakers and defibrillators have been implanted with minimal or no radiation exposure using an abdominal shield in and echocardiographic and electrocardiographic guidance. Similarly, ablation has been performed with minimal or no fluoroscopy using electroanatomic mapping.

FETAL ARRHYTHMIAS

Fetal arrhythmias can include supraventricular tachycardias, atrial flutter, and rarely ventricular tachycardia. Diagnosis is generally made using echocardiography and fetal electrocardiograms. Medications that have been used by administration to the mother include digoxin, propranolol, metoprolol, verapamil, procainamide, flecainide, sotalol, and amiodarone. Standard maternal monitoring for use of these drugs should be practiced.

Index

Note: Page numbers followed by *f* indicate figures and *t* indicate tables.

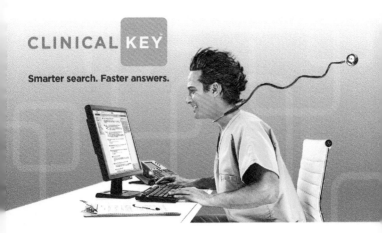

Printed and bound by CPI Group (UK) Ltd, Croydon, CR0 4YY

03/10/2024

01040451-0002